Non-Laryngeal Cancer and Voice

Non-Laryngeal
Cancer and Voice

Abdul-Latif Hamdan, MD, EMBA, MPH, FACS
Robert Thayer Sataloff, MD, DMA, FACS
Mary J. Hawkshaw, RN, BSN, CORLN, FCCP

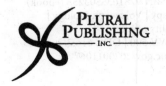

PLURAL
PUBLISHING
INC.

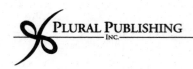

5521 Ruffin Road
San Diego, CA 92123

e-mail: information@pluralpublishing.com
Web site: https://www.pluralpublishing.com

Typeset in 10.5/13 Minion Pro by Achorn International
Printed in the United States of America by Integrated Books International

NOTICE TO THE READER
Care has been taken to confirm the accuracy of the indications, procedures, drug dosages, and diagnosis and remediation protocols presented in this book and to ensure that they conform to the practices of the general medical and health services communities. However, the authors, editors, and publisher are not responsible for errors or omissions or for any consequences from application of the information in this book and make no warranty, expressed or implied, with respect to the currency, completeness, or accuracy of the contents of the publication. The diagnostic and remediation protocols and the medications described do not necessarily have specific approval by the Food and Drug administration for use in the disorders and/or diseases and dosages for which they are recommended. Application of this information in a particular situation remains the professional responsibility of the practitioner. Because standards of practice and usage change, it is the responsibility of the practitioner to keep abreast of revised recommendations, dosages, and procedures.

Library of Congress Cataloging-in-Publication Data
Names: Hamdan, A. L. (Abdul Latif), author. | Sataloff, Robert Thayer,
  author. | Hawkshaw, Mary, author.
Title: Non-laryngeal cancer and voice / Abdul-Latif Hamdan, Robert Thayer
  Sataloff, Mary J. Hawkshaw.
Description: San Diego, CA : Plural Publishing, Inc., [2021] | Includes
  bibliographical references and index.
Identifiers: LCCN 2020011067 | ISBN 9781635503241 (paperback) |
  ISBN 1635503248 (paperback) | ISBN 9781635503258 (ebook)
Subjects: MESH: Dysphonia—therapy | Voice—physiology |
  Neoplasms—complications | Quality of Life
Classification: LCC RF510 | NLM WV 500 | DDC 616.2/2—dc23
LC record available at https://lccn.loc.gov/2020011067

Contents

Preface

Voice, a reflection of well-being, is often neglected in patients with non-laryngeal cancer who suffer a myriad of physical and emotional disturbances. A change in voice quality is rarely given deference in the context of what many physicians perceive as more disabling cancer-induced morbidities. However, dysphonia can be disabling in many patients who are professional voice users including not only singers, but also teachers, physicians, lawyers, and others. The quality-of-life impact of dysphonia is often substantial. The review presented in this book underscores the importance of identifying voice symptoms and signs in patients with cancer. These are very often masked by the overwhelming complaints of affected patients, impairments in other body systems caused by their disease, and the adverse effects of treatment. Dysphonia as a symptom amid the wide spectrum of cancer-related symptoms warrants special attention, particularly in professional voice users who rely on their voice to make a living. Meeting the vocal needs of cancer patients with dysphonia falls within the scope of caring for the whole cancer patient, and not only for the cancer.

This book reviews the literature on voice in cancer patients, with emphasis on both disease-induced and treatment-induced dysphonia. A better understanding of the link between cancer and voice can assist physicians in detecting phonatory disorders early in cancer patients. Proper and timely referral to laryngologists and voice specialists for comprehensive voice evalu-ation is crucial for adequate diagnosis and treatment. Cancer patients deserve equal attention to their vocal apparatus, similar to that directed to any other systems impacted by their primary disease.

The order of chapters of this book has been chosen in alignment with the frequency of cancers based on the estimated annual incidence listed in the Worldwide Cancer Data[4] and by the American Cancer Society.[14] Lung and breast cancers are considered the most common, followed by colorectal and prostate cancers. Cancers with a low incidence are not discussed in this book.

Cancer of the larynx or other areas of the vocal tract has effects on the voice that are intuitively obvious. However, the impact on voice of non-laryngeal cancers is less apparent. This book is intended as a resource for not only laryngologists, speech-language pathologists, and singing voice specialists, but also oncologists, surgeons, and others who treat patients who depend on their voices, especially professional voice users. The book also is designed to serve as a resource for voice professionals who develop common cancers outside the larynx and want a convenient overview of the disease and the voice-related consequences of the cancer and its treatment.

For non-laryngologists, the first 3 chapters cover basic information about the voice. Chapter 1 reviews clinical anatomy and physiology, Chapter 2 discusses the information obtained from the specialized histories for voice professionals, and Chapter 3 covers the state-of-the-art in physical examination of voice patients.

There are 2.1 million new cases of lung cancer diagnosed annually,[1] and the incidence has increased over the years in both genders. As discussed in Chapter 4, lung cancer and its treatment can affect the voice directly by impairing pulmonary function and thereby decreasing the voice power source (support), paralyzing the vocal folds, metastasizing (including to the larynx), and other mechanisms. Surgery routinely alters voice function, especially if part or all of a lung is resected. Of course, any surgery can alter voice if there are complications with intubation. Chemotherapy and radiation for lung cancer also can cause voice problems. Radiation not only alters laryngeal tissues directly if the larynx is included in the radiation field, but it also can cause recurrent laryngeal nerve paresis or paralysis.

Chapter 5 discusses breast cancer, the second most common cancer in the world and the most common malignancy in women.[2] In 2018, there were more than 2 million new cases.[1] Breast cancer can be particularly disturbing for some women, and the emotional reaction often is reflected in the voice. Breast cancer can metastasize to the vocal tract, and pulmonary metastases can cause recurrent laryngeal nerve paralysis. Vocal fold paralysis in breast cancer patients also can be caused by metastases to the skull base. Anxiety and depression are common in patients with breast cancer, and the consequences of anxiety and depression on voice are well known.[3] Generalized fatigue, pain, and sleep deprivation are common with breast cancer and commonly are associated with dysphonia. Radiation, chemotherapy, and particularly endocrine therapy for breast cancer frequently cause dysphonia. Surgical treatment also can affect the voice, especially if abdominal muscles are used for breast reconstruction, potentially affecting the efficiency of abdominal support.

Colorectal cancer is the third most common cancer in the world, with about 1.8 million new cases in 2018,[1] as reviewed in Chapter 6. In 2018, there were about 161 000 deaths from colon cancer.[4] Colorectal cancer is associated with severe reduction in quality of life. Abdominal discomfort that impairs support, and metastatic disease that can involve the vocal tract and causes vocal fold paralysis can cause dysphonia. Metastases can involve the larynx or structures close to the larynx, including the thyroid gland. Metastases to the neck and chest can cause vocal fold paralysis by compression or invasion. Colorectal cancer is treated by surgical resection with or without chemotherapy. The surgery may affect abdominal support muscle function, and chemotherapy can cause short-term and long-term side effects that result in dysphonia.

Prostate cancer, discussed in Chapter 7, is the second most common cancer in men, with approximately 174 615 new cases in the United States in 2019.[5] The disease usually affects men in their seventh decade, and less than 10% of those affected are below the age of 45 years.[6] Approximately 10% to 15% of patients with prostate cancer have metastasis at the time of diagnosis. Although metastatic disease to the larynx is uncommon, it can occur; and metastasis to the lungs can result in vagus nerve injury and consequent vocal fold paralysis. Metastasis to the thyroid gland also occurs. Like breast cancer, prostate cancer adversely affects mental well-being. Depression and anxiety are common.[7] Treatment for prostate cancer also can cause voice changes, particularly orchiectomy and hormone therapy. Surgery for prostate cancer has various potential adverse effects that can have psychological impact that may be reflected in the voice, including impotence. In 2019, Jarzemski et al studied the mental well-being of 100 patients with prostate cancer and found an association between physical symptoms and deferred memory, depression, and anxiety.[8] Some chemotherapy used for prostate cancer causes diarrhea, nausea, and vomiting, which can affect the voice in the short term. More research is needed to evaluate the long-term voice consequences of chemotherapy for prostate cancer.

Problems associated with thyroid disease in general, and thyroid cancer specifically, are covered in Chapter 8, and elsewhere.[9] It has been known for decades that even mild hypothyroidism can cause dysphonia, described typically as a sensation of a "veil over the voice." Thyroid cancer and its treatment routinely result in dysphonia. Voice changes may be caused by hypothyroidism, hyperthyroidism, recurrent or superior laryngeal nerve injury, surgical scar adherence to the trachea impairing laryngotracheal vertical motion, and other causes. When thyroid cancer presents with vocal fold paresis, treatment rarely results in restoration of normal neuromuscular function.[10,11]

Chapter 9 reviews non-Hodgkin lymphoma, which accounts for 4.2% of all cancers diagnosed in the United States, with approximately 74 200 new diagnoses in 2019.[12] It accounts for 90% of all lymphomas,[13] and it is more common in patients older than 65 years, affecting men more frequently than women.[14] Hodgkin lymphoma affects primarily the lymph nodes. Non-Hodgkin lymphoma affects lymph nodes, but it also has extranodal manifestations in 30% of patients,[15] most commonly affecting the Waldeyer ring, nasopharynx, oral cavity, salivary glands, thyroid, and paranasal sinuses.[16,17] Weight loss, fever, and night sweats are common, and these impairments of general health affect the voice adversely in the short term. Although uncommon, the larynx can be the target organ for non-Hodgkin lymphoma.[18] Hematopoietic laryngeal neoplasms account for less than 1% of all laryngeal cancers.[19] Non-Hodgkin lymphoma is classified into several subtypes that are not reviewed in detail in this book, but some can involve the larynx. These include diffuse large B-cell lymphoma (DLBCL), mucosa-associated lymphoid tissue (MALT) lymphoma, natural killer (NK) T-cell lymphoma, and T-cell lymphoma. In addition to involving the larynx directly, non-Hodgkin lymphoma can cause vocal fold paralysis by invasion or compression. Non-Hodgkin lymphoma also can cause paralysis through neurolymphomatosis or neoplastic meningitis. Chemotherapy is the primary treatment for non-Hodgkin lymphoma and may be combined with immunotherapy or radiation. Chemotherapy may have direct and indirect effects on the voice. Short-term effects are routine, and long-term effects may occur.[20] Vincristine, a chemotherapy agent used commonly for hematologic malignancies, can be complicated by neurotoxicity with axonal degeneration that can affect neural conduction in multiple cranial nerves, including the vagus nerve.[21,22] Radiation also is used commonly for lymphoma patients and can cause tissue toxicity and neurotoxicity.

In the United States in 2019, there were approximately 74 000 new cases of renal cell carcinoma,[23] discussed in Chapter 10. The incidence has risen over the last 2 decades, particularly in people between 70 and 79 years of age.[24] Renal cell carcinoma commonly has no symptoms until the disease is advanced, and incidental diagnosis is made in 50% of cases, with a minority of patients presenting with the classic triad of flank pain, mass, and hematuria.[25,26] Renal cell carcinoma is likely to metastasize, with metastatic disease identified at the time of diagnosis in 23% to 40% of patients; multiple metastases are common, particularly in younger patients.[27–30] Metastases to lungs and bones are most common,[31,32] but renal cell carcinoma metastasizes to the head and neck in about 15% of cases.[33,34] Laryngeal metastases have been reported. In addition to direct metastasis affecting the voice, metastasis to the lungs and to the structures in the neck can cause laryngeal nerve paralysis. Esophageal metastasis may result in similar problems, as well as weight loss and deterioration in general health that can cause dysphonia. Nearly half of patients with renal cell carcinoma have depression, and many have comorbid posttraumatic stress syndrome associated with excessive fatigue and sleep disturbance.[35] All of these problems can cause adverse voice changes. Various chemotherapy regimens used for renal cell carcinoma cause dysphonia, and dysphonia has been reported in up to 30% of patients treated with antiangiogenic therapy.[36] Fatigue is common in nearly all patients receiving chemotherapy and commonly is accompanied by dysphonia.

As reviewed in Chapter 11, gastric carcinoma is the fifth most common cancer in the world,[37] with approximately 27 500 cases worldwide diagnosed in 2019.[38] It is most common in people aged 70 years and older, and it occurs in men more than in women. It also is more common in overpopulated countries with low socioeconomic demographics.[39–41] Gastric cancer is notorious for causing weight loss and fatigue that can impair phonation. Like other cancers, depression and anxiety are common, and these also can have adverse effects on voice. Surgery is a mainstay of treatment. In addition to potentially impairing the support system, surgery for gastric cancer commonly causes reflux, sometimes severe reflux, that can damage the larynx. Gastric cancers commonly metastasize, and metastasis may involve the lungs and neck, causing compression or invasion of the vagus nerve resulting in vocal fold paralysis. Chemotherapy for gastric cancer causes problems as previously discussed with other cancers. However, antiangiogenic medications are increasingly and commonly used for gastric cancers, and they can cause severe ischemic vocal fold pathology.[42–45]

Chapter 12 provides an overview of liver cancer. The American Cancer Society estimated that there were 42 030 new cases of liver and intrahepatic bile duct cancer in the United States in 2019.[46] The prevalence of liver cancer increased by 75% worldwide between 1990 and 2015; in the United States, the number of cases more than tripled since 1980. Liver cancer is associated with alcohol, drug use, and fatty foods that can damage the liver. Cirrhosis, chronic infection with hepatitis B or C, and diabetes also increase the risk of liver cancer, as do obesity and unprotected sex. The liver performs more than 500 essential functions including clearing toxins; assisting digestion; storing vitamins and minerals from food; metabolizing carbohydrates, fats, and proteins; and filtering blood. The systemic effects of liver cancer can be profound. Typically, liver cancer presents with loss of appetite and weight, abdominal pain, nausea and vomiting, and jaundice. Hepatocellular carcinoma accounts for approximately 75% of all liver cancers, but other types include fibrolamellar, cholangiocarcinoma (bile duct cancer), angiosarcoma, and secondary liver cancer caused by metastasis from a cancer elsewhere. Although liver transplant is the ideal treatment, only a few patients with liver cancer are appropriate candidates. For most, immunotherapy, partial resection of the liver, chemotherapy, targeted therapy, and interventional radiology are used. Overall, the 5-year survival rate for liver cancer is 18%, although survival is better if the cancer is diagnosed at an early stage. Liver cancer and its treatment are almost always debilitating. In addition to weight loss, muscle wasting, fatigue, and psychological response to the disease may cause voice dysfunction for reasons discussed earlier in relation to other cancers.

Cancer almost always affects voice. In some cases, the cancer impairs the voice directly. In others, the cancer or its treatment causes debilitation, weight loss, depression, anxiety, and other reactions that interfere with optimal phonation. Dysphonia in cancer patients has a devastating impact on the physical and emotional aspects of their lives. Cancer patients need to be heard, and their voices warrant an attentive medical audience when affected. The authors hope that this book will not only provide useful information for our readers, but also highlight knowledge gaps and inspire further research.

References

1. World Health Organization. Cancer fact sheet. Updated September 12, 2018. Accessed July 1, 2019. https://www.who.int/news -room/fact-sheets/detail/cancer

2. Bonilla JM, Tabanera MT, Mendoza LR. Breast cancer in the 21st century: from early detection to new therapies. *Radiologia* (English Edition). 2017;59(5):368–379.

3. Rosen DC, Heuer RJ, Sasso DA, Sataloff RT. Psychological aspects of voice disorders. In: Hamdan AL, Sataloff RT, Hawkshaw M, eds. *Laryngeal Manifestations of Systemic Diseases*. San Diego, CA: Plural Publishing; 2018: 119–150.

4. World Cancer Research Fund. Colorectal cancer statistics. Published 2019. Accessed September 2, 2019. https://www.wcrf.org/diet andcancer/cancer-trends/colorectal-cancer -statistics

5. National Cancer Institute: Surveillance, Epidemiology, and End Results (SEER) Program. Cancer stat facts: Prostate cancer. Accessed September 2, 2019. https://seer.cancer.gov /statfacts/html/prost.html

6. Cancer Research UK. Prostate cancer statistics. Accessed September 2, 2019. https:// www.cancerresearchuk.org/health-profes sional/cancer-statistics/statistics-by-cancer -type/prostate-cancer#heading-Three

7. Salvo N, Zeng L, Zhang L, et al. Frequency of reporting and predictive factors for anxiety and depression in patients with advanced cancer. *Clin Oncol*. 2012;24(2):139–148.

8. Jarzemski P, Brzoszczyk B, Popiolek A, et al. Cognitive function, depression and anxiety in patients undergoing radical prostatectomy with and without adjuvant treatment. *Neuropsychiatr Dis Treat*. 2019;15:819–829.

9. Pfaff JA, Caruso-Sales H, Jaworek A, et al. The vocal effects of thyroid disorders and their treatment. In: Sataloff RT. *Professional Voice: The Science and Art of Clinical Care*. 4th ed. San Diego, CA: Plural Publishing; 2017:671–682.

10. Heman-Ackah Y, Joglekar S, Caroline M, et al. The prevalence of undiagnosed thyroid disease in patient with symptomatic vocal fold paresis. *J Voice*. 2011;25(4):496–500.

11. Caroline M, Joglekar S, Mandel S, Sataloff R, Heman-Ackah Y. The predictors of postoperative laryngeal nerve paresis in patients undergoing thyroid surgery: a pilot study. *J Voice*. 2010;26(2):262–266.

12. National Cancer Institute: Surveillance, Epidemiology, and End Results (SEER) Program. Cancer stat facts: Non-Hodgkin lymphoma. Accessed September 26, 2019. https://seer .cancer.gov/statfacts/html/nhl.html

13. Kim KH, Kim RB, Woo SH. Individual participant data meta-analysis of primary laryngeal lymphoma: Focusing on the clinical characteristics and prognosis. *Laryngoscope*. 2015;125(12):2741–2748.

14. American Cancer Society. Key statistics for non-Hodgkin lymphoma. Accessed October 1, 2019. https://www.cancer.org/cancer/non -hodgkin-lymphoma/about/key-statistics.html

15. Arican A, Dincol D, Akbulut H, et al. Clinicopathologic features and prognostic factors of primary extranodal non-Hodgkin's

lymphoma in Turkey. *Am J Clin Oncol.* 1999; 22(6):587–592.

16. Hermans R, Horvath M, De Schrijver T, Lemahieu SF, Baert AL. Extranodal non-Hodgkin lymphoma of the head and neck. *J Belge Radiol.* 1994;77(2):72–77.

17. Urquhart A, Berg T. Hodgkin's and non-Hodgkin's lymphoma of the head and neck. *Laryngoscope.* 2001;111(9):1565–1569.

18. Horny HP, Kaiserling E. Involvement of the larynx by hemopoietic neoplasms. An investigation of autopsy cases and review of the literature. *Pathol Res Pract.* 1995;191(2): 130–138.

19. Markou K, Goudakos J, Constantinidis J, Kostopoulos I, Vital V, Nikolaou A. Primary laryngeal lymphoma: report of 3 cases and review of the literature. *Head Neck.* 2010; 32(4):541–549.

20. Mattioni J, Opperman DA, Solimando DA Jr, Sataloff RT. Cancer chemotherapy: an overview and voice implications. In: Sataloff RT. *Professional Voice: The Science and Art of Clinical Care.* 3rd ed. San Diego, CA: Plural Publishing; 2017:1137–1140.

21. Oakes SG, Santone KS, Powis G. Effect of some anticancer drugs on the surface membrane electrical properties of differentiated murine neuroblastoma cells. *J Natl Cancer Inst.* 1987;79:155–161.

22. Bay A, Yilmaz C, Yilmaz N, Oner AF. Vincristine induced cranial polyneuropathy. *Indian J Pediatr.* 2006;73(6):531–533.

23. American Cancer Society. Cancer facts and figures 2019. Updated 2019. Accessed October 15, 2019. https://www.cancer.org /research/cancer-facts-statistics/all-cancer -facts-figures/cancer-facts-figures-2019.html

24. Rossi SH, Klatte T, Usher-Smith J, Stewart GD. Epidemiology and screening for renal cancer. *World J Urol.* 2018;36(9):1341–1353.

25. Welch HG, Skinner JS, Shroeck FR, Zhou W, Black WC. Regional variation of computed tomographic imaging in the United States and the risk of nephrectomy. *JAMA Intern Med.* 2018;178(2):221–227.

26. Ochsner MG. Renal cell carcinoma: five year follow-up study of 70 cases. *J Urol.* 1965;93: 361–363.

27. Ferlito A, Caruso G, Recher G. Secondary laryngeal tumors. Report of seven cases with review of the literature. *Arch Otolaryngol Head Neck Surg.* 1988;114(6):635–639.

28. Saitoh H. Distant metastasis of renal adenocarcinoma. *Cancer.* 1981;48(6):1487–1491.

29. Pagano S, Franzoso F, Ruggeri P. Renal cell carcinoma metastases. Review of unusual clinical metastases, metastatic modes and patterns and comparison between clinical and autopsy metastatic series. *Scand J Urol Nephrol.* 1996;30(3):165–172.

30. Greenberg RE, Cooper J, Krigel RL, Richter RM, Kessler H, Petersen RO. Hoarseness; a unique clinical presentation for renal cell carcinoma. *Urology.* 1992;40(2):159–161.

31. Hsiang-Che H, Chang KP, Ming Chen T, Kwai-Fong W, Ueng SH. Renal cell carcinoma metastases in the head and neck. *Chang Gung Med J.* 2006;29(4):59–65.

32. Wong JA, Rendon RA. Progression to metastatic disease from a small renal cell carcinoma prospectively followed with an active surveillance protocol. *Can Urol Assoc J.* 2007; 1(2):120–122.

33. Son PM, Norton KI, Shugar JM, et al. Metastatic hypernephroma to the head and neck. *AJNR Am J Neuroradiol.* 1987;8(6):1103–1106.

34. Boles R, Cerny J. Head and neck metastases from renal cell carcinoma. *Mich Med.* 1971; 70(16):616–618.

35. Thekdi SM, Milbury K, Spelman A, et al. Posttraumatic stress and depressive symptoms in renal cell carcinoma: association with quality of life and utility of single-item distress screening. *Psychooncol.* 2015;24(11): 1477–1484.

36. Saavedra E, Hollebecque A, Soria JC, Hartl DM. Dysphonia induced by anti-angiogenic compounds. *Invest New Drugs.* 2014;32(4): 774–782.

37. Bray F, Ferlay J, Soerjomataram I, Siegel RL, Torre LA, Jemal A. Global cancer statistics 2018: GLOBOCAN estimates of incidence and mortality worldwide for 36 cancers in 185 countries. *CA Cancer J Clin.* 2018;68(6): 394–424.

38. American Cancer Society. Key statistics about stomach cancer. Accessed November 5, 2019. https://www.cancer.org/cancer/stomach-cancer/about/key-statistics.html

39. Zeb A, Rasool A, Nasreen S. Occupation and cancer incidence in district Dir (NWFP), Pakistan, 2000–2004. *Asian Pac J Cancer Prev.* 2006;7(3):483–484.

40. Zhong C, Li NK, Bi JW, Wang BC. Sodium intake, salt taste and gastric cancer risk according to *Helicobacter pylori* infection, smoking, histological type and tumor site in China. *Asian Pac J Cancer Prev.* 2012;13(6): 2481–2484.

41. Torre LA, Bray F, Siegel RL, Ferlay J, Lortet-Tieulent J, Jemal A. Global cancer statistics, 2012. *CA Cancer J Clin.* 2015;65(2):87–108.

42. Hartl DM, Bahleda R, Hollebecque A, Bosq J, Massard C, Soria JC. Bevacizumab-induced laryngeal necrosis. *Ann Oncol.* 2012;23(1): 276–278.

43. Caruso AM, Meyer TK, Allen CT. Hoarseness after metastatic colon cancer treatment. *JAMA Otolaryngol Head Neck Surg.* 2014;140(9):881–882.

44. Shord SS, Bressler LR, Tierney LA, Cuellar S, George A. Understanding and managing the possible adverse effects associated with bevacizumab. *Am J Health Syst Pharm.* 2009; 66(11):999–1013.

45. Saavedra E, Hollebecque A, Soria JC, Hartl DM. Dysphonia induced by anti-angiogenic compounds. *Invest New Drugs.* 2014;32(4): 774–782.

46. American Cancer Society. Key statistics about liver cancer. Accessed November 21, 2019.https://www.cancer.org/cancer/liver-cancer/about/what-is-key-statistics.html

Contributors

Abdul-Latif Hamdan, MD, EMBA, MPH, FACS
Professor of Otolaryngology—Head and
Neck Surgery
Head, Division of Laryngology
Director of "Hamdan Voice Unit"
American University of Beirut Medical
Center
Beirut, Lebanon
Chapters 4, 5, 6, 7, 8, 9, 10, 11, and 12

Mary J. Hawkshaw, RN, BSN, CORLN, FCCP
Research Professor
Department of Otolaryngology—Head
and Neck Surgery
Drexel University College of Medicine
Philadelphia, Pennsylvania
Chapters 4, 5, 6, 7, 8, 9, 10, 11, and 12

Dahlia M. Sataloff, MD, FACS
Chairman, Department of Surgery
Pennsylvania Hospital
Professor of Clinical Surgery
University of Pennsylvania
Perelman School of Medicine
Philadelphia, Pennsylvania
Chapter 5

Robert Thayer Sataloff, MD, DMA, FACS
Professor and Chairman, Department
of Otolaryngology—Head and Neck
Surgery
Senior Associate Dean for Clinical
Academic Specialties
Drexel University College of Medicine
Philadelphia, Pennsylvania
Chapters 1, 2, 3, 4, 5, 6, 7, 8, 9, 10, 11, and 12

SECTION I

Basic Science

1

Anatomy and Physiology of the Voice

Robert Thayer Sataloff

To treat voice patients knowledgeably and responsibly, health care professionals must understand the medical aspects of voice disorders and their treatment. This requires core knowledge of the anatomy and physiology of phonation. The human voice consists of much more than simply the vocal folds, popularly known as the vocal cords. State-of-the-art voice diagnosis, nonsurgical therapy, and voice surgery depend on understanding the complex workings of the vocal tract. Psychotherapists specializing in the care of voice patients, especially voice professionals, should be familiar with at least the basics of the latest concepts in voice function. The physiology of phonation is much more complex than this brief chapter might suggest, and readers interested in acquiring more than a clinically essential introduction are encouraged to consult other literature.[1] This chapter is written to be accessible to patients as well as health care providers.

Anatomy

The larynx is essential to normal voice production, but the anatomy of the voice is not limited to the larynx. The vocal mechanism includes the abdominal and back musculature, rib cage, lungs, pharynx, oral cavity, and nose, among other structures. Each component performs an important function in voice production, although it is possible to produce voice even without a larynx, for example, in patients who have undergone laryngectomy. In addition, virtually all parts of the body play some role in voice production and may be responsible for voice dysfunction. Even something as remote as a sprained ankle may alter posture, thereby impairing abdominal, back, and thoracic muscle function, resulting in vocal inefficiency, weakness, and hoarseness.

The larynx is composed of four basic anatomical units: skeleton, intrinsic muscles, extrinsic muscles, and mucosa. The most important components of the laryngeal skeleton are the thyroid cartilage, cricoid cartilage, and two arytenoid cartilages (Figure 1–1). Intrinsic muscles of the larynx are connected to these cartilages (Figure 1–2). One of the intrinsic muscles, the *thyroarytenoid muscle* (its medial belly is also known as the vocalis muscle), extends on each side from the vocal process of the arytenoid cartilage to the inside of the thyroid

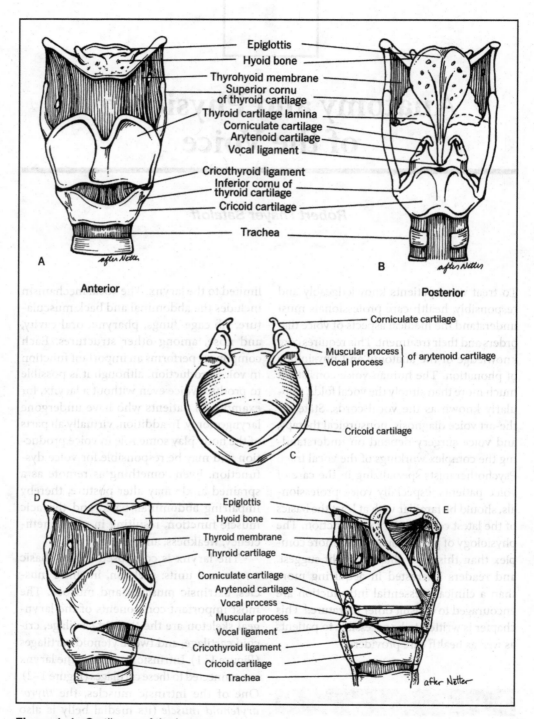

Figure 1–1. Cartilages of the larynx.

The labels in the figure read:

Epiglottis
Hyoid bone
Thyrohoid membrane
Superior cornu of thyroid cartilage
Thyroid cartilage lamina
Corniculate cartilage
Arytenoid cartilage
Vocal ligament
Cricothyroid ligament
Inferior cornu of thyroid cartilage
Cricoid cartilage
Trachea

A

Anterior

after Netter

Corniculate cartilage
Muscular process
Vocal process } of arytenoid cartilage
Cricoid cartilage

B

Posterior

after Netter

C

Epiglottis
Hyoid bone
Thyroid membrane
Thyroid cartilage
Corniculate cartilage
Arytenoid cartilage
Vocal process
Muscular process
Vocal ligament
Cricothyroid ligament
Cricoid cartilage
Trachea

D

E

after Netter

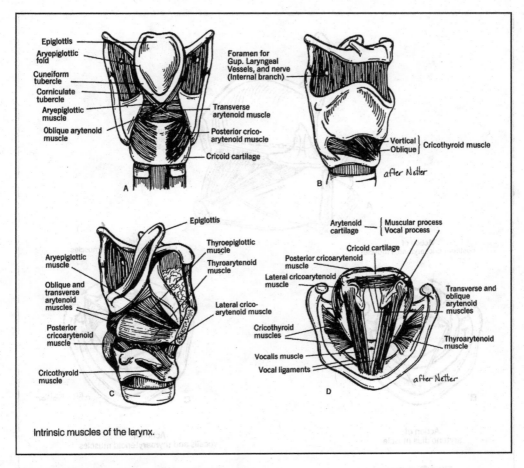

Figure 1–2. Intrinsic muscles of the larynx.

cartilage just below and behind the thyroid prominence ("Adam's apple"), forming the body of the vocal folds. The vocal folds act as the *oscillator* or *voice source* of the vocal tract. The space between the vocal folds is called the *glottis* and is used as an anatomical reference point. The intrinsic muscles alter the position, shape, and tension of the vocal folds, bringing them together (adduction), moving them apart (abduction), or stretching them by increasing longitudinal tension (Figure 1–3). They are able to do so because the laryngeal cartilages are connected by soft attachments that allow changes in their relative angles and dis-

tances, thereby permitting alteration in the shape and tension of the tissues suspended between them. The arytenoid cartilages on their elliptic cricoarytenoid joints are capable of motion in multiple planes, permitting complex vocal fold motion and alteration in the shape of the vocal fold edge associated with intrinsic muscle action (Figure 1–4). All but one of the muscles on each side of the larynx are innervated by one of the two *recurrent laryngeal nerves*. Because this nerve runs in a long course (especially on the left) from the neck down into the chest and then back up to the larynx (hence, the name *recurrent*), it is injured easily by

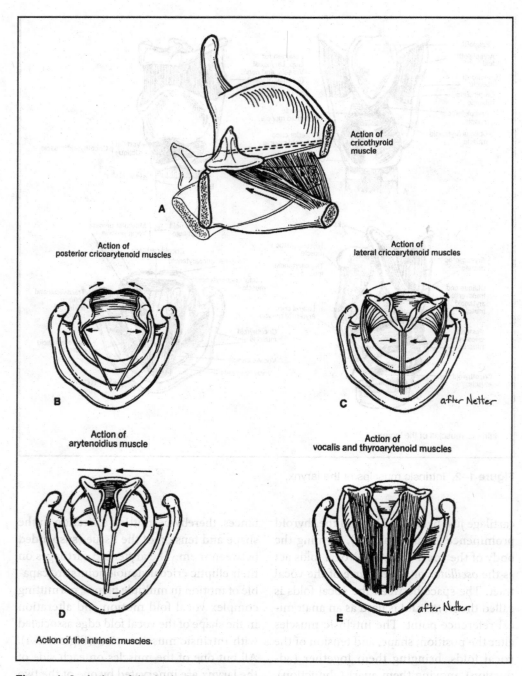

Action of
cricothyroid
muscle

Action of
posterior cricoarytenoid muscles

Action of
lateral cricoarytenoid muscles

after Netter

Action of
arytenoidius muscle

Action of
vocalis and thyroarytenoid muscles

after Netter

Action of the intrinsic muscles.

Figure 1–3. Action of the intrinsic muscles.

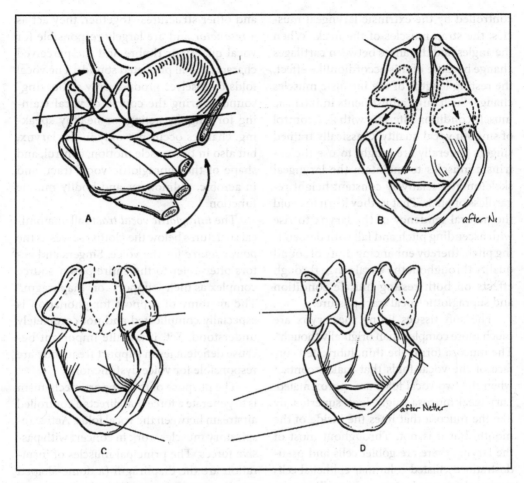

Figure 1–4. Complex arytenoid motion.

trauma, neck surgery, and chest surgery. Injury may result in vocal fold paresis or paralysis. The remaining muscle (*cricothyroid muscle*) is innervated by the superior laryngeal nerve on each side, which is especially susceptible to viral and traumatic injury. It causes changes in longitudinal tension that are important in voice projection and pitch control. The "false vocal folds" are located above the vocal folds, and unlike the true vocal folds, usually do not make contact during normal speaking or singing.[1] The neuroanatomy and neurophysiology of phonation are extremely complicated

and only partially understood. As the new field of neurolaryngology advances, a more thorough understanding of the subject is becoming increasingly important to medical and psychological clinicians. Readers interested in acquiring a deeper, scientific understanding of neurolaryngology are encouraged to consult other literature[2] and the publications cited therein.

Because the attachments of the laryngeal cartilages are flexible, the positions of the cartilages with respect to each other change when the laryngeal skeleton is elevated or lowered. Such changes in vertical height are controlled by the extrinsic laryngeal muscles, the strap muscles of the neck. When the angles and distances between cartilages change because of this accordionlike effect, the resting lengths of the intrinsic muscles change. Such large adjustments in intrinsic muscle condition interfere with fine control of smooth vocal quality. Classically trained singers generally are taught to use the extrinsic muscles to maintain the laryngeal skeleton at a relatively constant height regardless of pitch. That is, they learn to avoid the natural tendency of the larynx to rise with ascending pitch and fall with descending pitch, thereby enhancing unity of sound quality throughout the vocal range through effects on both resting muscle condition and supraglottic vocal tract posture.

The soft tissues lining the larynx are much more complex than originally thought. The mucosa forms the thin, lubricated surface of the vocal folds that makes contact when the two vocal folds are approximated. Laryngeal mucosa might look superficially like the mucosa that lines the inside of the mouth, but it is not. Throughout most of the larynx, there are goblet cells and pseudostratified ciliated columnar epithelial cells designed for producing and handling mucous secretions, similar to mucosal surfaces found throughout the respiratory tract. However, the mucosa overlying the vocal folds is different. First, it is stratified squamous epithelium, which is better suited to withstand the trauma of vocal fold contact. Second, the vocal fold is not simply muscle covered with mucosa. Rather, it consists of 5 layers as described by Hirano.[3] Mechanically, the vocal fold structures act more like 3 layers consisting of the *cover* (epithelium and superficial layer of the lamina propria), *transition* (intermediate and deep layers of the lamina propria), and *body* (the vocalis muscle).

The *supraglottic vocal tract* includes the pharynx, tongue, palate, oral cavity, nose, and other structures. Together, they act as a *resonator* and are largely responsible for vocal quality or timbre and the perceived character of all phonated sounds. The vocal folds themselves produce only a "buzzing" sound. During the course of vocal training for singing, acting, or healthy speaking, changes occur not only in the larynx, but also in the muscle motion, control, and shape of the supraglottic vocal tract, and in aerobic, pulmonary, and bodily muscle function.

The *infraglottic vocal tract* (all anatomical structures below the glottis) serves as the *power source* for the voice. Singers and actors often refer to the entire power source complex as their "support" or "diaphragm." The anatomy of support for phonation is especially complicated and not completely understood. Yet, it is quite important because deficiencies in support frequently are responsible for voice dysfunction.

The purpose of the support mechanism is to generate a force that directs a controlled airstream between the vocal folds. Active respiratory muscles work in concert with passive forces. The principal muscles of inspiration are the diaphragm (a dome-shaped muscle that extends along the bottom of the rib cage) and the external intercostal muscles (located between the ribs). During quiet respiration, expiration is largely passive. The lungs and rib cage generate passive expiratory forces under many common circumstances such as after a full breath.

Many of the muscles used for active expiration also are employed in "support" for phonation. Muscles of active expiration either raise the intra-abdominal pressure, forcing the diaphragm upward, or lower the ribs or sternum to decrease the dimensions of the thorax, or both, thereby compressing air in the chest. The primary muscles of expiration are "the abdominal muscles," but internal intercostals and other chest and back muscles also are involved. Trauma or surgery that alters the structure or function of these muscles or ribs undermines the power source of the voice, as do diseases, such as asthma, that impair expiration. Deficiencies in the support mechanism often result in compensatory efforts that utilize the laryngeal muscles, which are not designed for power functions. Such behavior can result in impaired voice quality, rapid fatigue, pain, and even structural pathology such as vocal fold nodules. Current expert treatment for such vocal problems focuses on correction of the underlying malfunction rather than surgery whenever possible, including attention to the psychological concomitants of the condition.

Physiology

The physiology of voice production is extremely complex. Volitional production of voice begins in the cerebral cortex (Figure 1–5). The command for vocalization involves complex interactions among brain centers for speech, as well as other areas. For singing, speech directives must be integrated with information from the centers for musical and artistic expression, which are discussed elsewhere.[1] The "idea" of the planned vocalization is conveyed to the precentral gyrus in the motor cortex that transmits another set of instructions to the motor nuclei in the brain stem and spinal cord. These areas send out the complicated messages necessary for coordinated activity of the larynx, thoracic and abdominal musculature, lungs, and vocal tract articulators, among other structures. Additional refinement of motor activity is provided by the extrapyramidal and autonomic nervous systems. These impulses combine to produce a sound that is transmitted not only to

the ears of the listener, but also to those of the speaker or singer. Auditory feedback is transmitted from the ear through the brain stem to the cerebral cortex, and within milliseconds adjustments are made that permit the vocalist to match the sound produced with the sound intended, integrating the acoustic properties of the performance environment. Tactile feedback from throat and other muscles involved in phonation also is believed to help in fine-tuning vocal output, although the mechanism and role of tactile feedback are not understood fully. Many trained singers and speakers cultivate the ability to use tactile feedback effectively because of expected interference with auditory feedback data from ancillary sound such as an orchestra or a band.

Phonation, the production of sound, requires interaction among the power source, oscillator, and resonator. The voice may be compared to a brass instrument such as a trumpet. Power is generated by the chest and abdominal and back musculature, and a high-pressure airstream is produced. The trumpeter's lips open and close against the mouthpiece producing a "buzz" similar to the sound produced by vocal folds when they come together and move apart (oscillate) during phonation. This sound then passes through the trumpet that has acoustic resonance characteristics that shape the sound we associate with trumpet music. If a trumpet mouthpiece is placed on a French horn, the sound we hear will sound like a French horn, not a trumpet. Quality characteristics are dependent on the resonator more than on the oscillatory source. The nonmouthpiece portions of a brass instrument are analogous to the supraglottic vocal tract.

During phonation, the infraglottic musculature must make rapid, complex adjustments because the resistance changes almost continuously as the glottis closes, opens,

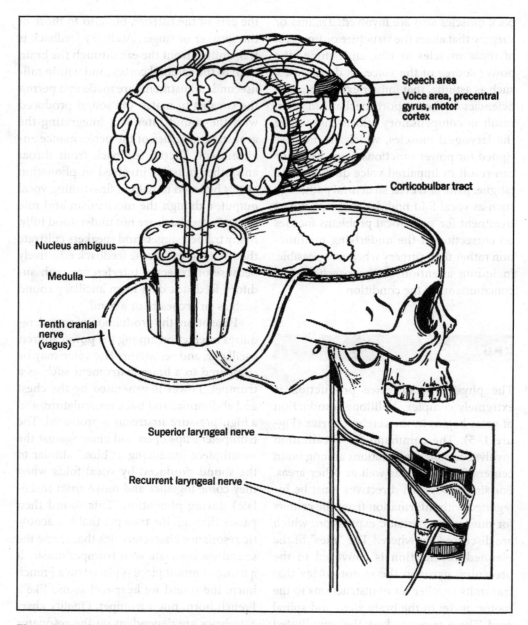

Figure 1–5. Simplified summary of pathway for volitional phonation.

and changes shape. At the beginning of each phonatory cycle, the vocal folds are approximated, and the glottis is obliterated. This permits infraglottic air pressure to build, typically to a level of about 7 cm of water for conversational speech. At that point, the vocal folds are convergent (Figure 1–6A). Because the vocal folds are closed, there is no airflow. The subglottic pressure then pushes the vocal folds progressively farther apart from the bottom up and from the back forward (Figure 1–6B)

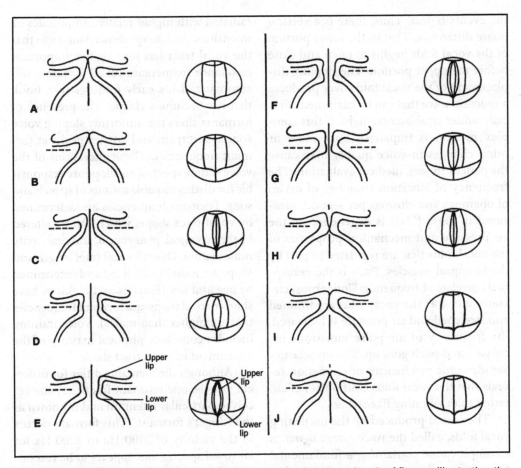

Figure 1–6. Frontal view (left) and view from above (right) in each pair of figures illustrating the normal pattern of vocal fold vibration. The vocal folds close and open from the inferior aspect of the vibratory margin upward, and from posterior to anterior.

until a space develops (Figures 1–6C, D) and air begins to flow. Bernoulli force created by the air passing between the vocal folds combines with the mechanical properties of the folds to begin closing the lower portion of the vocal folds almost immediately (Figures 1–6E, F, G, H), even while the upper edges are still separating. The principles and mathematics of Bernoulli force are complex. It is a flow effect more easily understood by familiar examples such as the sensation of pull exerted on a vehicle when passed by a truck at high speed or the inward motion

of a shower curtain when the water flows past it.

The upper portion of the vocal folds has elastic properties that also tend to make the vocal folds snap back to the midline. This force becomes more dominant as the upper edges are stretched and the opposing force of the airstream diminishes because of approximation of the lower edges of the vocal folds. The upper portions of the vocal folds are then returned to the midline (Figure 1–6I), completing the glottic cycle. Subglottal pressure then builds again (Figure 1–6J), and the events repeat. Thus, there is a vertical phase difference. That is, the lower portion of the vocal folds begins to open and close before the upper portion. The rippling displacement of the vocal fold cover produces a mucosal wave that can be examined clinically under stroboscopic light. If this complex motion is impaired, hoarseness or other changes in voice quality may cause the patient to seek medical evaluation. The frequency of vibration (number of cycles of openings and closings per second, measured in hertz [Hz]) is dependent on the air pressure and mechanical properties of the vocal folds that are regulated in part by the laryngeal muscles. Pitch is the perceptual correlate of frequency. Under most circumstances, as the vocal folds are thinned and stretched and air pressure is increased, the frequency of air pulse emissions increases, and pitch goes up. The myoelastic-aerodynamic mechanism of phonation reveals that the vocal folds emit pulses of air, rather than vibrating like strings.

The sound produced by the oscillating vocal folds, called the *voice source signal*, is a complex tone containing a fundamental frequency and many overtones, or higher harmonic partials. The amplitude of the partials decreases uniformly at approximately 12 dB per octave. Interestingly, the acoustic spectrum of the voice source is about the same in ordinary speakers as it is in trained singers and speakers. Voice quality differences in voice professionals occur as the voice source signal passes through their supraglottic vocal tract resonator system (Figure 1–7).

The pharynx, oral cavity, and nasal cavity act as a series of infinitely variable interconnected resonators, which are more complex than that in our trumpet example or other single resonators. As with other resonators, some frequencies are attenuated, and others are enhanced. Enhanced frequencies are radiated with higher relative amplitudes or intensities. Sundberg[4] showed long ago that the vocal tract has four or five important resonance frequencies called *formants* and summarized his early findings in a book that has become a classic. The presence of formants alters the uniformly sloping voice source spectrum and creates peaks at formant frequencies. These alterations of the voice source spectral envelope are responsible for distinguishable sounds of speech and song. Formant frequencies are determined by vocal tract shape, which can be altered by the laryngeal, pharyngeal, and oral cavity musculature. Overall vocal tract length and shape are individually fixed and determined by age and sex (females and children have shorter vocal tracts and formant frequencies that are higher than males). Voice training includes conscious physical mastery of the adjustment of vocal tract shape.

Although the formants differ for different vowels, one resonant frequency has received particular attention and is known as the "singer's formant." This formant occurs in the vicinity of 2300 Hz to 3200 Hz for all vowel spectra and appears to be responsible for the "ring" in a singer's or trained speaker's ("speaker's formant") voice. The ability to hear a trained voice clearly even over a loud choir or orchestra is dependent primarily on the presence of the singer's formant.[1] Interestingly, there is little or no significant difference in maximum vocal intensity between trained and untrained singers. The singer's formant also contributes substantially to the differences in fach (voice classification) among voice categories, occurring in basses at about 2400 Hz, baritones at 2600 Hz, tenors at 2800 Hz, mezzo-sopranos at 2900 Hz, and sopranos at 3200 Hz. It is frequently much less prominent in high soprano singing.[1]

The mechanisms that control two vocal characteristics are particularly important:

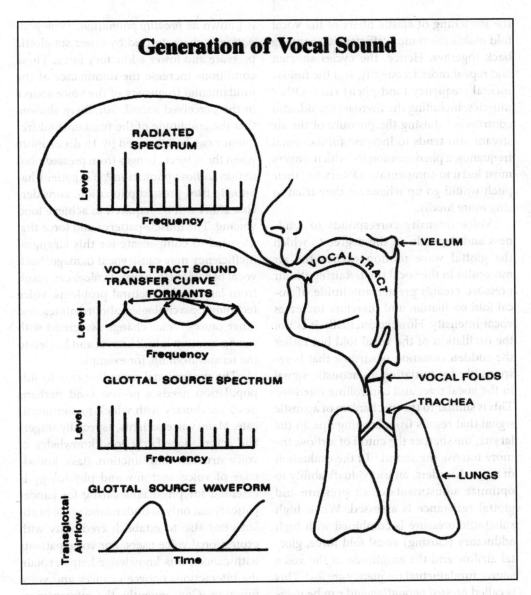

Figure 1–7. Determinants of the spectrum of a vowel (oral-output signal).

fundamental frequency and intensity. Fundamental frequency, which corresponds to pitch, can be altered by changing either air pressure or the mechanical properties of the vocal folds, although the latter is more efficient under most conditions. When the cricothyroid muscle contracts, it makes the

thyroid cartilage pivot on the cricothyroid joint and increases the distance between the thyroid and arytenoid cartilages, thus stretching the vocal folds. This increases the surface area exposed to subglottal pressure and makes the air pressure more effective in opening the glottis. In addition, the stretching of elastic fibers of the vocal fold makes them more efficient at snapping back together. Hence, the cycles shorten and repeat more frequently, and the fundamental frequency (and pitch) rises. Other muscles, including the thyroarytenoid, also contribute.[1] Raising the pressure of the air stream also tends to increase fundamental frequency, a phenomenon for which singers must learn to compensate. Otherwise, their pitch would go up whenever they tried to sing more loudly.

Voice intensity corresponds to loudness and depends on the degree to which the glottal wave motion excites the air molecules in the vocal tract. Raising the air pressure creates greater amplitude of vocal fold oscillation and therefore increases vocal intensity. However, actually it is not the oscillation of the vocal fold but rather the sudden cessation of airflow that is responsible for initiating an acoustic signal in the vocal tract and controlling intensity. This is similar to the mechanism of acoustic signal that results from buzzing lips. In the larynx, the sharper the cutoff of airflow, the more intense the sound.[1] In the evaluation of voice disorders, an individual's ability to optimize adjustments of air pressure and glottal resistance is assessed. When high subglottic pressure is combined with high adductory (closing) vocal fold force, glottal airflow and the amplitude of the voice source fundamental frequency are low. This is called *pressed phonation* and can be measured clinically through a technique known as flow glottography. Flow glottogram wave amplitude indicates the type of phonation being used, and the slope (closing rate) provides information about the sound pressure level or loudness. If adductory forces are so weak that the vocal folds do not make contact, the vocal folds become inefficient at resisting air leakage, and the voice source fundamental frequency is low. This is known as *breathy phonation. Flow phonation* is characterized by lower subglottic pressure and lower adductory force. These conditions increase the dominance of the fundamental frequency of the voice source in the perceived sound. Sundberg showed that the amplitude of the fundamental frequency can be increased by 15 dB or more when the subject changes from pressed phonation to flow phonation.[4] If a patient habitually uses pressed phonation, considerable effort will be required to achieve loud voicing. The muscle patterns and force that are used to compensate for this laryngeal inefficiency may cause vocal damage. Such vocal behavior (ie, pressed voice) can result from laryngeal structural problems, voice technique, psychological abnormalities, and other causes. Voice change associated with strong emotion is well known and has led to the term *choked up*, for example.

The professional providing care to this population needs a precise (and perhaps new) vocabulary with which to communicate. Many voice patients, especially singers and actors, have fairly good knowledge of voice structure and function. Basic knowledge of voice anatomy and physiology is essential for physicians caring for cancer patients not only to understand voice problems but also to establish credibility with professional voice users. For voice patients with cancer, this knowledge helps explain the interactions between cancer and voice function. Consequently, the effectiveness and credibility of the clinician are impaired substantially when the psychotherapist does not possess at least a basic understanding of the voice. Rapport is essential to therapeutic communication, regardless of the patient's psychological status. Being able to join, pace, and therefore communicate more effectively within the contextual world of the patient enhances treatment efficacy.

References

1. Sataloff RT. *Professional Voice: The Science and Art of Clinical Care*. 4th ed. San Diego, CA: Plural Publishing; 2017.
2. Sataloff RT. *Neurolaryngology*. San Diego, CA: Plural Publishing; 2017.
3. Hirano M. Phonosurgery: basic and clinical investigations. *Otologia* (Fukuoka). 1975; 21:239–442.
4. Sundberg J. *The Science of the Singing Voice*. DeKalb, IL: Northern Illinois University Press; 1987.

2

Patient History*

Robert Thayer Sataloff

A comprehensive history and physical examination usually reveal the cause of voice dysfunction. Effective history taking and physical examination depend on a practical understanding of the anatomy and physiology of voice production.[1-3] Because dysfunction in virtually any body system may affect phonation, medical inquiry must be comprehensive. The current standard of care for all voice patients evolved from advances inspired by medical problems of voice professionals such as singers and actors. Even minor problems may be particularly symptomatic in singers and actors because of the extreme demands they place on their voices. However, a great many other patients are voice professionals. They include teachers, salespeople, attorneys, clergy, physicians, politicians, telephone receptionists, and anyone else whose ability to earn a living is impaired in the presence of voice dysfunction. Because good voice quality is so important in our society, the majority of our patients are voice profes-

sionals, and all patients should be treated as such.

The scope of inquiry and examination for most patients is similar to that required for singers and actors, except that performing voice professionals have unique needs that require additional history and examination. Questions must be added regarding performance commitments, professional status and voice goals, the amount and nature of voice training, the performance environment, rehearsal practices, abusive habits during speech and singing, and many other matters. Such supplementary information is essential to proper treatment selection and patient counseling in singers and actors. However, analogous factors must also be taken into account for stockbrokers, factory shop foremen, elementary school teachers, homemakers with several noisy children, and many others. Physicians familiar with the management of these challenging patients are well equipped to evaluate all patients with voice complaints.

---

* Reprinted with permission from Hamdan AL, Sataloff RT, Hawkshaw MJ. *Obesity and Voice*. San Diego, CA: Plural Publishing; 2020.

Patient History

Obtaining extensive historical background information is necessary for thorough evaluation of the voice patient, and the otolaryngologist who sees voice patients (especially singers) only occasionally cannot reasonably be expected to remember all the pertinent questions. Although some laryngologists consider a lengthy inquisition helpful in establishing rapport, many of us who see a substantial number of voice patients each day within a busy practice need a thorough but less time-consuming alternative. A history questionnaire can be extremely helpful in documenting all the necessary information, helping the patient sort out and articulate his or her problems, and saving the clinician time recording information. The author has developed a questionnaire[4] that has proven helpful (Appendix 2–A). The patient is asked to complete the relevant portions of the form at home prior to his or her office visit or in the waiting room before seeing the doctor. A similar form has been developed for voice patients who are not singers.

No history questionnaire is a substitute for direct, penetrating questioning by the physician. However, the direction of most useful inquiry can be determined from a glance at the questionnaire, obviating the need for extensive writing, which permits the physician greater eye contact with the patient and facilitates rapid establishment of the close rapport and confidence that are so important in treating voice patients. The physician is also able to supplement initial impressions and historical information from the questionnaire with seemingly leisurely conversation during the physical examination. The use of the history questionnaire has added substantially to the efficiency, consistent thoroughness, and ease of managing these patients. A similar set of questions is also used by the speech-language pathologist with new patients and by many enlightened singing teachers when assessing new students.

How Old Are You?

Serious vocal endeavor may start in childhood and continue throughout a lifetime. As the vocal mechanism undergoes normal maturation, the voice changes. The optimal time to begin serious vocal training is controversial. For many years, most singing teachers advocated delay of vocal training and serious singing until near puberty in the female and after puberty and voice stabilization in the male. However, in a child with earnest vocal aspirations and potential, starting specialized training early in childhood is reasonable. Initial instruction should teach the child to vocalize without straining and to avoid all forms of voice abuse. It should not permit premature indulgence in operatic bravado. Most experts agree that taxing voice use and singing during puberty should be minimized or avoided altogether, particularly by the male. Voice maturation (attainment of stable adult vocal quality) may occur at any age from the early teenage years to the fourth decade of life. The dangerous tendency for young singers to attempt to sound older than their vocal years frequently causes vocal dysfunction.

All components of voice production are subject to normal aging. Abdominal and general muscular tone frequently decrease, lungs lose elasticity, the thorax loses its distensibility, the mucosa of the vocal tract atrophies, mucous secretions change character and quantity, nerve endings are reduced in number, and psychoneurologic functions change. Moreover, the larynx itself loses muscle tone and bulk and may show depletion of submucosal ground substance in the vocal folds. The laryngeal cartilages ossify, and the joints may become arthritic and stiff. Hormonal influence is altered. Vocal range, intensity, and quality all may be modified. Vocal fold atrophy may be the most striking alteration. The clinical effects of aging seem more pronounced in female singers, although vocal fold histologic changes may be more prominent in males. Excellent male singers occasionally extend their careers into their 70s or beyond.[5,6] However, some degree of breathiness, decreased range, and other evidence of aging should be expected in elderly voices. Nevertheless, many of the changes we typically associate with elderly singers (wobble, flat pitch) are due to lack of conditioning, rather than inevitable changes of biological aging. These aesthetically undesirable concomitants of aging can often be reversed.

What Is Your Voice Problem?

Careful questioning as to the onset of vocal problems is needed to separate acute from chronic dysfunction. Often an upper respiratory tract infection will send a patient to the physician's office, but penetrating inquiry, especially in singers and actors, may reveal a chronic vocal problem that is the patient's real concern. Identifying acute and chronic problems before beginning therapy is important so that both patient and physician may have realistic expectations and make optimal therapeutic selections.

The specific nature of the vocal complaint can provide a great deal of information. Just as dizzy patients rarely walk into the physician's office complaining of "rotary vertigo," voice patients may be unable to articulate their symptoms without guidance. They may use the term *hoarseness* to describe a variety of conditions that

the physician must separate. Hoarseness is a coarse or scratchy sound that is most often associated with abnormalities of the leading edge of the vocal folds, such as laryngitis or mass lesions. Breathiness is a vocal quality characterized by excessive loss of air during vocalization. In some cases, it is due to improper technique. However, any condition that prevents full approximation of the vocal folds can be responsible. Possible causes include vocal fold paralysis, a mass lesion separating the leading edges of the vocal folds, arthritis of the cricoarytenoid joint, arytenoid dislocation, scarring of the vibratory margin, senile vocal fold atrophy (presbyphonia), psychogenic dysphonia, malingering, and other conditions.

Fatigue of the voice is the inability to continue to speak or sing for extended periods without change in vocal quality, control, or both. The voice may show fatigue by becoming hoarse, losing range, changing timbre, breaking into different registers, or exhibiting other uncontrolled aberrations. A well-trained singer should be able to sing for several hours without vocal fatigue.

Voice fatigue may occur through more than one mechanism. Most of the time, it is assumed to be due to muscle fatigue. This is often the case in patients who have voice fatigue associated with muscle tension dysphonia. The mechanism is most likely to be peripheral muscle fatigue and due to chemical changes (or depletion) in the muscle fibers. "Muscle fatigue" may also occur on a central (neurologic) basis. This mechanism is common in certain neuropathic disorders, such as multiple sclerosis; may occur with myasthenia gravis (actually neuromuscular junction pathology); or may be associated with paresis from various causes. However, the voice may also fatigue due to changes in the vibratory margin of the vocal fold. This phenomenon may be described as "lamina propria" fatigue (our descriptive, not universally used). It, too, may be related to chemical or fluid changes in the lamina propria or cellular damage associated with conditions such as phonotrauma and dehydration. Excessive voice use, suboptimal tissue environment (eg, dehydration, effects of pollution, etc), lack of sufficient time of recovery between phonatory stresses, and genetic or structural tissue weaknesses that predispose to injury or delayed recovery from trauma all may be associated with lamina propria fatigue.

Although it has not been proven, this author (RTS) suspects that fatigue may also be related to the linearity of vocal fold vibrations. However, briefly, voices have linear and nonlinear (chaotic) characteristics. As the voice becomes more trained, vibrations become more symmetrical, and the system becomes more linear. In many pathologic voices, the nonlinear components appear to become more prominent. If a voice is highly linear, slight changes in the vibratory margin may have little effect on the output of the system. However, if the system has substantial nonlinearity due to vocal fold pathology, poor tissue environment, or other causes, slight changes in the tissue (slight swelling, drying, surface cell damage) may cause substantial changes in the acoustic output of the system (the butterfly effect), causing vocal quality changes and fatigue much more quickly with much smaller changes in initial condition in more linear vocal systems.

Fatigue is often caused by misuse of abdominal and neck musculature or oversinging, singing too loudly, or singing too long. However, we must remember that vocal fatigue may be a sign not only of general tiredness or vocal abuse (sometimes secondary to structural lesions or glottal closure problems) but also of serious illnesses such as myasthenia gravis. So, the importance of this complaint should not be understated.

Volume disturbance may manifest as the inability to sing loudly or the inability to sing softly. Each voice has its own dynamic range. Within the course of training, singers learn to sing more loudly by singing more efficiently. They also learn to sing softly, a more difficult task, through years of laborious practice. Actors and other trained speakers go through similar training. Most volume problems are secondary to intrinsic limitations of the voice or technical errors in voice use, although hormonal changes, aging, and neurologic disease are other causes. Superior laryngeal nerve paralysis impairs the ability to speak or sing loudly. This is a frequently unrecognized consequence of herpes infection (cold sores) and Lyme disease and may be precipitated by any viral upper respiratory tract infection.

Most highly trained singers require only about 10 minutes to half an hour to "warm up the voice." Prolonged warm-up time, especially in the morning, is most often caused by reflux laryngitis. Tickling or choking during singing is most often a symptom of an abnormality of the vocal fold's leading edge. The symptom of tickling or choking should contraindicate singing until the vocal folds have been examined. Pain while singing can indicate vocal fold lesions, laryngeal joint arthritis, infection, or gastric acid reflux irritation of the arytenoid region. However, pain is much more commonly caused by voice abuse with excessive muscular activity in the neck rather than an acute abnormality on the leading edge of a vocal fold. In the absence of other symptoms, these patients do not generally require immediate cessation of singing pending medical examination. However, sudden onset of pain (usually sharp pain) while singing may be associated with a mucosal tear or a vocal fold hemorrhage and warrants voice conservation pending laryngeal examination.

Do You Have Any Pressing Voice Commitments?

If a singer or professional speaker (eg, actor, politician) seeks treatment at the end of a busy performance season and has no pressing engagements, management of the voice problem should be relatively conservative and designed to ensure long-term protection of the larynx, the most delicate part of the vocal mechanism. However, the physician and patient rarely have this luxury. Most often, the voice professional needs treatment within a week of an important engagement and sometimes within less than a day. Younger singers fall ill shortly before performances, not because of hypochondria or coincidence, but rather because of the immense physical and emotional stress of the preperformance period. The singer is frequently working harder and singing longer hours than usual. Moreover, he or she may be under particular pressure to learn new material and to perform well for a new audience. The singer may also be sleeping less than usual because of additional time spent rehearsing or because of the discomforts of a strange city. Seasoned professionals make their living by performing regularly, sometimes several times a week. Consequently, any time they get sick is likely to precede a performance. Caring for voice complaints in these situations requires highly skilled judgment and bold management.

Tell Me About Your Vocal Career, Long-Term Goals, and the Importance of Your Voice Quality and Upcoming Commitments

To choose a treatment program, the physician must understand the importance of the patient's voice and his or her long-term career plans, the importance of the upcoming vocal commitment, and the consequences of canceling the engagement. Injudicious prescription of voice rest can be almost as damaging to a vocal career as injudicious performance. For example, although a singer's voice is usually his or her most important commodity, other factors distinguish the few successful artists from the multitude of less successful singers with equally good voices. These include musicianship, reliability, and "professionalism." Canceling a concert at the last minute may seriously damage a performer's reputation. Reliability is especially critical early in a singer's career. Moreover, an expert singer often can modify a performance to decrease the strain on his or her voice. No singer should be allowed to perform in a manner that will permit serious injury to the vocal folds, but in the frequent borderline cases, the condition of the larynx must be weighed against other factors affecting the singer as an artist.

How Much Voice Training Have You Had?

Establishing how long a singer or actor has been performing seriously is important, especially if his or her active performance career predates the beginning of vocal training. Active untrained singers and actors frequently develop undesirable techniques that are difficult to modify. Extensive voice use without training or premature training with inappropriate repertoire may underlie persistent vocal difficulties later in life. The number of years a performer has been training his or her voice may be a fair index of vocal proficiency. A person who has studied voice for 1 or 2 years is somewhat more likely to have gross technical difficulties than is someone who has been studying for 20 years. However, if training has been intermittent or discontinued, technical problems are common, especially among singers. In addition, methods of technical voice use vary among voice teachers. Hence, a student who has had many teachers in a relatively brief period of time commonly has numerous technical insecurities or deficiencies that may be responsible for vocal dysfunction. This is especially true if the singer has changed to a new teacher within the preceding year. The physician must be careful not to criticize the patient's current voice teacher in such circumstances. It often takes years of expert instruction to correct bad habits.

All people speak more often than they sing, yet most singers report little speech training. Even if a singer uses the voice flawlessly while practicing and performing, voice abuse at other times can cause damage that affects singing.

Under What Kinds of Conditions Do You Use Your Voice?

The Lombard effect is the tendency to increase vocal intensity in response to increased background noise. A well-trained singer learns to compensate for this tendency and to avoid singing at unsafe volumes. Singers of classical music usually have such training and frequently perform with only a piano, a situation in which the balance can be controlled well. However, singers performing in large halls, with orchestras, or in operas early in their careers tend to over-sing and strain their voices. Similar problems occur during outdoor concerts because of the lack of auditory feedback. This phenomenon is seen even more among "pop" singers. Pop singers are

in a uniquely difficult position; often, despite little vocal training, they enjoy great artistic and financial success and endure extremely stressful demands on their time and voices. They are required to sing in large halls or outdoor arenas not designed for musical performance, amid smoke and other environmental irritants, accompanied by extremely loud background music. One frequently neglected key to survival for these singers is the proper use of monitor speakers. These direct the sound of the singer's voice toward the singer on the stage and provide auditory feedback. Determining whether the pop singer uses monitor speakers and whether they are loud enough for the singer to hear is important.

Amateur singers are often no less serious about their music than are professionals, but generally they have less ability to compensate technically for illness or other physical impairment. Rarely does an amateur suffer a great loss from postponing a performance or permitting someone to sing in his or her place. In most cases, the amateur singer's best interest is served through conservative management directed at long-term maintenance of good vocal health.

A great many of the singers who seek physicians' advice are primarily choral singers. They often are enthusiastic amateurs, untrained but dedicated to their musical recreation. They should be handled as amateur solo singers, educated specifically about the Lombard effect, and cautioned to avoid the excessive volume so common in a choral environment. One good way for a singer to monitor loudness is to cup a hand to his or her ear. This adds about 6 dB[7] to the singer's perception of his or her own voice and can be a very helpful guide in noisy surroundings. Young professional singers are often hired to augment amateur choruses. Feeling that the professional quartet has been hired to "lead" the rest of the choir, they often make the mistake of trying to accomplish that goal by singing louder than others in their sections. These singers should be advised to lead their section by singing each line as if they were soloists giving a voice lesson to the people standing next to them and as if there were a microphone in front of them recording their choral performance for their voice teacher. This approach usually not only preserves the voice but also produces a better choral sound.

How Much Do You Practice and Exercise Your Voice? How, When, and Where Do You Use Your Voice?

Vocal exercise is as essential to the vocalist as exercise and conditioning of other muscle systems is to the athlete. Proper vocal practice incorporates scales and specific exercises designed to maintain and develop the vocal apparatus. Simply acting or singing songs or giving performances without routine studious concentration on vocal technique is not adequate for the vocal performer. The physician should know whether the vocalist practices daily, whether he or she practices at the same time daily, and how long the practice lasts. Actors generally practice and warm up their voices for 10 to 30 minutes daily, although more time is recommended. Most serious singers practice for at least 1 to 2 hours per day. If a singer routinely practices in the late afternoon or evening but frequently performs in the morning (religious services, school classes, teaching voice, choir rehearsals, etc), one should inquire into the warm-up procedures preceding such performances as well as cool-down procedures after voice use. Singing "cold," especially early in the morning, may result in the use of minor muscular alterations to compensate for vocal insecurity produced by inadequate

preparation. Such crutches can result in voice dysfunction. Similar problems may result from instances of voice use other than formal singing. Schoolteachers, telephone receptionists, salespeople, and others who speak extensively also often derive great benefit from 5 or 10 minutes of vocalization of scales first thing in the morning. Although singers rarely practice their scales too long, they frequently perform or rehearse excessively. This is especially true immediately before a major concert or audition, when physicians are most likely to see acute problems. When a singer has hoarseness and vocal fatigue and has been practicing a new role for 14 hours a day for the last 3 weeks, no simple prescription will solve the problem. However, a treatment regimen can usually be designed to carry the performer safely through his or her musical obligations.

The physician should be aware of common habits and environments that are often associated with abusive voice behavior and should ask about them routinely. Screaming at sports events and at children is among the most common. Extensive voice use in noisy environments also tends to be abusive. These include noisy rooms, cars, airplanes, sports facilities, and other locations where background noise or acoustic design impairs auditory feedback. Dry, dusty surroundings may alter vocal fold secretions through dehydration or contact irritation, altering voice function. Activities such as cheerleading, teaching, choral conducting, amateur singing, and frequent communication with hearing-impaired persons are likely to be associated with voice abuse, as is extensive professional voice use without formal training. The physician should inquire into the patient's routine voice use and should specifically ask about any activities that frequently lead to voice change such as hoarseness or discomfort in the neck or throat. Laryngologists should ask specifically about other activities that may be abusive to the vocal folds, such as weight lifting, aerobics, and the playing of some wind instruments.

Are You Aware of Misusing or Abusing Your Voice During Singing?

A detailed discussion of vocal technique in singing is beyond the scope of this chapter but is discussed in other chapters. The most common technical errors involve excessive muscle tension in the tongue, neck, and larynx; inadequate abdominal support; and excessive volume. Inadequate preparation can be a devastating source of voice abuse and may result from limited practice, limited rehearsal of a difficult piece, or limited vocal training for a given role. The latter error is common. In some situations, voice teachers are at fault; both the singer and teacher must resist the impulse to "show off " the voice in works that are either too difficult for the singer's level of training or simply not suited to the singer's voice. Singers are habitually unhappy with the limitations of their voices. At some time or another, most baritones wish they were tenors and walk around proving they can sing high Cs in "Vesti la giubba." Singers with other vocal ranges have similar fantasies. Attempts to make the voice something that it is not, or at least that it is not yet, frequently are harmful.

Are You Aware of Misusing or Abusing Your Voice During Speaking?

Common patterns of voice abuse and misuse will not be discussed in detail in this chapter. Voice abuse and/or misuse should be sus-

pected particularly in a patient who complains of voice fatigue associated with voice use, whose voice is worse at the end of a working day or week, and who is chronically hoarse. Technical errors in voice use may be the primary etiology of a voice complaint, or the technical error may develop secondarily due to a patient's effort to compensate for voice disturbance from another cause.

Dissociation of one's speaking and singing voices is probably the most common cause of voice abuse problems in excellent singers. Too frequently, all the expert training in support, muscle control, and projection is not applied to a singers' speaking voice. Unfortunately, the resultant voice strain affects the singing voice as well as the speaking voice. Such damage is especially likely to occur in noisy rooms and in cars, where the background noise is louder than it seems. Backstage greetings after a lengthy performance can be particularly devastating. The singer usually is exhausted and distracted, the environment is often dusty and dry, and generally a noisy crowd is present. Similar conditions prevail at postperformance parties, where smoking and alcohol worsen matters. These situations should be avoided by any singer with vocal problems and should be controlled through awareness at other times.

Three particularly abusive and potentially damaging vocal activities are worthy of note. *Cheerleading* requires extensive screaming under the worst possible physical and environmental circumstances. It is a highly undesirable activity for anyone considering serious vocal endeavor. This is a common conflict in younger singers because the teenager who is the high school choir soloist often is also student council president, yearbook editor, captain of the cheerleaders, and so on.

Conducting, particularly choral conducting, can also be deleterious. An enthusiastic conductor, especially of an amateur group, frequently sings all 4 parts intermittently, at volumes louder than the entire choir, during lengthy rehearsals. Conducting is a common avocation among singers but must be done with expert technique and special precautions to prevent voice injury. Hoarseness or loss of soft voice control after conducting a rehearsal or concert suggests voice abuse during conducting. The patient should be instructed to record his or her voice throughout the vocal range singing long notes at dynamics from soft to loud to soft. Recordings should be made prior to rehearsal and following rehearsal. If the voice has lost range, control, or quality during the rehearsal, voice abuse has occurred. A similar test can be used for patients who sing in choirs, teach voice, or perform other potentially abusive vocal activities. Such problems in conductors can generally be managed by additional training in conducting techniques and by voice training, including warm-up and cool-down exercises.

Teaching singing may also be hazardous to vocal health. It can be done safely but requires skill and thought. Most teachers teach while seated at the piano. Late in a long, hard day, this posture is not conducive to maintenance of optimal abdominal and back support. Usually, teachers work with students continually positioned to the right or left of the keyboard. This may require the teacher to turn his or her neck at a particularly sharp angle, especially when teaching at an upright piano. Teachers also often demonstrate vocal works in their students' vocal ranges rather than their own, illustrating bad as well as good technique. If a singing teacher is hoarse or has neck discomfort, or his or her soft singing control deteriorates at the end of a teaching day (assuming that the teacher warms up before beginning to teach voice lessons), voice abuse should be suspected. Helpful

modifications include teaching with a grand piano, sitting slightly sideways on the piano bench, or alternating student position to the right and left of the piano to facilitate better neck alignment. Retaining an accompanist so that the teacher can stand rather than teach from sitting behind a piano, and many other helpful modifications, are possible.

Do You Have Pain When You Talk or Sing?

Odynophonia, or pain caused by phonation, can be a disturbing symptom. It is not uncommon, but relatively little has been written or discussed on this subject. A detailed review of odynophonia is beyond the scope of this publication. However, laryngologists should be familiar with the diagnosis and treatment of at least a few of the most common causes, at least, as discussed elsewhere in this book.

What Kind of Physical Condition Are You In?

Phonation is an athletic activity that requires good conditioning and coordinated interaction of numerous physical functions. Maladies of any part of the body may be reflected in the voice. Failure to maintain good abdominal muscle tone and respiratory endurance through exercise is particularly harmful because deficiencies in these areas undermine the power source of the voice. Patients generally attempt to compensate for such weaknesses by using inappropriate muscle groups, particularly in the neck, causing vocal dysfunction. Similar problems may occur in the well-conditioned vocalist in states of fatigue. These are compounded by mucosal changes that accompany excessively long hours of hard work. Such problems may be seen even in the best singers shortly before important performances in the height of the concert season.

A popular but untrue myth holds that great opera singers must be obese. However, the vivacious, gregarious personality that often distinguishes the great performer seems to be accompanied frequently by a propensity for excess, especially culinary excess. This excess is as undesirable in the vocalist as it is in most other athletic artists, and it should be prevented from the start of one's vocal career. Appropriate and attractive body weight has always been valued in the pop music world and is becoming particularly important in the opera world as this formerly theater-based art form moves to television and film media. However, attempts at weight reduction in an established speaker or singer are a different matter. The vocal mechanism is a finely tuned, complex instrument and is exquisitely sensitive to minor changes. Substantial fluctuations in weight frequently cause deleterious alterations of the voice, although these are usually temporary. Weight reduction programs for people concerned about their voices must be monitored carefully and designed to reduce weight in small increments over long periods. A history of sudden recent weight change may be responsible for almost any vocal complaint.

Have You Noted Voice or Bodily Weakness, Tremor, Fatigue, or Loss of Control?

Even minor neurologic disorders may be extremely disruptive to vocal function. Specific questions should be asked to rule out neuromuscular and neurologic diseases such as myasthenia gravis, Parkinson dis-

ease, tremors, other movement disorders, spasmodic dysphonia, multiple sclerosis, central nervous system neoplasm, and other serious maladies that may be present with voice complaints.

Do You Have Allergy or Cold Symptoms?

Acute upper respiratory tract infection causes inflammation of the mucosa, alters mucosal secretions, and makes the mucosa more vulnerable to injury. Coughing and throat clearing are particularly traumatic vocal activities and may worsen or provoke hoarseness associated with a cold. Postnasal drip and allergy may produce the same response. Infectious sinusitis is associated with discharge and diffuse mucosal inflammation, resulting in similar problems, and may actually alter the sound of a voice, especially the patient's own perception of his or her voice. Futile attempts to compensate for disease of the supraglottic vocal tract in an effort to return the sound to normal frequently result in laryngeal strain. The expert singer or speaker should compensate by monitoring technique by tactile rather than by auditory feedback, or singing "by feel" rather than "by ear."

Do You Have Breathing Problems, Especially After Exercise?

Voice patients usually volunteer information about upper respiratory tract infections and postnasal drip, but the relevance of other maladies may not be obvious to them. Consequently, the physician must seek out pertinent history.

Respiratory problems are especially important in voice patients. Even mild respiratory dysfunction may adversely affect the power source of the voice.[8] Occult asthma may be particularly troublesome.[9] A complete respiratory history should be obtained in most patients with voice complaints, and pulmonary function testing is often advisable.

Have You Been Exposed to Environmental Irritants?

Any mucosal irritant can disrupt the delicate vocal mechanism. Allergies to dust and mold are aggravated commonly during rehearsals and performances in concert halls, especially older theaters and concert halls, because of numerous curtains, backstage trappings, and dressing room facilities that are rarely cleaned thoroughly. Nasal obstruction and erythematous conjunctivae suggest generalized mucosal irritation. The drying effects of cold air and dry heat may also affect mucosal secretions, leading to decreased lubrication, a "scratchy" voice, and a tickling cough. These symptoms may be minimized by nasal breathing, which allows inspired air to be filtered, warmed, and humidified. Nasal breathing, whenever possible, rather than mouth breathing, is proper vocal technique. While the performer is backstage between appearances or during rehearsals, inhalation of dust and other irritants may be controlled by wearing a protective mask, such as those used by carpenters, or a surgical mask that does not contain fiberglass. This is especially helpful when sets are being constructed in the rehearsal area.

A history of recent travel suggests other sources of mucosal irritation. The air in airplanes is extremely dry, and airplanes are noisy.[10] One must be careful to avoid talking loudly and to maintain good hydration and nasal breathing during air travel. Environmental changes can also be disruptive. Las Vegas is infamous for the mucosal irritation caused by its dry atmosphere and smoke-filled rooms. In fact, the resultant complex of hoarseness, vocal "tickle," and fatigue is referred to as "Las Vegas voice." A history of recent travel should also suggest jet lag and generalized fatigue, which may be potent detriments to good vocal function.

Environmental pollution is responsible for the presence of toxic substances and conditions encountered daily. Inhalation of toxic pollutants may affect the voice adversely by direct laryngeal injury, by causing pulmonary dysfunction that results in voice maladies, or through impairments elsewhere in the vocal tract. Ingested substances, especially those that have neurolaryngologic effects, may also adversely affect the voice. Nonchemical environmental pollutants such as noise can also cause voice abnormalities. Laryngologists should be familiar with the laryngologic effects of the numerous potentially irritating substances and conditions found in the environment. We must also be familiar with special pollution problems encountered by performers. Numerous materials used by artists to create sculptures, drawings, and theatrical sets are toxic and have adverse voice effects. In addition, performers are exposed routinely to chemicals encountered through stage smoke and pyrotechnic effects. Although it is clear that some of the "special effects" may result in serious laryngologic consequences, much additional study is needed to clarify the nature and scope of these occupational problems.

Do You Smoke, Live With a Smoker, or Work Around Smoke?

The effects of smoking on voice performance were reviewed recently in the *Journal of Singing*,[11] and that review is recapitulated here. Smoking tobacco is the number one cause of preventable death in the United States as well as the leading cause of heart disease, stroke, emphysema, and cancer. The Centers for Disease Control and Prevention (CDC) attribute approximately 442 000 premature (shortened life expectancy) deaths annually in the United States to smoking, which is more than the combined incidence of deaths caused by highway accidents, fires, murders, illegal drugs, suicides, and AIDS.[12] Approximately 4 million deaths per year worldwide result from smoking, and if this trend continues, by 2030, this figure will increase to about 10 million deaths globally.[13] In addition to causing life-threatening diseases, smoking impairs many body systems, including the vocal tract. Harmful consequences of smoking or being exposed to smoke adversely influence voice performance.

Singers need good vocal health to perform well. Smoking tobacco can irritate the mucosal covering of the vocal folds, causing redness and chronic inflammation, and can have the same effect on the mucosal lining of the lungs, trachea, nasopharynx (behind the nose and throat), and mouth. In other words, the components of voice production—the generator, the oscillator, the resonator, and the articulator—all can be compromised by the harmful effects of tobacco use. The onset of effects from smoking may be immediate or delayed.

Individuals who have allergies and/or asthma are usually more sensitive to cigarette smoke with potential for an immediate adverse reaction involving the lungs, larynx, nasal cavities, and/or eyes. Chronic use of tobacco, or exposure to it, causes the toxic chemicals in tobacco to accumulate in the body, damaging the delicate linings of the vocal tract, as well as the lungs, heart, and circulatory system.

The lungs are critical components of the power source of the vocal tract. They help generate an airstream that is directed superiorly through the trachea toward the undersurface of the vocal folds. The vocal folds respond to the increase in subglottic pressure by producing sounds of variable intensities and frequencies. The number of times per second the vocal folds vibrate influences the pitch, and the amplitude of the mucosal wave influences the loudness of the sound. The sound produced by the vibration (oscillation) of the vocal folds passes upward through the oral cavity and nasopharynx where it resonates, giving the voice its richness and timbre, and eventually it is articulated by the mouth, teeth, lips, and tongue into speech or song.

Any condition that adversely affects lung function such as chronic exposure to smoke or uncontrolled asthma can contribute to dysphonia by impairing the strength, endurance, and consistency of the airsteam responsible for establishing vocal fold oscillation. Any lesion that compromises vocal fold vibration and glottic closure can cause hoarseness and breathiness. Inflammation of the cover layer of the vocal folds and/or the mucosal lining of the nose, sinuses, and oral nasopharyngeal cavities can affect the quality and clarity of the voice.

Tobacco smoke can damage the lungs' parenchyma and the exchange of air through respiration. Cigarette manufacturers add hundreds of ingredients to their tobacco products to improve taste, to make smoking seem milder and easier to inhale, and to prolong burning and shelf life.[14] More than 7000 chemical compounds have been identified in tobacco smoke, and more than 250 of these compounds are carcinogens.[15] The tobacco plant, *Nicotiana tabacum*, is grown for its leaves, which can be smoked, chewed, or sniffed with various effects. The nicotine in tobacco is the addictive component and rivals crack cocaine in its ability to enslave its users. Most smokers want to stop, yet only a small percentage are successful in quitting cigarettes; the majority who quit relapse into smoking once again.[16] Tar and carbon monoxide are among the disease-causing components in tobacco products. The tar in cigarettes exposes the individual to a greater risk of bronchitis, emphysema, and lung cancer. These chemicals affect the entire vocal tract as well as the cardiovascular system (Table 2–1).

Cigarette smoke in the lungs can lead also to increased vascularity, edema, and excess mucous production, as well as epithelial tissue and cellular changes. The toxic agents in cigarette smoke have been associated with an increase in the number and severity of asthma attacks, chronic bronchitis, emphysema, and lung cancer, all of which can interfere with the lungs' ability to generate the stream of air needed for voice production.

Chronic bronchitis due to smoking has been associated with an increase in the number of goblet (mucous) cells, an increase in the size (hyperplasia) of the mucosal-secreting glands, and a decrease in the number of ciliated cells, the cells used to clean the lungs. Chronic cough and sputum production are also seen more commonly in smokers compared with nonsmokers. Also, the heat and chemicals of unfiltered cigarette and marijuana smoke are especially irritating to the lungs and larynx.

An important component of voice quality is the symmetrical, unencumbered vibration of the true vocal folds. Anything that prevents the epithelium covering the vocal folds from vibrating or affects the loose connective tissue under the epithelium (in the superficial layer of the lamina propria known as the Reinke space) can cause dysphonia. Cigarette smoking can cause the epithelium of the true vocal folds to become red and swollen, develop whitish discolorations (leukoplakia), undergo chronic inflammatory changes, or develop squamous metaplasia or dysplasia (tissue changes from normal to a potentially malignant state). In chronic smokers, the voice may become husky due to the accumulation of fluid in the Reinke space (Reinke edema). These alterations in structure can interfere with voice production by changing the biomechanics of the vocal folds and their vibratory characteristics. In severe cases, cancer can deform and paralyze the vocal folds.

Vocal misuse often follows in an attempt to compensate for dysphonia and an alerted self-perception of one's voice. The voice may feel weak, breathy, raspy, or strained. There may be a loss of range, vocal breaks, long warm-up time, and fatigue. The throat may feel raw, achy, or tight. As the voice becomes unreliable, bad habits increase as the individual struggles harder and harder to compensate vocally. As selected sound waves move upward, from the larynx toward and through the pharynx, nasopharynx, mouth, and nose (the resonators), sounds gain a unique richness and timbre. Exposing the pharynx to cigarette smoke aggravates the linings of the oropharynx, mouth, nasopharynx, sinuses, and nasal cavities. The resulting erythema, swelling, and inflammation predispose one to nasal congestion and impaired mucosal function; there may be predisposition to sinusitis and pharyngitis, in which the voice may become hyponasal, the sinus achy, and the throat painful.

Although relatively rare in the United States, cancer of the nasopharynx has been associated with cigarette smoking,[17] and one of the presenting symptoms is unilateral hearing loss due to fluid in the middle ear caused by eustachian tube obstruction from the cancer. Smoking-induced cancers of the oral cavity, pharynx, larynx, and lung are common throughout the world, including in the United States.

The palate, tongue, cheeks, lips, and teeth articulate the sound modified by the

Table 2–1. Chemical Additives Found in Tobacco and Commercial Products

Tobacco Chemical Additives	Also Found In
Acetic acid	Vinegar, hair dye
Acetone	Nail polish remover
Ammonia	Floor cleaner, toilet cleaner
Arsenic	Poison
Benzene	A leukemia-producing agent in rubber cement
Butane	Cigarette lighter fluid
Cadmium	Batteries, some oil paints
Carbon monoxide	Car exhaust
DDT	Insecticides
Ethanol	Alcohol
Formaldehyde	Embalming fluid, fabric, laboratory animals
Hexamine	Barbecue lighter
Hydrazine	Jet fuel, rocket fuel
Hydrogen cyanide	Gas chamber poison
Methane	Swamp gas
Methanol	Rocket fuel
Naphthalene	Explosives, mothballs, paints
Nickel	Electroplating
Nicotine	Insecticides
Nitrobenzene	Gasoline additive
Nitrous oxide phenols	Disinfectant
Phenol	Disinfectants, plastics
Polonium-210	A radioactive substance
Stearic acid	Candle wax
Styrene	Insulation materials
Toluene	Industrial solvent, embalmer's glue
Vinyl chloride	Plastic manufacturing, garbage bags

resonators into speech. Cigarettes, cigar, or pipe smoking may cause a "black hairy tongue," precancerous oral lesions (leukoplakia), and/or cancer of the tongue and lips.[18] Any irritation that causes burning or inflammation of the oral mucosa can affect phonation, and all tobacco products are capable of causing these effects.

Smokeless "spit" tobacco is highly addictive, and users who dip 8 to 10 times a day may get the same nicotine exposure as those who smoke 1½ to 2 packs of cigarettes per day.[19] Smokeless tobacco has been associated with gingivitis, cheek carcinoma, and cancer of the larynx and hypopharynx.

Exposure to environmental tobacco smoke (ETS), also called secondhand smoke, sidestream smoke, or passive smoke, accounts for an estimated 3000 lung cancer deaths and approximately 35 000 deaths in the United States from heart disease in nonsmoking adults.[20]

Secondhand smoke is the "passive" inhalation of tobacco smoke from environmental sources such as smoke given off by pipes, cigars, or cigarettes (sidestream), or the smoke exhaled from the lungs of smokers and inhaled by other people (mainstream). This passive smoke contains a mixture of thousands of chemicals, some of which are known to cause cancer. The National Institutes of Health (NIH) lists ETS as a "known" carcinogen, and the more you are exposed to secondhand smoke, the greater your risk.[21]

Infants and young children are particularly affected by secondhand smoke with increased incidences of otitis media (ear infections), bronchitis, and pneumonia. If small children are exposed to secondhand smoke, the child's resulting illness can have a stressful effect on the parent who frequently catches the child's illness. Both the illness and the stress of caring for the sick child may interfere with voice performance. People who are exposed routinely to secondhand smoke are at risk for lung cancer, heart disease, respiratory infection, and an increased number of asthma attacks.[22]

There is an intricate relationship between the lungs, larynx, pharynx, nose, and mouth in the production of speech and song. Smoking can have deleterious effects on any part of the vocal tract, causing the respiratory system to lose power, damaging the vibratory margins of the vocal folds, and detracting from the richness and beauty of a voice.

The deleterious effects of tobacco smoke on mucosa are indisputable. Anyone concerned about the health of his or her voice should not smoke. Smoking causes erythema, mild edema, and generalized inflammation throughout the vocal tract. Both smoke itself and the heat of the cigarette appear to be important. Marijuana produces a particularly irritating, unfiltered smoke that is inhaled directly, causing considerable mucosal response. Voice patients who refuse to stop smoking marijuana should at least be advised to use a water pipe to cool and partially filter the smoke. Some vocalists are required to perform in smoke-filled environments and may suffer the same effects as the smokers themselves. In some theaters, it is possible to place fans upstage or direct the ventilation system so as to create a gentle draft toward the audience, clearing the smoke away from the stage. "Smoke eaters" installed in some theaters are also helpful.

Do Any Foods Seem to Affect Your Voice?

Various foods are said to affect the voice. Traditionally, singers avoid milk and ice cream before performances. In many people, these foods seem to increase the amount and viscosity of mucosal secretions. Allergy and casein have been implicated, but no satisfactory explanation has been established.

In some cases, restriction of these foods from the diet before a voice performance may be helpful. Chocolate may have the same effect and should be viewed similarly. Chocolate also contains caffeine, which may aggravate reflux or cause tremor. Voice patients should be asked about eating nuts. This is important not only because some people experience effects similar to those produced by milk products and chocolate but also because they are extremely irritating if aspirated. The irritation produced by aspiration of even a small organic foreign body may be severe and impossible to correct rapidly enough to permit performance. Highly spiced foods may also cause mucosal irritation. In addition, they seem to aggravate reflux laryngitis. Coffee and other beverages containing caffeine also aggravate gastric reflux and may promote dehydration and/or alter secretions and necessitate frequent throat clearing in some people. Fad diets, especially rapid weight-reducing diets, are notorious for causing voice problems. Eating a full meal before a speaking or singing engagement may interfere with abdominal support or may aggravate upright reflux of gastric juice during abdominal muscle contraction. Lemon juice and herbal teas are considered beneficial to the voice. Both may act as demulcents, thinning secretions, and may very well be helpful.

Do You Have Morning Hoarseness, Bad Breath, Excessive Phlegm, a Lump in Your Throat, or Heartburn?

Reflux laryngitis is especially common among singers and trained speakers because of the high intra-abdominal pressure associated with proper support and because of lifestyle. Singers frequently perform at night. Many vocalists refrain from eating before performances because a full stomach can compromise effective abdominal support. They typically compensate by eating heartily at postperformance gatherings late at night and then go to bed with a full stomach.

Chronic irritation of arytenoid and vocal fold mucosa by reflux of gastric secretions may occasionally be associated with dyspepsia or pyrosis. However, the key features of this malady are bitter taste and halitosis on awakening in the morning, a dry or "coated" mouth, often a scratchy sore throat or a feeling of a "lump in the throat," hoarseness, and the need for prolonged vocal warm-up. The physician must be alert to these symptoms and ask about them routinely; otherwise, the diagnosis will often be overlooked, because people who have had this problem for many years or a lifetime do not even realize it is abnormal.

Do You Have Trouble With Your Bowels or Belly?

Any condition that alters abdominal function, such as muscle spasm, constipation, or diarrhea, interferes with support and may result in a voice complaint. These symptoms may accompany infection, anxiety, various gastroenterological diseases, and other maladies.

Are You Under Particular Stress or in Therapy?

The human voice is an exquisitely sensitive messenger of emotion. Highly trained voice professionals learn to control the effects of anxiety and other emotional stress on their voices under ordinary circumstances. However, in some instances, this training may break down or a performer may be inadequately prepared to control the voice under specific stressful conditions. Preperformance anxiety is the most common example, but insecurity, depression, and other emotional disturbances are also generally reflected in the voice. Anxiety reactions are mediated in part through the autonomic nervous system and result in a dry mouth, cold clammy skin, and thick secretions. These reactions are normal, and good vocal training coupled with assurance that no abnormality or disease is present generally overcome them. However, long-term, poorly compensated emotional stress and exogenous stress (from agents, producers, teachers, parents, etc) may cause substantial vocal dysfunction and may result in permanent limitations of the vocal apparatus. These conditions must be diagnosed and treated expertly. Hypochondriasis is uncommon among professional singers, despite popular opinion to the contrary.

Publications have highlighted the complexity and importance of psychological factors associated with voice disorders.[23] A comprehensive discussion of this subject is also presented elsewhere in this book. It is important for the physician to recognize that psychological problems may not only cause voice disorders but also delay recovery from voice disorders that were entirely organic in etiology. Professional voice users, especially singers, have enormous psychological investment and personality identifications associated with their voices. A condition that causes voice loss or permanent injury often evokes the same powerful psychological responses seen following death of a loved one. This process may be initiated even when physical recovery is complete if an incident (injury or surgery) has made the vocalist realize that voice loss is possible. Such a "brush with death" can have profound emotional consequences in some patients. It is essential for laryngologists to be aware of these powerful factors and manage them properly if optimal therapeutic results are to be achieved expeditiously.

Do You Have Problems Controlling Your Weight? Are You Excessively Tired? Are You Cold When Other People Are Warm?

Endocrine problems warrant special attention. The human voice is extremely sensitive to endocrinologic changes. Many of these are reflected in alterations of fluid content of the lamina propria just beneath the laryngeal mucosa. This causes alterations in the bulk and shape of the vocal folds and results in voice change. Hypothyroidism[24–28] is a well-recognized cause of such voice disorders, although the mechanism is not fully understood. Hoarseness, vocal fatigue, muffling of the voice, loss of range, and a sensation of a lump in the throat may be present even with mild hypothyroidism. Even when thyroid function test results are within the low-normal range, this diagnosis should be entertained, especially if thyroid-stimulating hormone levels are in the high-normal range or are elevated. Thyrotoxicosis may result in similar voice disturbances.[25]

Do You Have Menstrual Irregularity, Cyclical Voice Changes Associated With Menses, Recent Menopause, or Other Hormonal Changes or Problems?

Voice changes associated with sex hormones are commonly encountered in clinical practice and have been investigated more thoroughly than have other hormonal changes.[29,30] Although a correlation appears to exist between sex hormone levels and depth of male voices (higher testosterone and lower estradiol levels in basses than in tenors),[29] the most important hormonal considerations in males occur during or related to puberty.[31,32] Voice problems related to sex hormones are more common in female singers.[33–49]

Do You Have Jaw Joint or Other Dental Problems?

Dental disease, especially temporomandibular joint (TMJ) dysfunction, introduces muscle tension in the head and neck, which is transmitted to the larynx directly through the muscular attachments between the mandible and the hyoid bone and indirectly as generalized increased muscle tension. These problems often result in decreased range, vocal fatigue, and change in the quality or placement of a voice. Such tension often is accompanied by excess tongue muscle activity, especially pulling of the tongue posteriorly. This hyperfunctional behavior acts through hyoid attachments to disrupt the balance between the intrinsic and extrinsic laryngeal musculature. TMJ problems are also problematic for wind instrumentalists and some string players, including violinists. In some cases, the problems may actually be caused by instrumental technique. The history should always include information about musical activities, including instruments other than the voice.

Do You or Your Blood Relatives Have Hearing Loss?

Hearing loss is often overlooked as a source of vocal problems. Auditory feedback is fundamental to speaking and singing. Interference with this control mechanism may result in altered vocal production, particularly if the person is unaware of the hearing loss. Spouses, friends and others who accompany patients to appointments may be asked whether they suspect hearing loss in the patient. The author obtains hearing tests routinely in new voice patients. Distortion, particularly pitch distortion (diplacusis), may also pose serious problems for the singer. This appears to be due not only to aesthetic difficulties in matching pitch but also to vocal strain that accompanies pitch shifts.[50]

In addition to determining whether the patient has hearing loss, and related symptoms such as tinnitus and vertigo, inquiry should be made about hearing impairment occurring in family members, roommates, and other close associates. Speaking loudly to people who are hard of hearing can cause substantial, chronic vocal strain. This possibility should be investigated routinely when evaluating voice patients.

Have You Suffered Whiplash or Other Bodily Injury?

Various bodily injuries outside the confines of the vocal tract may have profound effects on the voice. Whiplash, for example, commonly causes changes in technique, with consequent voice fatigue, loss of range, difficulty singing softly, and other problems. These problems derive from the neck muscle spasm, abnormal neck posturing secondary to pain, and consequent hyperfunctional voice use. Lumbar, abdominal, head, chest, supraglottic, and extremity injuries may also affect vocal technique and be responsible for the dysphonia that prompted the voice patient to seek medical attention.

Did You Undergo Any Surgery Prior to the Onset of Your Voice Problems?

A history of laryngeal surgery in a voice patient is a matter of great concern. It is important to establish exactly why the surgery was done, by whom it was done, whether intubation was necessary, and whether voice therapy was instituted preoperatively or postoperatively if the lesion was associated with voice abuse (vocal nodules). If the vocal dysfunction that sent the patient to the physician's office dates from the immediate postoperative period, surgical trauma must be suspected.

Otolaryngologists frequently are asked about the effects of tonsillectomy on the voice. Singers, especially, may consult the physician after tonsillectomy and complain of vocal dysfunction. Certainly, removal of tonsils can alter the voice.[51,52] Tonsillectomy changes the configuration of the supraglottic vocal tract. In addition, scarring alters pharyngeal muscle function, which is trained meticulously in the professional singer. Singers must be warned that they may have permanent voice changes after tonsillectomy; however, these can be minimized by dissecting in the proper plane to lessen scarring. The singer's voice generally requires 3 to 6 months to stabilize or return to normal after surgery, although it is generally safe to begin limited singing within 2 to 4 weeks following surgery. As with any procedure for which general anesthesia may be needed, the anesthesiologist should be advised preoperatively that the patient is a professional singer. Intubation and extubation should be performed with great care, and the use of nonirritating plastic rather than rubber or ribbed metal endotracheal tubes is preferred. Use of a laryngeal mask may be advisable for selected procedures for mechanical reasons, but this device is often not ideal for tonsillectomy, and it can cause laryngeal injury such as arytenoid dislocation.

Surgery of the neck, such as thyroidectomy, may result in permanent alterations in the vocal mechanism through scarring of the extrinsic laryngeal musculature. The cervical (strap) muscles are important in maintaining laryngeal position and stability

of the laryngeal skeleton, and they should be retracted rather than divided whenever possible. A history of recurrent or superior laryngeal nerve injury may explain a hoarse, breathy, or weak voice. However, in rare cases, even a singer can compensate for recurrent laryngeal nerve paralysis and have a nearly normal voice.

Thoracic and abdominal surgery interferes with respiratory and abdominal support. After these procedures, singing and projected speaking should be prohibited until pain has subsided and healing has occurred sufficiently to allow normal support. Abdominal exercises should be instituted before resumption of vocalizing. Singing and speaking without proper support are often worse for the voice than not using the voice for performance at all.

Other surgical procedures may be important factors if they necessitate intubation or if they affect the musculoskeletal system so that the person has to change stance or balance. For example, balancing on one foot after leg surgery may decrease the effectiveness of the support mechanism.

What Medications and Other Substances Do You Use?

A history of alcohol abuse suggests the probability of poor vocal technique. Intoxication results in incoordination and decreased awareness, which undermine vocal discipline designed to optimize and protect the voice. The effect of small amounts of alcohol is controversial. Although many experts oppose its use because of its vasodilatory effect and consequent mucosal alteration, many people do not seem to be adversely affected by small amounts of alcohol, such as a glass of wine with a meal. However, some people have mild sensitivities to certain wines or beers. Patients who develop nasal congestion and rhinorrhea after drinking beer, for example, should be made aware that they probably have a mild allergy to that particular beverage and should avoid it before voice commitments.

Patients frequently acquire antihistamines to help control "postnasal drip" or other symptoms. The drying effect of antihistamines may result in decreased vocal fold lubrication, increased throat clearing, and irritability leading to frequent coughing. Antihistamines may be helpful to some voice patients, but they must be used with caution.

When a voice patient seeking the attention of a physician is already taking antibiotics, it is important to find out the dose and the prescribing physician, if any, as well as whether the patient frequently treats himself or herself with inadequate courses of antibiotics often supplied by colleagues. Singers, actors, and other speakers sometimes have a "sore throat" shortly before important vocal presentations and start themselves on inappropriate antibiotic therapy, which they generally discontinue after their performance.

Diuretics are also popular among some performers. They are often prescribed by gynecologists at the vocalist's request to help deplete excess water in the premenstrual period. They are not effective in this scenario, because they cannot diurese the protein-bound water in the laryngeal ground substance. Unsupervised use of these drugs may cause dehydration and consequent mucosal dryness.

Hormone use, especially use of oral contraceptives, must be mentioned specifically during the physician's inquiry. Women frequently do not mention them routinely when asked whether they are taking any medication. Vitamins are also frequently not mentioned. Most vitamin therapy seems to have little effect on the voice. However, high-dose vitamin C (5–6 g/d), which some

people use to prevent upper respiratory tract infections, seems to act as a mild diuretic and may lead to dehydration and xerophonia.[53]

Cocaine use is common, especially among pop musicians. This drug can be extremely irritating to the nasal mucosa, causes marked vasoconstriction, and may alter the sensorium, resulting in decreased voice control and a tendency toward vocal abuse.

Many pain medications (including aspirin and ibuprofen), psychotropic medications, and others may be responsible for a voice complaint. So far, no adverse vocal effects have been reported with selective COX-2 inhibiting anti-inflammatory medications (which do not promote bleeding, as do other nonsteroidal anti-inflammatory medicines and aspirin), such as celecoxib (Celebrex; Pfizer, Inc, New York, New York) and valdecoxib (Bextra; Pharmacia Corp, New York, New York). However, this group of drugs has been demonstrated to have other side effects and should, in our view, only be taken under the care of a physician.[54] The effects of other new medications such as sildenafil citrate (Viagra; Pfizer, Inc) and medications used to induce abortion remain unstudied and unknown, but it seems plausible that such medication may affect voice function, at least temporarily. Laryngologists should be familiar with the laryngologic effects of the many substances ingested medically and recreationally.

References

1. Sataloff RT. Professional singers: the science and art of clinical care. *Am J Otolaryngol.* 1981;2:251–266.
2. Sataloff RT. The human voice. *Sci Am.* 1992; 267:108–115.

3. Sundberg J. *The Science of the Singing Voice.* DeKalb, IL: Northern Illinois University Press; 1987.

4. Sataloff RT. Efficient history taking in professional singers. *Laryngoscope.* 1984;94: 1111–1114.

5. Ackerman R, Pfan W. Gerontology studies on the susceptibility to voice disorders in professional speakers. *Folia Phoniatr (Basel).* 1974;26:95–99.

6. von Leden H. Speech and hearing problems in the geriatric patient. *J Am Geriatr Soc.* 1977;25:422–426.

7. Schiff M. *Comment.* Presented at: Seventh Symposium on Care of the Professional Voice; June 15–16, 1978; The Juilliard School, New York, NY.

8. Spiegel JR, Cohn JR, Sataloff RT, et al. Respiratory function in singers: medical assessment, diagnoses, treatments. *J Voice.* 1988;2:40–50.

9. Cohn JR, Sataloff RT, Spiegel JR, et al. Airway reactivity-induced asthma in singers (ARIAS). *J Voice.* 1991;5:332–337.

10. Feder RJ. The professional voice and airline flight. *Otolaryngol Head Neck Surg.* 1984;92:251–254.

11. Anticaglia A, Hawkshaw M, Sataloff RT. The effects of smoking on voice performance. *J Singing.* 2004;60:161–167.

12. Centers for Disease Control and Prevention (CDC). Annual smoking-attributable, mortality, years of potential life lost, and economic costs, United States—1995–1999. *MMWR Morb Mortal Wkly Rep.* 2002;51(14):300–303.

13. World Health Organization. *World Health Report 1999.* Geneva, Switzerland: World Health Organization; 1999.

14. US Department of Health Services (USDHHS). *Tobacco Products Fact Sheet.* Washington, DC: Government Printing Office; 2000.

15. National Cancer Institute. Harms of Cigarette Smoking and Health Benefits of Quitting. http://www.cancer.gov/about-cancer /causes-prevention/risk/tobacco/cessation -fact-sheet

16. Centers for Disease Control and Prevention. Cigarette smoking among adults—United States, 1993. *MMWR Morb Mortal Wkly Rep.* 1994;3:925–929.

17. Chow WH, McLaughlin JK, Hrubec Z, et al. Tobacco use and nasopharyngeal carcinoma in a cohort of US veterans. *Int J Cancer.* 1993;55(4):538–540.

18. Casiglia J, Woo, SB. A comprehensive view of oral cancer. *Gen Dent.* 2001;49(1): 72–82.

19. Centers for Disease Control and Prevention. Determination of nicotine pH and moisture content of six U.S. commercial moist snuff products. *MMWR Morb Mortal Wkly Rep.* 1999;48(19):398.

20. American Cancer Society. *Cancer Facts and Figures 2002.* Atlanta, GA: American Cancer Society; 2002.

21. National Toxicology Program (NTP). *Report on Carcinogens.* 14th ed. Research Triangle Park, NC: US Department Health and Human Services, Public Health Service, National Toxicology Program; 2002. http://ntp .niehs.nih.gov/go/rpck/

22. Academy of Pediatrics, Committee on Environmental Health. Environmental tobacco smoke; a hazard to children. *Pediatrics.* 1997; 99(4):639–642.

23. Rosen DC, Sataloff RT. *Psychology of Voice Disorders.* San Diego, CA: Singular Publishing; 1997.

24. Gupta OP, Bhatia PL, Agarwal MK, et al. Nasal pharyngeal and laryngeal manifestations of hypothyroidism. *Ear Nose Throat J.* 1997;56:10–21.

25. Malinsky M, Chevrie-Muller, Cerceau N. Etude clinique et electrophysiologique des alterations de la voix au cours des thyrotoxioses. *Ann Endocrinol (Paris).* 1997;38: 171–172.

26. Michelsson K, Sirvio P. Cry analysis in congenital hypothyroidism. *Folia Phoniatr (Basel).* 1976;28:40–47.

27. Ritter FN. The effect of hypothyroidism on the larynx of the rat. *Ann Otol Rhinol Laryngol.* 1964;67:404–416.

28. Ritter FN. Endocrinology. In: Paparella M, Shumrick D, eds. *Otolaryngology.* Vol. I. Philadelphia, PA: Saunders; 1973:727–734.

29. Meuser W, Nieschlag E. Sex hormones and depth of voice in the male [in German]. *Dtsch Med Wochenschr.* 1977:102:261–264.

30. Schiff M. The influence of estrogens on connective tissue. In: Asboe-Hansen G, ed. *Hormones and Connective Tissue.* Copenhagen, Denmark: Munksgaard Press; 1967: 282–341.

31. Brodnitz F. The age of the castrato voice. *J Speech Hear Disord.* 1975;40:291–295.

32. Brodnitz F. Hormones and the human voice. *Bull NY Acad Med.* 1971;47:183–191.

33. Carroll C. Personal communication with Dr. Hans von Leden; 1992; Arizona State University at Tempe.

34. von Gelder L. Psychosomatic aspects of endocrine disorders of the voice. *J Commun Disord.* 1974;7:257–262.

35. Lacina O. Der Einfluss der Menstruation auf die Stimme der Sangerinnen. *Folia Phoniatr (Basel).* 1968;20:13–24.

36. Wendler J. The influence of menstruation on the voice of the female singer. *Folia Phoniatr (Basel).* 1972;24:259–277.

37. Brodnitz F. Medical care preventive therapy (panel). In: Lawrence VL, ed. *Transcripts of the Seventh Annual Symposium, Care of the Professional Voice.* Vol. 3. New York, NY: The Voice Foundation; 1978:86.

38. Dordain M. Etude Statistique de l'influence des contraceptifs hormonaux sur la voix. *Folia Phoniatr (Basel).* 1972;24:86–96.

39. Pahn J, Goretzlehner G. Voice changes following the use of oral contraceptives [in German]. *Zentralbl Gynakol.* 1978;100:341–346.

40. Schiff M. "The pill" in otolaryngology. *Trans Am Acad Ophthalmol Otolaryngol.* 1968; 72:76–84.

41. von Deuster CV. Irreversible vocal changes in pregnancy [in German]. *HNO.* 1977;25: 430–432.

42. Flach M, Schwickardi H, Simen R. Welchen Einfluss haben Menstruation and Schwangerschaft auf die augsgebildete Gesangsstimme? *Folia Phoniatr (Basel).* 1968;21:199–210.

43. Arndt HJ. Stimmstorungen nach Behandlung mit Androgenen und anabolen Hor-

monen. *Munch Med Wochenschr.* 1974;116: 1715–1720.

44. Bourdial J. Les troubles de la voix provoques par la therapeutique hormonale androgene. *Ann Otolaryngol Chir Cervicofac.* 1970;87: 725–734.

45. Damste PH. Virilization of the voice due to anabolic steroids [in Dutch]. *Ned Tijdschr Geneeskd.* 1963;107:891–892.

46. Damste PH. Voice changes in adult women caused by virilizing agents. *J Speech Hear Disord.* 1967;32:126–132.

47. Saez S, Francoise S. Recepteurs d'androgenes: mise en evidence dans la fraction cytosolique de muqueuse normale et d'epitheliomas phryngolarynges humains. *C R Acad Sci Hebd Seances Acad Sci D.* 1975;280:935–938.

48. Vuorenkoski V, Lenko HL, Tjernlund P, et al. Fundamental voice frequency during normal and abnormal growth, and after androgen treatment. *Arch Dis Child.* 1978;53: 201–209.

49. Imre V. Hormonell bedingte Stimmstorungen. *Folia Phoniatr (Basel).* 1968;20:394–404.

50. Sundberg J, Prame E, Iwarsson J. Replicability and accuracy of pitch patterns in professional singers. In: Davis PJ, Fletcher NH, eds. *Vocal Fold Physiology: Controlling Chaos and Complexity.* San Diego, CA: Singular Publishing; 1996:291–306.

51. Gould WJ, Alberti PW, Brodnitz F, Hirano M. Medical care preventive therapy [Panel]. In: Lawrence VL, ed. *Transcripts of the Seventh Annual Symposium, Care of the Professional Voice.* Vol. 3. New York, NY: The Voice Foundation; 1978:74–76.

52. Wallner LJ, Hill BJ, Waldrop W, Monroe C. Voice changes following adenotonsillectomy. *Laryngoscope.* 1968;78:1410–1418.

53. Lawrence VL. Medical care for professional voice (panel). In: Lawrence VL, ed. *Transcripts from the Annual Symposium, Care of the Professional Voice.* Vol. 3. New York, NY: The Voice Foundation; 1978:17–18.

54. Cannon CP. COX-2 inhibitors and cardiovascular risk. *Science.* 2012;336(6087): 1386–1387.

APPENDIX 2–A

Patient History Form for Professional Voice Users

Name _____ Age _____ Sex _____ Race _____

Height _____ Weight _____ Date _____

How long have you had your present voice problem?

    Who noticed it?

    Do you know what caused it?   Yes   No

    If so, what?

    Did it come on slowly or suddenly?   Slowly   Suddenly

    Is it getting: Worse   Better   Same?

Which symptoms do you have? (Please check all that apply.)

    Hoarseness (coarse or scratchy sound)

    Fatigue (voice tires or changes quality after speaking for a short period of time)

    Volume disturbance (trouble speaking) softly, loudly

    Loss of range: high, low

    Prolonged warm-up time (over ½ hour to warm up)

    Breathiness

    Tickling or choking sensation while speaking

    Pain in throat while speaking

    Other (Please specify):

Have you ever had training for your singing voice?

    Yes   No

Have there been periods of months or years without lessons in that time?

    Yes   No

How long have you studied with your present teacher?

    Teacher's name:

    Teacher's address:

    Teacher's telephone number:

Please list previous teachers and years during which you studied with them:

In what capacity do you use your voice professionally?
    Actor
    Announcer (television/radio/sports arena)
    Attorney
    Clergy
    Politician
    Salesperson
    Teacher
    Telephone operator or receptionist
    Other (Please specify):

Do you have an important performance in the near future?
    Yes   No
    Date(s):

Do you do regular voice exercises?
    Yes   No
    If yes, describe:

Do you play a musical instrument?
    Yes   No
    If yes, please check all that apply:
        Keyboard (Piano, Organ, Harpsichord, Other _____)
        Violin, Viola, Cello
        Bass
        Plucked Strings (Guitar, Harp, Other _____)
        Brass
        Wind with single reed
        Wind with double reed
        Flute, Piccolo
        Percussion
        Bagpipe
        Accordion
        Other (Please specify):

Do you warm up your voice before practice or performance?

Yes   No

Do you cool down after using it?

Yes   No

How much are you speaking at present (average hours per day)?

Rehearsal   Performance   Other

Please check all that apply to you:

Voice worse in the morning

Voice worse later in the day, after it has been used

Sing performances or rehearsals in the morning

Speak extensively (teacher, clergy, attorney, telephone, work, etc)

Cheerleader

Speak extensively backstage or at postperformance parties

Choral conductor

Frequently clear your throat

Frequent sore throat

Jaw joint problems

Bitter or acid taste; bad breath or hoarseness first thing in the morning

Frequent "heartburn" or hiatal hernia

Frequent yelling or loud talking

Frequent whispering

Chronic fatigue (insomnia)

Work around extreme dryness

Frequent exercise (weight lifting, aerobics, etc)

Frequently thirsty, dehydrated

Hoarseness first thing in the morning

Chest cough

Eat late at night

Ever use antacids

Under particular stress at present (personal or professional)

Frequent bad breath

Live, work, or perform around smoke and fumes

Traveled recently:

When:

Where:

Your family doctor's name, address, and telephone number:

Your laryngologist's name, address, and telephone number:

Recent cold?

Yes   No

Current cold?

Yes   No

Have you been evaluated by an allergist?

Yes   No

If yes, what allergies do you have?

[none, dust, mold, trees, cats, dogs, foods, other]

If yes, give name and address of allergist:

Are you allergic to any medications?   Yes No

If yes, please list:

How many packs of cigarettes do you smoke per day?

Smoking history:

Never

Quit. When?

Smoked about _____ packs per day for _____ years.

Smoke _____ packs per day. Have smoked for _____ years.

Do you work in a smoky environment?

Yes   No

How much alcohol do you drink?

none   rarely   a few times per week   daily

If daily, or a few times per week, on the average, how much do you consume?

1   2   3   4   5   6   7   8   9   10 more   glasses per   day   week of   beer   wine   liquor

Did you drink more heavily in the past?

Yes   No

How many cups of coffee, tea, cola, or other caffeine-containing drinks do you drink per day?

List other recreational drugs you use:

marijuana   amphetamines   barbiturates   heroin   other _____

Have you noticed any of the following? (Check all that apply.)

Hypersensitivity to heat or cold

Excessive sweating

Change in weight: gained/lost _____ lb. in _____ weeks/_____ months

Change in your voice

Change in skin or hair

Palpitation (fluttering) of the heart

Emotional lability (swings of mood)

Double vision

Numbness of the face or extremities

Tingling around the mouth or face

Blurred vision or blindness

Weakness or paralysis of the face

Clumsiness in arms or legs

Confusion or loss of consciousness

Difficulty with speech

Difficulty with swallowing

Seizure (epileptic fit)

Pain in the neck or shoulder

Shaking or tremors

Memory change

Personality change

For females:

Are you pregnant?   Yes   No

Are your menstrual periods regular?   Yes   No

Have you undergone hysterectomy?   Yes   No

Were your ovaries removed?   Yes   No

At what age did you reach puberty? _____

Have you gone through menopause?   Yes   No

Have you ever consulted a psychologist or psychiatrist?

Yes   No

Are you currently under treatment?

Yes   No

Have you injured your head or neck (whiplash, etc)?

Yes   No

Describe any serious accidents related to this visit:

Are you involved in legal action involving problems with your voice?

Yes   No

List names of spouse and children:

Brief summary of ENT problems, some of which may not be related to your present complaint.

Hearing loss	Nosebleeds
Ear pain	Mouth sores
Ear noises	Trouble swallowing
Facial pain	Trouble breathing
Lump in face or head	Eye problem
Lump in neck	Excess eye skin
Dizziness	Excessive facial skin
Stiff neck	Jaw joint problem
Facial paralysis	Other (please specify):
Nasal obstruction	
Nasal deformity	

Do you have or have you ever had:

Diabetes	Heart attack
Seizures	Angina
Hypoglycemia	Irregular heartbeat
Psychological therapy or counseling	Rheumatic fever
Thyroid problems	Other heart problems
Frequent bad headaches	Unexplained weight loss
Syphilis	Cancer of _____
Ulcers	Other tumor _____
Gonorrhea	Blood transfusions
Herpes	Hepatitis
Urinary problems	Tuberculosis
Cold sores (fever blisters)	AIDS
Arthritis or skeletal	Glaucoma
High blood pressure problems	Meningitis
Severe low blood pressure	Multiple sclerosis
Cleft palate	Other illnesses (Please specify):
Intravenous antibiotics or diuretics	
Asthma, lung or breathing problems	

Do any blood relatives have:

Diabetes

Hypoglycemia

Cancer

Heart disease

Other major medical problems such as those listed above.

Please specify:

Describe serious accident unless directly related to your doctor's visit here.

None

Occurred with head injury, loss of consciousness, or whiplash

Occurred without head injury, loss of consciousness, or whiplash

Describe:

List all current medications and doses (include birth control pills and vitamins).

    None

    Aspirin

    Codeine

    Medication for allergies

    Novocaine

    Penicillin

    Sulfamides

    Tetracycline

    Erythromycin

    Keflex/Ceclor/Ceftin

    Iodine

    X-ray dyes

    Adhesive tape

    Other (Please specify):

List operations:

    Tonsillectomy (age _____)

    Adenoidectomy (age _____)

    Appendectomy (age _____)

    Heart surgery (age _____)

    Other (Please specify):

List toxic drugs or chemicals to which you have been exposed:

    Streptomycin, Neomycin, Kanamycin

    Lead

    Mercury

    Other (Please list):

Have you had x-ray treatments to your head or neck (including treatments for acne or ear problems as a child), treatments for cancer, etc?

    Yes   No

Describe serious health problems of your spouse or children:

3

Physical Examination*

Robert Thayer Sataloff

Physical Examination

A detailed history frequently reveals the cause of a voice problem even before a physical examination is performed. However, a comprehensive physical examination, often including objective assessment of voice function, also is essential.[1-3] In response to feedback from readers of the previous editions, this chapter has been expanded to include a brief overview of objective voice assessment, and other subjects covered more comprehensively in subsequent chapters. This overview is provided here for the reader's convenience.

Physical examination must include a thorough ear, nose, and throat evaluation and assessment of general physical condition. A patient who is extremely obese or appears fatigued, agitated, emotionally stressed, or otherwise generally ill has increased potential for voice dysfunction. This could be due to any number of factors: altered abdominal support, loss of fine motor control of laryngeal muscles, decreased bulk of the submucosal vocal

fold ground substance, change in the character of mucosal secretions, or other similar mechanisms. Any physical condition that impairs the normal function of the abdominal musculature is suspect as cause for dysphonia. Some conditions, such as pregnancy, are obvious; however, a sprained ankle or broken leg that requires the singer to balance in an unaccustomed posture may distract him or her from maintaining good abdominal support and thereby may result in voice dysfunction. A tremorous neurologic disorder, endocrine disturbances such as thyroid dysfunction or menopause, the aging process, and other systemic conditions also may alter the voice. The physician must remember that maladies of almost any body system may result in voice dysfunction and must remain alert for conditions outside the head and neck. If the patient uses his or her voice professionally for singing, acting, or other vocally demanding professions, physical examination should also include assessment of the patient during typical professional vocal tasks. For example, a singer should be asked to sing.

---

* Reprinted with permission from Hamdan AL, Sataloff RT, Hawkshaw MJ. *Obesity and Voice*. San Diego, CA: Plural Publishing; 2020.

Complete Ear, Nose, and Throat Examination

Examination of the ears must include assessment of hearing acuity. Even a relatively slight hearing loss may result in voice strain as a singer tries to balance his or her vocal intensity with that of associate performers. Similar effects are encountered among speakers, but they are less prominent in the early stages of hearing loss. This is especially true of hearing losses acquired after vocal training has been completed. The effect is most pronounced with sensorineural hearing loss. Diplacusis, distortion of pitch perception, makes vocal strain even worse. With conductive hearing loss, singers tend to sing more softly than appropriate rather than too loudly, and this is less harmful.

During an ear, nose, and throat examination, the conjunctivae and sclerae should be observed routinely for erythema that suggests allergy or irritation, for pallor that suggests anemia, and for other abnormalities such as jaundice. These observations may reveal the problem reflected in the vocal tract even before the larynx is visualized. Hearing loss in a spouse may be problematic as well if the voice professional strains vocally to communicate.

The nose should be assessed for patency of the nasal airway, character of the nasal mucosa, and nature of secretions, if any. A patient who is unable to breathe through the nose because of anatomic obstruction is forced to breathe unfiltered, unhumidified air through the mouth. Pale, gray allergic mucosa or swollen infected mucosa in the nose suggests abnormal mucosa elsewhere in the respiratory tract.

Examination of the oral cavity should include careful attention to the tonsils and lymphoid tissue in the posterior pharyngeal wall, as well as to the mucosa. Diffuse lymphoid hypertrophy associated with a complaint of "scratchy" voice and irritative cough may indicate infection. The amount and viscosity of mucosal and salivary secretions also should be noted. Xerostomia is particularly important. The presence of scalloping of the lateral aspects of the tongue should be noted. This finding is caused commonly by tongue thrust and may be associated with inappropriate tongue tension and muscle tension dysphonia. Dental examination should focus not only on oral hygiene but also on the presence of wear facets suggestive of bruxism. Bruxism is a clue to excessive tension and may be associated with dysfunction of the temporomandibular joints, which should also be assessed routinely. Thinning of the enamel of the central incisors in a normal or underweight patient may be a clue to bulimia. However, it may also result from excessive ingestion of lemons, which some singers eat to help thin their secretions.

The neck should be examined for masses, restriction of movement, excess muscle tension and/or spasm, and scars from prior neck surgery or trauma. Laryngeal vertical mobility is also important. For example, tilting of the larynx produced by partial fixation of cervical muscles cut during previous surgery may produce voice dysfunction, as may fixation of the trachea to overlying neck skin. Particular attention should be paid to the thyroid gland. Examination of posterior neck muscles and range of motion should not be neglected. The cranial nerves should also be examined. Diminished fifth nerve sensation, diminished gag reflex, palatal deviation, or other mild cranial nerve deficits may indicate cranial polyneuropathy. Postviral, infectious neuropathies may involve the superior laryngeal nerve(s) and cause weakness of the vocal fold muscle secondary to decreased neural input, fatigability, and loss of range and projection in the voice. The recurrent laryngeal nerve is also affected in some cases. More serious neurologic disease may also be associated with such symptoms and signs.

Laryngeal Examination

Examination of the larynx begins when the singer or other voice patient enters the physician's office. The range, ease, volume, and quality of the speaking voice should be noted. If the examination is not being conducted in the patient's native language, the physician should be sure to listen to a sample of the patient's mother tongue, as well. Voice use is often different under the strain or habits of foreign language use. Rating scales of the speaking voice may be helpful.[4,5] The classification proposed by the Japanese Society of Logopedics and Phoniatrics is one of the most widely used. It is known commonly as the GRBAS (grade, roughness, breathiness, asthenia, and strain) voice rating scale and is discussed below in the section on psychoacoustic evaluation.[6]

Physicians are not usually experts in voice classification. However, the physicians should at least be able to discriminate substantial differences in range and timbre, such as between bass and tenor, or alto and soprano. Although the correlation between speaking and singing voices is not perfect, a speaker with a low, comfortable bass voice who reports that he is a tenor may be misclassified and singing inappropriate roles with consequent voice strain. This judgment should be deferred to an expert, but the observation should lead the physician to make the appropriate referral. Excessive volume or obvious strain during speaking clearly indicates that voice abuse is present and may be contributing to the patient's singing complaint. The speaking voice can be evaluated more consistently and accurately using standardized reading passages, and

such assessments are performed routinely by speech-language pathologists, by phoniatricians, and sometimes by laryngologists.

The definition of "register" or "registration" is controversial, and many different terms are used by musicians and scientists. Often, the definitions are unclear. Terms to describe register include chest, creek, falsetto, head, heavy, light, little, low, middle, modal, normal, pulse, upper, vocal fry, voce di petto, voce di mista, voce di testa, and whistle (also called flageolet and flute register). A register is a range of frequencies that has a consistent quality or timbre. The break between registers is an area of instability called the passaggio. During vocal training, singers are taught to integrate qualities of their various registers and to smooth and obscure the transition between registers. Registers occur not only in voices but also in some instruments, notably the organ. Vocal register changes are associated with changes in laryngeal musculature and in vocal fold shape. For example, in chest register, contraction of the thyroarytenoid muscles causes thickening of the vocal folds, with a square-shaped glottis and large vibratory margin contact area. In falsetto in men and head voice in women, cricothyroid muscle contraction is dominant, vocal folds are elongated, and the contact area is much thinner and more triangular than in chest voice. Vertical phase differences are diminished in head voice in comparison with chest voice. Controversy remains on the use of traditional terms in males such as chest, middle, head, and falsetto register, or chest and head register in females. Voice scientists commonly prefer terms such as modal register. In any case, health care professionals should understand that there is a difference between the terms *register* and *range*. For example, if a singer complains of an inability to sing high notes, this should be described as a loss of upper range, not a loss of upper register. Register and range difficulties should be noted.

Vibrato is a fluctuation of the fundamental frequency of a note. It is produced by the vocal mechanism under neural control and is present naturally in adult voices. The primary components of vibrato include rate (the number of frequency fluctuations per second), extent (number of hertz of fluctuation above and below the center frequency), regularity (consistency of frequency variations from one cycle to the next), and waveform. Rate and extent have been studied most extensively and are arguably the most important components in determining how the vibrato is perceived. Natural vibrato generally is about 6 Hz. Vibrato rate is slower in males than in females, and vocal pitch and effort do not have a substantial influence on vibrato. However, singers are able to alter vibrato rate and pitch oscillation voluntarily for stylistic purposes. The athletic choice of vibrato rate varies over time. For example, vibrato rates of 6 to 7 Hz were popular in classical Western (operatic) singing in the early 20th century, but a vibrato rate of 5.5 to 6 Hz was considered more attractive by the end of the 20th century. In general, pitch fluctuation covers about 1 semitone (half a semitone above and half a semitone below the center frequency) at present. A prominent wobble, as may be heard in some elderly singers who are not in ideal physical and vocal condition generally, is referred to as a tremolo. The excessive pitch (and sometimes intensity) fluctuations are caused by muscle activity, sometimes with a respiratory component, and are superimposed on the individual's vibrato in most cases, rather than actually being a widened, distorted vibrato. The true source of natural vibrato is uncertain, although the larynx, pharynx, tongue, and other components of the vocal tract may move in concert with vibrato, as well as with tremolo. Vibrato is thought to

be due primarily to phonatory structural activity rather than to the respiratory source. The presence of vibrato abnormalities or tremolo should be documented.

Any patient with a voice complaint should be examined by indirect laryngoscopy at least. It is not possible to judge voice range, quality, or other vocal attributes by inspection of the vocal folds. However, the presence or absence of nodules, mass lesions, contact ulcers, hemorrhage, erythema, paralysis, arytenoid erythema (reflux), and other anatomic abnormalities must be established. Erythema and edema of the laryngeal surface of the epiglottis are seen often in association with muscle tension dysphonia and with frequent coughing or clearing of the throat. It is caused by direct trauma from the arytenoids during these maneuvers. The mirror or a laryngeal telescope often provides a better view of the posterior portion of the endolarynx than is obtained with flexible endoscopy. Stroboscopic examination adds substantially to diagnostic abilities (Figure 3–1), as discussed later. Another occasionally helpful adjunct is the operating microscope. Magnification allows visualization of small mucosal disruptions and hemorrhages that may be significant but overlooked otherwise. This technique also allows photography of the larynx with a microscope camera. Magnification may also be achieved through magnifying laryngeal mirrors or by wearing loupes. Loupes usually provide a clearer image than do most of the magnifying mirrors available.

A laryngeal telescope may be combined with a stroboscope to provide excellent visualization of the vocal folds and related structures. The author usually uses a 70° laryngeal telescope, although 90° telescopes are required for some patients. The combination of a telescope and stroboscope provides optimal magnification and optical

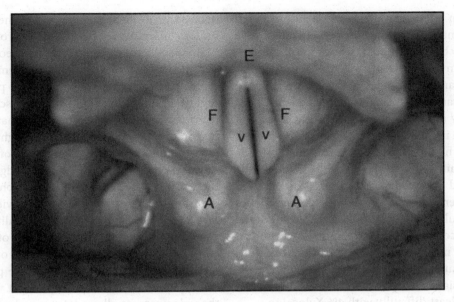

Figure 3–1. Normal larynx showing the true vocal folds (V), false vocal folds (F), arytenoids (A), and epiglottis (E).

quality for assessment of vocal fold vibration. However, it is generally performed with the tongue in a fixed position, and the nature of the examination does not permit assessment of the larynx during normal phonatory gestures.

Flexible fiberoptic laryngoscopy can be performed as an office procedure and allows inspection of the vocal folds in patients whose vocal folds are difficult to visualize indirectly. In addition, it permits observation of the vocal mechanism in a more natural posture than does indirect laryngoscopy, permitting sophisticated dynamic voice assessment. In the hands of an experienced endoscopist, this method may provide a great deal of information about both speaking and singing techniques. The combination of a fiberoptic laryngoscope with a laryngeal stroboscope may be especially useful. This system permits magnification, photography, and detailed inspection of vocal fold motion. Sophisticated systems that permit flexible or rigid fiber-

optic strobovideolaryngoscopy are currently available commercially. They are invaluable assets for routine clinical use. The video system also provides a permanent record, permitting reassessment, comparison over time, and easy consultation. A refinement not currently available commercially is stereoscopic fiberoptic laryngoscopy, accomplished by placing a laryngoscope through each nostril, fastening the 2 together in the pharynx, and observing the larynx through the eyepieces.[7] This method allows visualization of laryngeal motion in 3 dimensions. However, it is used primarily in a research setting.

Rigid endoscopy under general anesthesia may be reserved for the rare patient whose vocal folds cannot be assessed adequately by other means or for patients who need surgical procedures to remove or biopsy laryngeal lesions. In some cases, this may be done with local anesthesia, avoiding the need for intubation and the traumatic coughing and vomiting that may occur even after general anesthesia administered by mask. Coughing after general anesthesia may be minimized by using topical anesthesia in the larynx and trachea. However, topical anesthetics may act as severe mucosal irritants in a small number of patients. They may also predispose the patient to aspiration in the postoperative period. If a patient has had difficulty with a topical anesthetic administered in the office, it should not be used in the operating room. When used in general anesthesia cases, topical anesthetics should usually be applied at the end of the procedure. Thus, if inflammation occurs, it will not interfere with performance of microsurgery. Postoperative duration of anesthesia is also optimized. The author has had the least difficulty with 4% Xylocaine.

Objective Tests

Reliable, valid, objective analysis of the voice is extremely important and is an essential part of a comprehensive physical examination.[2] It is as valuable to the laryngologist as audiometry is to the otologist.[8,9] Familiarity with some of the measures and technological advances currently available is helpful. This information is included here as a brief overview for the convenience of the reader.

Strobovideolaryngoscopy

Integrity of the vibratory margin of the vocal fold is essential for the complex motion required to produce good vocal quality. Under continuous light, the vocal folds vibrate approximately 250 times per second while phonating at middle C. Naturally, the human eye cannot discern the necessary

details during such rapid motion. The vibratory margin may be assessed through high-speed photography, strobovideolaryngoscopy, high-speed video, videokymography, electroglottography (EGG), or photoglottography. Strobovideolaryngoscopy provides the necessary clinical information in a practical fashion. Stroboscopic light allows routine slow-motion evaluation of the mucosal cover layer of the leading edge of the vocal fold. This state-of-the-art physical examination permits detection of vibratory asymmetries, structural abnormalities, small masses, submucosal scars, and other conditions that are invisible under ordinary light.[10,11] Documentation of the procedure by coupling stroboscopic light with the video camera allows later reevaluation by the laryngologist or other health care providers.

Stroboscopy does not provide a true slow-motion image, as obtained through high-speed photography (Figure 3–2). The stroboscope actually illuminates different points on consecutive vocal fold waves, each of which is retained on the retina for 0.2 seconds. The stroboscopically lighted portions of the successive waves are fused visually, and thus the examiner is actually evaluating simulated cycles of phonation. The slow-motion effect is created by having the stroboscopic light desynchronized with the frequency of vocal fold vibration by approximately 2 Hz. When vocal fold vibration and the stroboscope are synchronized exactly, the vocal folds appear to stand still, rather than move in slow motion (Figure 3–3). In most instances, this approximation of slow motion provides all the clinical information necessary. Our routine stroboscopy protocol is described elsewhere.[11] We use a modification of the standardized method of subjective assessment of strobovideolaryngoscopic images, as proposed by Bless et al[12] and Hirano.[13] Characteristics evalu-

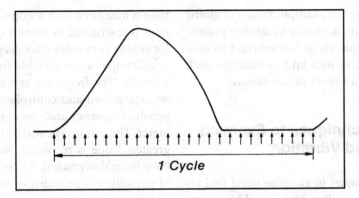

Figure 3–2. The principle of ultra–high-speed photography. Numerous images are taken during each vibratory cycle. This technique is a true slow-motion representation of each vocal fold vibration.

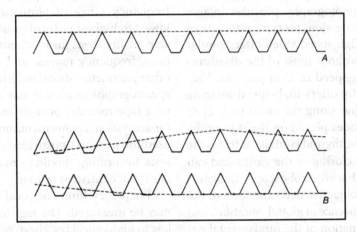

Figure 3–3. The principle of stroboscopy. The stroboscopic light illuminates portions of successive cycles. The eye fuses the illuminated points into an illusion of slow motion. **A.** If the stroboscope is synchronized with vocal fold vibration, a similar point is illuminated on each successive cycle and the vocal fold appears to stand still. **B.** If the stroboscope is slightly desynchronized, each cycle is illuminated at a slightly different point, and the slow-motion effect is created.

ated include the fundamental frequency, the symmetry of movements, periodicity, glottic closure, the amplitude of vibration, the mucosal wave, the presence of nonvibrating portions of the vocal fold, and other unusual findings. With practice, perceptual judgments of stroboscopic images provide a great deal of information. However, it is easy for the inexperienced observer to draw unwarranted conclusions because of normal variations in vibration. Vibrations depend on fundamental frequency, intensity, and vocal register. For example, failure of glottic closure occurs normally in falsetto phonation. Consequently, it is important to note these characteristics and to examine each voice under a variety of conditions.

Other Techniques to Examine Vocal Fold Vibration

Other techniques to examine vocal fold vibration include ultra–high-speed photography, electroglottography (EGG), photoelectroglottography and ultrasound glottography, and most recently videokymography[14] and high-speed video (digital or analog). Ultra–high-speed photography provides images that are in true slow motion, rather than simulated. High-speed video offers similar advantages without most of the disadvantages of high-speed motion pictures. Videokymography offers high-speed imaging of a single line along the vocal fold. EGG uses 2 electrodes placed on the skin of the neck above the thyroid laminae. It traces the opening and closing of the glottis and can be compared with stroboscopic images.[15] EGG allows objective determination of the presence or absence of glottal vibrations and easy determination of the fundamental period of vibration and is reproducible. It reflects the glottal condition more accurately during its closed phase. Photo electroglottography and ultrasound glottography are less useful clinically.[16]

Measures of Phonatory Ability

Objective measures of phonatory ability are easy to use, readily available to the laryngologist, helpful in the treatment of professional vocalists with specific voice disorders, and quite useful in assessing the results of surgical therapies. Maximum phonation time is measured with a stopwatch. The patient is instructed to sustain the vowel /a/ for as long as possible after deep inspiration, vocalizing at a comfortable frequency and intensity. The frequency and intensity may be determined and controlled by an inexpensive frequency analyzer and sound-level meter. The test is repeated 3 times, and the greatest value is recorded. Normal values have been determined.[16] Frequency range of phonation is recorded in semitones and documents the vocal range from the lowest note in the modal register (excluding vocal fry) to the highest falsetto note. This is the physiologic frequency range of phonation and disregards quality. The musical frequency range of phonation measures lowest to highest notes of musically acceptable quality. Tests for maximum phonation time, frequency ranges, and many of the other parameters discussed later (including spectrographic analysis) may be preserved on a tape recorder or digitized and stored for analysis at a convenient future time and used for pre- and posttreatment comparisons. Recordings should be made in a standardized, consistent fashion.

Frequency limits of vocal register also may be measured. The registers are (from low to high) vocal fry, chest, mid, head, and falsetto. However, classification of registers is controversial, and many other classifications are used. Although the classification listed earlier is common among musicians, at present, most voice scientists prefer to classify registers as pulse, modal, and loft. Overlap of frequency among registers occurs routinely.

Testing the speaking fundamental frequency often reveals excessively low pitch, an abnormality associated with chronic voice abuse and development of vocal nodules. This parameter may be followed objectively throughout a course of voice therapy. Intensity range of phonation (IRP) has proven a less useful measure than frequency range. It varies with fundamental frequency (which should be recorded) and is greatest in the middle frequency range. It is recorded in sound pressure level (SPL) (re 0.0002 microbar). For healthy adults who are not professional vocalists, measuring at a single fundamental frequency, IRP averages 54.8 dB for males and 51 dB for females.[17] Alterations of intensity are common in voice disorders, although IRP is not the most sensitive test to detect them. Information from these tests may be combined in fundamental frequency-intensity profile,[16] also called a *phonetogram*.

Glottal efficiency (ratio of the acoustic power at the level of the glottis to subglottal power) provides useful information but is not clinically practical because measuring acoustic power at the level of the glottis is difficult. Subglottic power is the product of subglottal pressure and airflow rate. These can be determined clinically. Various alternative measures of glottic efficiency have been proposed, including the ratio of radiated acoustic power to subglottal power,[18] airflow intensity profile,[19] and ratio of the root mean square value of the AC component to the mean volume velocity (DC component).[20] Although glottal efficiency is of great interest, none of these tests is particularly helpful under routine clinical circumstances.

Aerodynamic Measures

Traditional pulmonary function testing provides the most readily accessible measure of respiratory function. The most common parameters measured include (1) tidal volume, the volume of air that enters the lungs during inspiration and leaves during expiration in normal breathing; (2) functional residual capacity, the volume of air remaining in the lungs at the end of inspiration during normal breathing, which can be divided into expiratory reserve volume (maximal additional volume that can be exhaled) and residual volume (the volume of air remaining in the lungs at the end of maximal exhalation); (3) inspiratory capacity, the maximal volume of air that can be inhaled starting at the functional residual capacity; (4) total lung capacity, the volume of air in the lungs following maximal inspiration; (5) vital capacity, the maximal volume of air that can be exhaled from the lungs following maximal inspiration; (6) forced vital capacity, the rate of airflow with rapid, forceful expiration from total lung capacity to residual volume; (7) FEV_1, the forced expiratory volume in 1 second; FEV_3, the forced expiratory volume in 3 seconds; and (9) maximal midexpiratory flow, the mean rate of airflow over the middle half of the forced vital capacity (between 25% and 75% of the forced vital capacity).

For singers and professional speakers with an abnormality caused by voice abuse, abnormal pulmonary function tests may confirm deficiencies in aerobic conditioning or reveal previously unrecognized asthma.[21] Flow glottography with computer inverse filtering is also a practical and valuable diagnostic for assessing flow at the vocal fold level, evaluating the voice source, and imaging the results of the balance between adductory forces and subglottal pressure.[22] It also has therapeutic value as a biofeedback tool.

The spirometer, readily available for pulmonary function testing, can also be used for measuring airflow during phonation. However, the spirometer does not allow simultaneous display of acoustic signals, and its frequency response is poor. A pneumotachograph consists of a laminar air resistor, a differential pressure transducer, and an amplifying and recording system. It allows measurement of airflow and simultaneous recording of other signals when coupled with a polygraph. A hotwire anemometer allows determination of airflow velocity by measuring the electrical drop across the hot wire. Modern hotwire anemometers containing electrical feedback circuitry that maintains the temperature of the hot wire provide a flat response up to 1 kHz and are useful clinically.

The 4 parameters traditionally measured in the aerodynamic performance of a voice are subglottal pressure (P_{sub}), supraglottal pressure (P_{sup}), glottal impedance, and the volume velocity of airflow at the glottis. These parameters and their rapid variations can be measured under laboratory circumstances. However, clinically their mean value is usually determined as follows:

$$P_{sub} - P_{sup} = MFR \times GR$$

where *MFR* is the mean (root mean square) flow rate, and *GR* is the mean (root mean square) glottal resistance. When vocalizing the open vowel /a/, the supraglottic pressure equals the atmospheric pressure, reducing the equation to

$$P_{sub} = MFR \times GR$$

The mean flow rate is a useful clinical measure. While the patient vocalizes the vowel /a/, the mean flow rate is calculated by dividing the total volume of air used during phonation by the duration of phonation. The subject phonates at a comfortable pitch and loudness either over a determined period of time or for a maximum sustained period of phonation.

Air volume is measured by the use of a mask fitted tightly over the face or by phonating into a mouthpiece while wearing a nose clamp. Measurements may be made using a spirometer, pneumotachograph, or hotwire anemometer. The normal values for mean flow rate under habitual phonation, with changes in intensity or register, and under various pathologic circumstances, were determined in the 1970s.[16] Normal values are available for both adults and children. Mean flow rate also can be measured and is a clinically useful parameter to follow during treatment for vocal nodules, recurrent laryngeal nerve paralysis, spasmodic dysphonia, and other conditions.

Glottal resistance cannot be measured directly, but it may be calculated from the mean flow rate and mean subglottal pressure. Normal glottal resistance is 20 to 100 dyne s/cm^5 at low and medium pitches and 150 dyne s/cm^5 at high pitches.[18] The normal values for subglottal pressure under various healthy and pathologic voice conditions have also been determined by numerous investigators.[16] The phonation quotient is the vital capacity divided by the maximum phonation time. It has been shown to correlate closely with maximum flow rate[23] and is a more convenient measure. Normative data determined by various authors have been published.[16] The phonation quotient provides an objective measure of the effects of treatment and is particularly useful in cases of recurrent laryngeal nerve paralysis and mass lesions of the vocal folds, including nodules.

Acoustic Analysis

Acoustic analysis equipment can determine frequency, intensity, harmonic spectrum, cycle-to-cycle perturbations in frequency (jitter), cycle-to-cycle perturbations in amplitude (shimmer), harmonics/noise ratios, breathiness index, and many other parameters. The DSP Sona-Graph Sound Analyzer Model 5500 (Kay Elemetrics, Lincoln Park, New Jersey) is an integrated voice analysis system. It is equipped for sound spectrography capabilities. Spectrography provides a visual record of the voice. The acoustic signal is depicted using time (*x*-axis), frequency (*y*-axis), and intensity (*z*-axis), shading of light versus dark. Using the bandpass filters, generalizations about quality, pitch, and loudness can be made. These observations are used in formulating the voice therapy treatment plan. Formant structure and strength can be determined using the narrowband filters, of which a variety of configurations are possible. In clinical settings in which singers and other professional voice users are evaluated and treated routinely, this feature is extremely valuable. A sophisticated voice analysis program (an optional program) may be combined with the Sona-Graph and is an especially valuable addition to the clinical laboratory. The voice analysis program (Computer Speech Lab; Kay Elemetrics) measures speaking fundamental frequency, frequency perturbation (jitter), amplitude perturbation (shimmer), and harmonics-to-noise ratio and provides many other useful values. An EGG may be used in conjunction with the Sona-Graph to provide some of these voicing parameters. Examining the EGG waveform alone is possible with this setup, but its clinical usefulness has not yet been established. An important feature of the Sona-Graph is the long-term average (LTA) spectral capability, which permits analysis of longer voice samples (30–90 seconds). The LTA analyzes only voiced speech segments and may be useful in screening for hoarse or breathy voices. In addition, computer interface capabilities (also an optional program) have solved many data storage and file maintenance problems.

In analyzing acoustic signals, the microphone may be placed at the level of the mouth or positioned in or over the trachea, although intratracheal recordings are used for research purposes only. The position should be standardized in each office or laboratory.[24] Various techniques are being developed to improve the usefulness of acoustic analysis. Because of the enormous amount of information carried in the acoustic signal, further refinements in objective acoustic analysis should prove particularly valuable to the clinician.

Laryngeal Electromyography

Electromyography (EMG) requires an electrode system, an amplifier, an oscilloscope, a loudspeaker, and a recording system.[25] Electrodes are placed transcutaneously into laryngeal muscles. EMG can be extremely valuable in confirming cases of vocal fold paresis, in differentiating paralysis from arytenoid dislocation, distinguishing recurrent laryngeal nerve paralysis from combined recurrent and superior nerve paralysis, diagnosing other more subtle neurolaryngologic pathology, and documenting functional voice disorders and malingering. It is also recommended for needle localization when using botulinum toxin for treatment of spasmodic dysphonia and other conditions.

Psychoacoustic Evaluation

Because the human ear and brain are the most sensitive and complex analyzers of sound currently available, many researchers have tried to standardize and quantify psychoacoustic evaluation. Unfortunately, even definitions of basic terms such as hoarseness and breathiness are still controversial. Psychoacoustic evaluation protocols and interpretations are not standardized. Consequently, although subjective psychoacoustic analysis of voice is of great value to the individual skilled clinician, it remains generally unsatisfactory for comparing research among laboratories or for reporting clinical results.

The GRBAS scale[6] helps standardize perceptual analysis for clinical purposes. It rates the voice on a scale from 0 to 3, with regrading to grade, roughness, breathiness, asthenia, and strain. Grade 0 is normal, 1 is slightly abnormal, 2 is moderately abnormal, and 3 is extremely abnormal. Grade refers to the degree of hoarseness or voice abnormality. Roughness refers to the acoustic/auditory impression of irregularity of vibration and corresponds with gear and shimmer. Breathiness refers to the acoustic/auditory impression of air leakage and corresponds to turbulence. Asthenic evaluation assesses weakness or lack of power and corresponds to vocal intensity and energy in higher harmonics. Strain refers to the acoustic/auditory impression of hyperfunction and may be related to fundamental frequency, noise in the high-frequency range, and energy in higher harmonics. For example, a patient's voice might be graded as G2, R2, B1, A1, S2.

Outcomes Assessment

Measuring the impact of a voice disorder has always been challenging. However, recent advances have begun to address this problem. Validated instruments such as the voice handicap index (VHI)[26] are currently in clinical use and are likely to be used widely in future years.

Voice Impairment and Disability

Quantifying voice impairment and assigning a disability rating (percentage of whole person) remain controversial. This subject is still not addressed comprehensively even in the most recent editions (2008, 6th edi-

tion) of the American Medical Association's *Guides to the Evaluation of Permanent Impairment (AMA Guides)*. The *Guides* still do not take into account the person's profession when calculating disability. Alternative approaches have been proposed,[27] and advances in this complex arena are anticipated over the next few years.

Evaluation of the Singing Voice

The physician must be careful not to exceed the limits of his or her expertise, especially in caring for singers. However, if voice abuse or technical error is suspected, or if a difficult judgment must be reached on whether to allow a sick singer to perform, a brief observation of the patient's singing may provide invaluable information. This is accomplished best by asking the singer to stand and sing scales either in the examining room or in the soundproof audiology booth. Similar maneuvers may be used for professional speakers, including actors (who can vocalize and recite lines), clergy and politicians (who can deliver sermons and speeches), and virtually all other voice patients. The singer's stance should be balanced, with the weight slightly forward. The knees should be bent slightly, and the shoulders, torso, and neck should be relaxed. The singer should inhale through the nose whenever possible allowing filtration, warming, and humidification of inspired air. In general, the chest should be expanded, but most of the active breathing is abdominal. The chest should not rise substantially with each inspiration, and the supraclavicular musculature should not be involved obviously in inspiration. Shoulders and neck muscles should not be tensed even with deep inspiration. Abdominal musculature should be contracted shortly before the initiation of the tone. This may be evaluated visually or by palpation (Figure 3–4). Muscles of the neck and face should be relaxed. Economy is a basic principle of all art forms. Wasted energy and motion and muscle tension are incorrect and usually deleterious.

The singer should be instructed to sing a scale (a 5-note scale is usually sufficient) on the vowel /a/, beginning on any comfortable note. Technical errors are usually most obvious as contraction of muscles in the neck and chin, retraction of the lower lip, retraction of the tongue, or tightening of the muscles of mastication. The singer's mouth should be open widely but comfortably. When singing /a/, the singer's tongue should rest in a neutral position with the tip of the tongue lying against the back of the singer's mandibular incisors. If the tongue pulls back or demonstrates obvious muscular activity as the singer performs the scales, improper voice use can be confirmed on the basis of positive evidence (Figure 3–5). The position of the larynx should not vary substantially with pitch changes. Rising of the larynx with ascending pitch is evidence of technical dysfunction. This examination also gives the physician an opportunity to observe any dramatic differences between the qualities and ranges of the patient's speaking voice and the singing voice. A physical examination summary form has proven helpful in organization and documentation.[3]

Remembering the admonition not to exceed his or her expertise, the physician who examines many singers can often glean valuable information from a brief attempt to modify an obvious technical error. For example, deciding whether to allow a singer with mild or moderate laryngitis to perform is often difficult. On one hand, an expert singer has technical skills that allow him or her to compensate safely. On the other hand, if a singer does not sing with correct technique and does not have the discipline to modify volume, technique, and repertoire as necessary, the risk of vocal injury may be increased substantially even by mild inflammation of the vocal folds. In borderline circumstances, observation of the singer's technique may greatly help the physician in making a judgment.

If the singer's technique appears flawless, the physician may feel somewhat more secure in allowing the singer to proceed with performance commitments. More commonly, even good singers demonstrate technical errors when experiencing voice difficulties. In a vain effort to compensate for dysfunction at the vocal fold level, singers often modify their technique in the neck and supraglottic vocal tract. In the

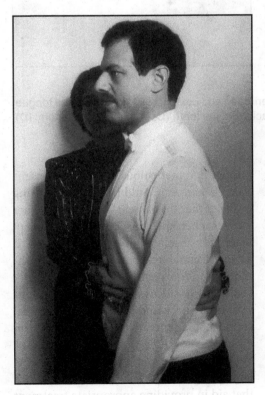

Figure 3–4. Bimanual palpation of the support mechanism. The singer should expand posteriorly and anteriorly with inspiration. Muscles should tighten prior to onset of sung tone.

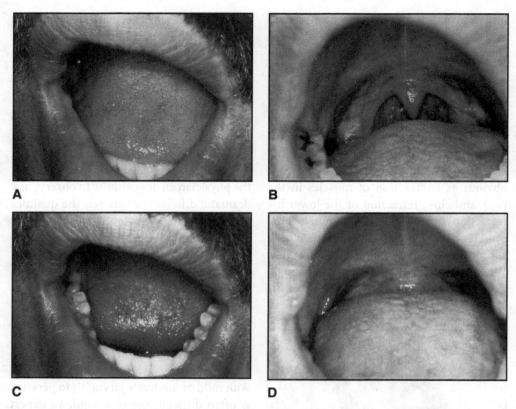

Figure 3–5. Proper relaxed position of the anterior (**A**) and posterior (**B**) portions of the tongue. Common improper use of the tongue pulled back from the teeth (**C**) and raised posteriorly (**D**).

good singer, this usually means going from good technique to bad technique. The most common error involves pulling back the tongue and tightening the cervical muscles. Although this increased muscular activity gives the singer the illusion of making the voice more secure, this technical maladjustment undermines vocal efficiency and increases vocal strain. The physician may ask the singer to hold the top note of a 5-note scale; while the note is being held, the singer may simply be told, "Relax your tongue." At the same time, the physician points to the singer's abdominal musculature. Most good singers immediately correct to good technique. If they do, and if upcoming performances are particularly important, the singer may be able to perform with a re-

minder that meticulous technique is essential. The singer should be advised to "sing by feel rather than by ear," consult his or her voice teacher, and conserve the voice except when it is absolutely necessary to use it. If a singer is unable to correct from bad technique to good technique promptly, especially if he or she uses excessive muscle tension in the neck and ineffective abdominal support, it is generally safer not to perform with even a mild vocal fold abnormality. With increased experience and training, the laryngologist may make other observations that aid in providing appropriate treatment recommendations for singer patients. Once these skills have been mastered for the care of singers, applying them to other patients is relatively easy, so long as the laryngologist takes the time to understand the demands of the individual's professional, avocational, and recreational vocal activities.

If treatment is to be instituted, making at least a tape recording of the voice is advisable in most cases and essential before any surgical intervention. The author routinely uses strobovideolaryngoscopy for diagnosis and documentation in virtually all cases as well as many of the objective measures discussed. Pretreatment testing is extremely helpful clinically and medicolegally.

Additional Examinations

A general physical examination should be performed whenever the patient's systemic health is questionable. Debilitating conditions such as mononucleosis may be noticed first by the singer as vocal fatigue. A neurologic assessment may be particularly revealing. The physician must be careful not to overlook dysarthrias and dysphonias, which are characteristic of movement disorders and of serious neurologic disease. Dysarthria is a defect in rhythm, enunciation, and articulation that usually results from neuromuscular impairment or weakness such as may occur after a stroke. It may be seen with oral deformities or illness, as well. Dysphonia is an abnormality of vocalization usually caused by problems at the laryngeal level.

Physicians should be familiar with the 6 types of dysarthria, their symptoms, and their importance.[28,29] Flaccid dysarthria occurs in lower motor neuron or primary muscle disorders such as myasthenia gravis and tumors or strokes involving the brainstem nuclei. Spastic dysarthria occurs in upper motor neuron disorders (pseudobulbar palsy) such as multiple strokes and cerebral palsy. Ataxic dysarthria is seen with cerebellar disease, alcohol intoxication, and

multiple sclerosis. Hypokinetic dysarthria accompanies Parkinson disease. Hyperkinetic dysarthria may be spasmodic, as in the Gilles de la Tourette disease, or dystonic, as in chorea and cerebral palsy. Mixed dysarthria occurs in amyotrophic lateral sclerosis (ALS) or Lou Gehrig disease. The preceding classification actually combines dysphonic and dysarthric characteristics but is very useful clinically. The value of a comprehensive neurolaryngologic evaluation[30] cannot be overstated. More specific details of voice changes associated with neurologic dysfunction and their localizing value are available elsewhere.[2,31]

It is extremely valuable for the laryngologist to assemble an arts-medicine team that includes not only a speech-language pathologist, singing voice specialist, acting voice specialist, and voice scientist but also medical colleagues in other disciplines. Collaboration with an expert neurologist, pulmonologist, endocrinologist, psychologist, psychiatrist, internist, physiatrist, and others with special knowledge of, and interest in, voice disorders is invaluable in caring for patients with voice disorders. Such interdisciplinary teams have not only changed the standard of care in voice evaluation and treatment but are also largely responsible for the rapid and productive growth of voice as a subspecialty.

References

1. Sataloff RT. Professional singers: the science and art of clinical care. *Am J Otolaryngol.* 1981;2:251–266.
2. Rubin JS, Sataloff RT, Korovin GS. *Diagnosis and Treatment of Voice Disorders.* 3rd ed. San Diego, CA: Plural Publishing; 2006.
3. Sataloff RT. The professional voice: part II, physical examination. *J Voice.* 1987;1:91–201.
4. Fuazawa T, Blaugrund SM, El-Assuooty A, Gould WJ. Acoustic analysis of hoarse voice:

a preliminary report. *J Voice*. 1988;2(2): 127–131.

5. Gelfer M. Perceptual attributes of voice: development and use of rating scales. *J Voice*. 1988;2(4):320–326.

6. Hirano M. *Clinical Examination of the Voice*. New York, NY: Springer-Verlag; 1981:83–84.

7. Fujimura O. Stereo-fiberoptic laryngeal observation. *J Acoust Soc Am*. 1979;65:70–72.

8. Sataloff RT, Spiegel JR, Carroll LM, Darby KS, Hawkshaw MJ, Rulnick RK. The clinical voice laboratory: practical design and clinical application. *J Voice*. 1990;4:264–279.

9. Sataloff RT, Heuer RH, Hoover C, Baroody MM. Laboratory assessment of voice. In: Gould WJ, Sataloff RT, Spiegel JR. eds. *Voice Surgery*. St. Louis, MO: Mosby; 1993:203–216.

10. Sataloff RT, Spiegel JR, Carroll LM, Schiebel BR, Darby KS, Rulnick RK. Strobovideolaryngoscopy in professional voice users: results and clinical value. *J Voice*. 1986;1:359–364.

11. Sataloff RT, Spiegel JR, Hawkshaw MJ. Strobovideolaryngoscopy: results and clinical value. *Ann Otol Rhinol Laryngol*. 1991;100:725–727.

12. Bless D, Hirano M, Feder RJ. Video stroboscopic evaluation of the larynx. *Ear Nose Throat J*. 1987;66:289–296.

13. Hirano M. Phonosurgery: basic and clinical investigations. *Otologia (Fukuoka)*. 1975;21: 239–442.

14. Svec J, Shutte H. Videokymography: high-speed line scanning of vocal fold vibration. *J Voice*. 1996;10:201–205.

15. Leclure FLE, Brocaar ME, Verscheeure J. Electroglottography and its relation to glottal activity. *Folia Phoniatr (Basel)*. 1975;27: 215–224.

16. Hirano M. *Clinical Examination of the Voice*. New York, NY: Springer-Verlag; 1981:25–27, 85–98.

17. Coleman RJ, Mabis JH, Hinson JK. Fundamental frequency sound pressure level profiles of adult male and female voices. *J Speech Hear Res*. 1977;20:197–204.

18. Isshiki N. Regulatory mechanism of voice intensity variation. *J Speech Hear Res*. 1964;7: 17–29.

19. Saito S. Phonosurgery: basic study on the mechanisms of phonation and endolaryngeal microsurgery. *Otologia (Fukuoka)*. 1977;23: 171–384.

20. Isshiki N. Functional surgery of the larynx. *Report of the 78th Annual Convention of the Oto-Rhino-Laryngological Society of Japan*. Fukuoka, Japan: Kyoto University; 1977.

21. Cohn JR, Sataloff RT, Spiegel JR, Fish JE, Kennedy K. Airway reactivity-induced asthma in singers (ARIAS). *J Voice*. 1991;5:332–337.

22. Sundberg J. *The Science of the Singing Voice*. Dekalb, IL: Northern Illinois University Press; 1987:11, 66, 77–89.

23. Hirano M, Koike Y, von Leden H. Maximum phonation time and air usage during phonation. *Folia Phoniatr (Basel)*. 1968;20:185–201.

24. Price DB, Sataloff RT. A simple technique for consistent microphone placement in voice recording. *J Voice*. 1988;2:206–207.

25. Sataloff RT, Mandel S, Heman-Ackah Y, Mañon-Espaillat R, Abaza M. *Laryngeal Electromyography*. 2nd ed. San Diego, CA: Plural Publishing; 2006.

26. Benninger MS, Gardner GM, Jacobson BH. New dimensions in measuring voice treatment outcomes. In: Sataloff RT. *Professional Voice: The Science and Art of Clinical Care*. 3rd ed. San Diego, CA: Plural Publishing; 2005:471–478.

27. Sataloff RT. Voice and speech impairment and disability. In: Sataloff RT. *Professional Voice: The Science and Art of Clinical Care*. 3rd ed. San Diego, CA: Plural Publishing; 2005:1427–1432.

28. Darley FL, Aronson AE, Brown JR. Differential diagnostic of patterns of dysarthria. *J Speech Hear Res*. 1969;12(2):246–249.

29. Darley FL, Aronson AE, Brown JR. Clusters of deviant speech dimensions in the dysarthrias. *J Speech Hear Res*. 1969;12(3):462–496.

30. Rosenfield DB. Neurolaryngology. *Ear Nose Throat J*. 1987;66:323–326.

31. Raphael BN, Sataloff RT. Increasing vocal effectiveness. In: Sataloff RT. *Professional Voice: Science and Art of Clinical Care*. 3rd ed. San Diego, CA: Plural Publishing; 2005:993–1004.

SECTION II

Non-Laryngeal Cancer

4

Lung Cancer and Voice

Abdul-Latif Hamdan, Robert Thayer Sataloff, and
Mary J. Hawkshaw

Lung Cancer: Incidence and Clinical Presentation

Lung cancer is the most common malignancy worldwide. There are 2.1 million newly diagnosed cases yearly.[1] Its incidence over the years has increased in both genders, with higher rates being observed in less-developed countries.[2,3] This rise has been linked to both educational and socioeconomic factors. Individuals with little education and low income are more likely to smoke and hence be affected in comparison to highly educated individuals with high income.[3] An equally important factor is ethnicity. Non-Hispanics are more affected than Hispanics, and African Americans are more affected than white Americans.[4,5] Lung cancer accounts for 25% of annual cancer mortalities, with an overall 5-year survival that does not exceed 18%.[1,6] In the United States, it is the leading cause of death with a projected estimation of 606 880 mortalities in 2019.[7,8]

Lung cancer refers to all malignancies "that originate in the airways or pulmonary parenchyma."[7] Various histologic types exist. Non-small cell lung carcinoma (NSCLC) accounts for 80% to 85% of reported cases and includes mainly squamous cell carci-noma, adenocarcinoma, and large cell carcinoma. Small cell lung carcinoma (SCLC) accounts for the remaining 15% of the cases reported.[4] The most important risk factors are smoking, a history of radiation therapy to the chest, and exposure to environmental toxins such as asbestos and polycyclic aromatic hydrocarbon.[8] Additional risk factors include pulmonary fibrosis, infection with human immunodeficiency virus (HIV) and alcohol consumption. Genetic predisposition also affects prevalence and overall prognosis.[8] Another important risk factor is radon exposure which is the second leading cause of lung cancer in smokers and the first in nonsmokers.[9]

The clinical manifestations in patients with lung cancer include symptoms referable to the intrathoracic and extrathoracic impact of the disease. Based on a study on 2293 patients with NSCLC, the most common intrathoracic symptoms were cough and dyspnea occurring in 54.7% and 45.3% of cases, respectively[10] (Figure 4–1). In a review by Chute et al, additional symptoms included chest pain and hemoptysis in 27% of the cases. These symptoms were associated with the overall stage of the disease rather than the cell type.[11] The prevalence and nature of symptoms also may vary with the location of the lesion. In patients with

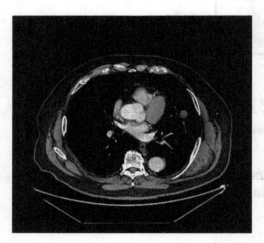

Figure 4–1. Clinical presentation of lung carcinoma. A 70-year-old man presented to the pulmonary clinic with history of cough and dyspnea not responding to medical treatment. A computed tomography scan of the chest was done and showed an 18-mm nodule with irregular borders in the left upper lobe. Biopsy of the lesion showed adenocarcinoma.

central pulmonary lesions, symptoms related to airway obstruction such as dyspnea and cough are common. Airway obstructive symptoms are invariably associated with endobronchial growth that can lead to intraluminal and/or extraluminal obstruction. Patients with peripheral pulmonary lesions may present with dull and persistent chest pain.[12] This is associated with the presence of pleural plaques, pleural effusion, and/or local extension of the tumor to the chest wall or mediastinum[13,14] (Figure 4–2). Less commonly described symptoms are shoulder and radicular pain along the neural distribution of the ulnar nerve together with paresthesia, often referred to as Pancoast syndrome. Symptoms related to impingement on the cervical sympathetic chain, pericardial invasion, and/or vascular compression as in patients with superior vena cava syndrome also may be present.[15-17] In addition, lung cancer may lead to a constel-

lation of nonspecific symptoms secondary to spread of the disease to other organs such as bones, liver, adrenals, and brain in up to 40% of cases.[18] In a study on the utility of percutaneous computed tomography (CT)–guided biopsy in patients with SCLC, 17% had evidence of adrenal gland metastasis despite normal radiologic findings.[19] Adrenal gland metastasis is usually asymptomatic, unlike bone metastasis that can present with severe back and chest pain. Bone metastasis is known to affect 20% of patients with NSCLC and 30% to 40% of patients with SCLC.[20,21]

Complaints related to the laryngopharyngeal complex are not uncommon in patients with lung cancer. The prevalence and increased burden of swallowing dysfunction in patients with lung cancer have been described by many authors with emphasis on early diagnosis. According to numerous studies, dysphagia and dyspepsia are common along the full course of

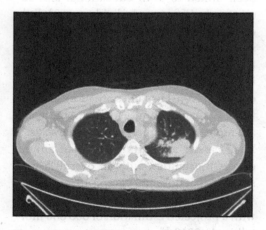

Figure 4–2. Clinical presentation of lung carcinoma. A 44-year-old man, a heavy smoker, presented with history of persistent chest pain not responding to anti-inflammatory medications. A computed tomography of the chest was requested and showed a peripheral lung tumor abutting the chest wall (axial view; lung window).

the disease despite their low prevalence at the time of presentation.[22-27] In the report by Stankey et al, dysphagia is often attributed to esophageal compression within the mediastinum by enlarged lymph nodes.[25] This pathophysiologic mechanism is in accordance with the high prevalence of mediastinal disease that has been reported in 92% of patients with lung cancer.[26] Other causes of esophageal compression may include lymphadenopathy at the subcarinal level, thoracic inlet, or neck. Cervical adenopathy has been reported in 15% to 20% of affected patients.[23] Direct tumor invasion also may lead to dysphagia with subsequent achalasia or vocal fold impairment.[26,27] Camidge expanded further on the possible mechanisms of dysphagia in lung cancer and reported brainstem lesions with damage to the nucleus ambiguus as a potential cause.[26] Based on a review by Counsell et al, lung cancer accounts for almost 50% of secondary intracranial tumors,[28] and cerebral metastasis may be present in 1 out of 5 patients with lung cancer at necropsy.[23] Swallowing obstructive symptoms also may be secondary to metastasis to the gastrointestinal system.[29] Gastrointestinal metastasis can be found in up to 14% of patients with lung cancer, with the middle third of the esophagus being most commonly affected.[30] Other suggested mechanisms for dysphagia in patients with lung cancer include associated systemic disorders, secondary primary tumors, increasing palliative care, and treatment-related causes such as radiation-induced esophageal stenosis.[26]

Phonatory symptoms in patients with lung cancer are common, as well. This chapter reviews the literature on the prevalence and pathophysiology of dysphonia in patients with lung cancer, including disease-related and therapy-induced changes in voice quality. Understanding the pathophysiology of dysphonia in patients with lung cancer is essential in the workup and management of affected patients.

Voice Disorders in Patients With Lung Cancer

Voice symptoms are not infrequent in patients with lung cancer. These may occur either at the time of presentation or along the course of the disease.[23,31-33] In the review by Midthun et al in 2019, hoarseness is listed as a main symptom secondary to the intrathoracic expansion of the disease, in addition to the commonly described respiratory symptoms in patients diagnosed with lung cancer.[8] Based on the National Institute for Health and Care Excellence, hoarseness is one of the characteristic symptoms of lung cancer in addition to cough, dyspnea, and hemoptysis.[34] Similarly, in a cross-sectional study of 40 patients with proven lung cancer and no brain metastasis, Lee et al reported mild-to-moderate voice disorders in 90% of cases,[35] although only 27.5% had elevated voice handicap index (VHI) despite the elevated perceptual rating of voice quality in most patients. Moreover, there was a significant correlation between patients' and physicians' ratings of voice, and the Medical Research Council (MRC) dyspnea scale,[36] which is a self-report of consequences of dyspnea. There was a significant correlation also between the total VHI score and the Eastern Cooperative Oncology Group (ECOG) performance status scale which reflects the overall level of patient's function.[37] The results of Lee et al's investigation highlight the systemic disabling effects of dysphonia in patients with lung cancer. When present, dysphonia may impact the quality of life markedly as evidenced by an increase in the VHI score in 1 out of 4 affected patients. Higher scores were reported on the physical and functional subscales in comparison to the emotional scale.[35]

Why Dysphonia in Patients With Lung Cancer?

Disease-Related Dysphonia

Disease-related dysphonia in lung cancer patients is multifaceted. The change in voice quality can be secondary to local growth of the tumor, its metastasis within the chest and neck, or to the presence of metastatic laryngeal tumors.[35] Mediastinal lymph-adenopathy or tumor extension within the chest and neck can lead to compression of contiguous neural structures such as the recurrent laryngeal nerves. Similarly, hematogenous spread of the disease may result in both laryngeal and systemic complaints.[8] Disease-related psychogenic disorders also can affect voice adversely. Important etiologies in that regard include affective mood disorders such as anxiety and depression that are commonly present in affected patients. Preexisting psychogenic diseases may impact voice quality in addition to disease prognosis and treatment outcome.[38,39] A thorough understanding of how lung cancer as a disease entity can lead to dysphonia is essential for clinicians.

Vocal Fold Paralysis in Patients With Lung Cancer

Patients with vocal fold paralysis and no clear etiology at the time of presentation are invariably suspected to have an extralaryngeal malignancy. Their workup usually includes CT of the neck and chest in order to evaluate the course of the recurrent laryngeal nerves.[40] In the imaging study by Glazer et al, lung cancer was reported as a

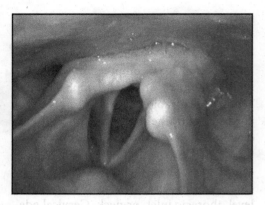

Figure 4–3. Disease-induced dysphonia. A 65-year-old man presented with dysphonia and aspiration of 2 months' duration. On laryngeal examination he had a left vocal fold paralysis in the paramedian position with incomplete closure of the vocal folds during phonation.

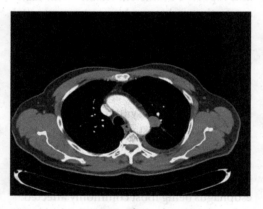

Figure 4–4. Further workup of the patient with computed tomography of the neck and chest revealed a 3.1 × 2.3 cm mass in the left upper lobe inseparable from the aortic arch. Biopsy of the lesion showed adenocarcinoma.

predominant etiology of vocal fold paralysis, in addition to other neoplasms in the mediastinum and neck[41] (Figures 4–3 and 4–4). The paralysis may be either unilateral or bilateral as described by Baumann and Heffner in their case report of bronchogenic carcinoma presenting with respiratory failure.[42] The true prevalence of lung cancer as the cause of unilateral vocal fold paralysis remains unknown, given the large disparity among reports.[43–49] In a review by Gauri et al, recurrent laryngeal nerve paralysis was present in 20% of patients with bronchogenic carcinoma. Other neurologic manifestations included paraneoplastic syndrome and phrenic nerve paralysis.[43] In another review by Terris et al which included 113 patients, lung cancer accounted for 41% (14 out of 34 cases) of the neoplastic causes of vocal fold paralysis.[44] In a study by Kraus et al on 63 patients with glottic incompetence secondary to intrathoracic malignancies, lung cancer was the primary pathology in 49 cases.[48] In an investigation by Benninger et al on the changing etiology of vocal fold immobility, non-laryngeal malignancies accounted for 24.7% of the cases. Pulmonary and mediastinal tumors were the most common causes (80%) in this subgroup of patients.[45] In the study by Havas et al in 1999, lung cancer was among the various etiologies of vocal fold paralysis in a group of 108 patients.[46] Similarly, in a review by Loughran et al on the etiology of unilateral vocal fold paralysis in 77 patients, bronchogenic carcinoma accounted for 43% of the cases.[47] In another review of 57 patients undergoing vocal fold medialization, NSCLC and SCLC were the primary causes of vocal fold paralysis in 47 cases.[49] In a study on 92 cases of vocal fold paralysis out of which 31.5% were idiopathic, Koc et al reported lung cancer as the prime etiology in only 6.5% of cases.[50] In a more recent investigation on 168 patients with unilateral vocal fold paralysis, Bilici et al described lung cancer as the most common cause ($n = 28$) among the occult cause group, where chest lesions were found in 52 cases.[51]

In conclusion, there is enough evidence in the literature to support the paramount role of lung cancer in the etiology of vocal fold paralysis. A patient with lung cancer complaining of dysphonia should be investigated for the presence of vocal fold paralysis with a strong assumption that the primary disease might be the cause of the paralysis. Similarly, a patient with unexplained vocal fold paralysis should be evaluated for lung cancer as a possible cause.

Pulmonary Morbidities Associated With Lung Cancer

Many patients with lung cancer have multiple pulmonary and nonpulmonary morbidities that require palliative care.[52] In a report by Cesario in 2007 on pulmonary function and rehabilitation in patients with lung cancer, the authors reported a decrease in forced expiratory volume (FEV), forced expiratory volume during the first second (FEV1), 6-minute walking test, and PaO_2[53] (Figure 4–5). The reduced lung function in affected subjects is often associated with chronic lung diseases, most common of which is chronic obstructive pulmonary disease (COPD). This association is not surprising given the common habit of smoking between lung cancer patients and COPD patients.[54] COPD is a chronic inflammatory disease of the lower airway that leads to loss of lung tissue with subsequent airway obstruction.[55] In a review on the prevalence of COPD in patients with lung cancer, Loganathan et al reported 72.8% in men and 52.5% in women. The gender difference was significant after adjusting for age and smoking in the analysis of both subgroups.[56] Similarly, based on a study on the prognostic impact of comorbidities in patients with lung cancer, Read et al reported COPD in 50% to 70% of patients with lung cancer.[57] The presence of COPD in patients with lung cancer was associated with worse prognosis and poorer outcome following oncologic surgery. In a meta-analysis looking at the impact of COPD on the prognosis of patients with lung cancer, Lin et al showed that the coexistence of COPD leads to an increased rate of postoperative complications such as bronchopleural fistula, pneumonia, and prolonged mechanical ventilation.[58] Moreover, the 5-year overall survival was markedly affected. The meta-analysis included 29 studies with more than 70 000 patients.

COPD also has been found to be an independent risk factor for lung cancer.[59,60] Numerous studies have shown that the incidence of lung cancer is higher in patients with COPD, almost twice in comparison to patients with no COPD.[61] This link between COPD and lung cancer has been attributed to the common local and systemic inflammatory response that can potentially lead to genetic errors or mutations during the cell repair mechanism with subsequent alterations in cell cycle regulation and apoptosis.[62-66] In keeping with the

aforementioned, Zhu et al described abnormalities in cell biobehavioral inflammatory biomarkers in subjects with chronic lung diseases and highlighted the predictive role of these alterations in the development of lung cancer.[67]

Given the paramount role of breathing in phonation and the aforementioned disease-induced respiratory impairment, patients with lung cancer are at a high risk to develop dysphonia. The reduction in breathing capacity and expiratory flow can lead to many vocal symptoms such as voice fatigue and loss of power.[68-70] This in turn may result in hyperfunctional laryngeal behavior manifested by an increase in both intrinsic and extrinsic laryngeal muscle tension. The presence of COPD can further accentuate the prevalence and severity of phonatory complaints. Ryu et al demonstrated that COPD is an independent risk factor

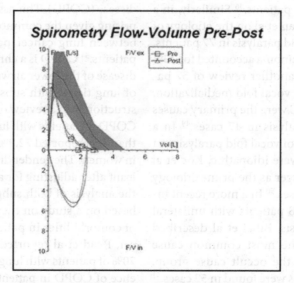

Figure 4–5. Disease-induced respiratory impairment. Pulmonary function test of a 77-year-old diagnosed case of lung adenocarcinoma showing mild obstructive pulmonary disease with reduction in forced vital capacity.

for dysphonia in elderly patients undergoing laryngoscopy.[71] The dysphonia is partially due to the increased usage of steroid inhalers in affected subjects.[72] More details on the association between COPD and voice can be found in the chapter on Laryngeal Manifestations of Respiratory Disorders.[73]

In conclusion, pulmonary impairment in patients with lung cancer is irrefutable. Its impact on phonation remains hypothetical given the lack of any study on the cause-effect relation between pulmonary impairment and dysphonia in patients with lung cancer without vocal fold paralysis or laryngeal tumor. Nevertheless, the well-documented benefits of pulmonary rehabilitation on breathing in patients with lung cancer[74,75] suggest value to the integration of voice therapy in the treatment of patients with lung cancer and dysphonia. Future research is warranted.

Overall Body Fatigability and Weakness in Patients With Lung Cancer

Patients with lung cancer have multiple non-pulmonary comorbidities that can markedly impact body function and subsequently voice. Affected individuals are subject to systemic lipolysis and proteolysis that may result in marked weight loss and overall body fatigue. Symptoms related to muscle weakness and endurance may lead to physical inactivity that improves with physiotherapy.[76,77] Given that muscle function is an important determinant of voice production, its disturbance may impact phonation adversely and result in voice symptoms. Based on a review on the current concepts of voice fatigue by Welham and Maclagan, muscle fatigue is listed as a cause of voice fatigue, as are respiratory dysfunction and dehydration.[68] The impact of disease-induced muscular impairment in patients with lung cancer is even

more accentuated in professional voice users in whom optimal physical endurance and exercise tolerance are paramount for performance.[78] Several means to address this functional disability have been emphasized by many authors. In a review on the effect of chest physiotherapy in patients with lung cancer, Ozalevli et al reported an improvement in physical mobility and energy. The study was conducted on 18 patients with advanced lung cancer for whom functional capacity was measured using the 6-minute walking test.[76] In another review by Cheville et al, improvement in patients' fatigue, mobility, and sleep quality following a rapid and easy strength training exercise program has been demonstrated in patients with stage IV lung cancer.[77] In view of the aforementioned, and given the well-known impact of body fatigue on voice, it is clear that physical training should have a favorable effect on voice of lung cancer patients with dysphonia. The potential benefit of incorporating voice therapy and rehabilitation in the physical training program of affected patients remains unknown and warrants investigation.

In conclusion, lung cancer is associated with body fatigue, and body fatigue is associated with dysphonia. The impact of body fatigue on voice in patients with lung cancer without laryngeal pathology has not been investigated. Future studies on the association between body fatigue and dysphonia in lung cancer patients accounting for confounding variables should be encouraged.

Distress, Anxiety, and Depression in Patients With Lung Cancer

In addition to physical incapacity, patients with lung cancer are subject to emotional and psychological liabilities. The burden of the disease inflicted by symptoms of pain, dyspnea, and anorexia, especially in the absence of effective palliative care, commonly lead to affective and psychosocial distress.[79] In a study by Tishelman on 400 patients diagnosed with inoperable lung cancer and stratified according to time closest to death, the authors reported an association between disease-related symptoms and distress in all subgroups.[80] Similarly, in an investigation by Zabora et al on the prevalence of psychosocial distress in 4496 patients with different types of cancer, the overall reported rate was 35.1% with the highest figure being in patients with lung cancer (43.4%).[81] It is important to note that symptoms of distress can be heterogeneous and often masked by the clinical presentation of the disease itself, social status, and the preexistence of affective or mood disorders that warrant psychological assessment and intervention.[82–84] Moreover, emotional distress in patients with lung cancer can lead to anxiety and depression. Anxiety defined as a "fearful anticipation of an imminent but intangible danger"[85] is present in a substantial number of patients with lung carcinoma. Similarly, depression described as "persistent sadness and loss of interest in activities that you normally enjoy" may either precede or follow the diagnosis of cancer.[86] In 1985, Hughes reported depressive illness in 21 out of 134 patients diagnosed with lung cancer. The prevalence of depressive illness correlated with disease metastasis and prior history of psychiatric diseases.[87] Montazeri et al reported anxiety and depression in 10% and 12%, respectively, of patients with lung cancer at their first visit to pulmonary physicians. The authors also reported higher levels of anxiety and depression in those with low quality of life.[88] Other precipitating factors include absence of social support, poor knowledge of the disease, and personality traits.[88] Brintzenhofe-Szoc examined the prevalence of anxiety and depression in an outpatient tertiary cancer center and reported overall depression and anxiety

symptoms in 18.3% and 24%, respectively. Higher rates of mixed anxiety/depression were described in patients with lung cancer.[89] These findings were supported in a study by Arrieta et al which also revealed depression and anxiety in 32.9% and 34.1% of patients with advanced NSCLC.[90]

The emotional distress, anxiety, and depression present in patients with lung cancer not only negatively impact quality of life, prognosis, and treatment adherence as reported by Arrieta et al,[90] but also phonation. The association between the emotional status and voice is irrefutable. As a personal trait, the voice signal very often reflects the state of distress, anxiety, and depression of the speaker. In a study by Mendoza and Carballo looking at the effect of stress on voice in 82 subjects who were asked to perform 4 different vocal tasks under stressful conditions, the authors showed an increase in fundamental frequency (F0) and perturbation parameters, and a decrease in spectral noise. The stress-induced tasks included recital of the alphabet in reverse order, in addition to delayed auditory feedback. Enrolled subjects were also informed that their performance was linked to their grades.[91] Van Lierde et al reported the impact of stress on subjective and objective voice measures in 54 female subjects who were asked to read a public speech before a large audience. There was a decrease in the fundamental frequency, highest intensity, and maximum phonation time, and an increase in the perceived breathiness and strain. However, there was no effect on vocal asthenia, roughness, pitch, and intensity.[92] In a review by Giddens et al on vocal indices of stress, the authors reported a consistent trend for an increase in F0 which was attributed partially to excessive tension within the cricothyroid muscle.[93] In keeping with this, in a study on 201 patients stratified as high-grade and low-grade anxiety, Gomes et al showed a correlation between anxiety and voice symptoms. Subjects with a higher grade of anxiety had vocal symptoms more frequently than those with a low grade of anxiety. The authors used the State Trait Anxiety Inventory (STAI) to measure anxiety, and the Voice Symptom scale and the Vocal Screening-Protocol as self-assessment tools for voice. Thirteen vocal risk factors have been associated with anxiety.[94]

In conclusion, anxiety and depression are common in lung cancer patients. Although these are clearly associated with dysphonia, the prevalence of dysphonia in patients with lung cancer and anxiety and depression versus those without remains unknown. Future investigation is needed.

Age: A Predisposing Demographic Variable for Dysphonia

Lung cancer occurs predominantly in the elderly.[95] In a study on lung cancer and its burden, Owonikoko et al reported that half affected patients were above the age of 70 years. The analysis was carried on 316 682 patients who were stratified into 3 age groups, less than 70 years old, 70 to 79 years, and older than 80 years.[96] With aging, there are physiological changes that affect the various components of the phonatory apparatus. There is reduction in vital capacity and expiratory flow leading to a decrease in breath support. These respiratory changes are partially attributed to the reduced elasticity of lung tissue and the decrease in the contractile force of respiratory muscles, and they impact phonation negatively.[97] At the level of the larynx, there is laryngeal descent that results in elongation of the vocal tract with subsequent redistribution in the position and dispersion of the various harmonics. Xue and Hao reported lengthening of the oral cavity and an increase in the volume of the vocal tract as a sequel to aging in a

group of elderly subjects.[98] Subsequent to these anatomical changes, there is lowering of the spectral peaks, more in women compared with men, as reported by Linville and Rens.[99] There are also physiologic and constitutional changes in the vocal folds. There is atrophy of the vocal fold epithelium with evidence of desquamation on electron microscopic examination.[100] Moreover, the extracellular matrix of the lamina propria is remodeled with alteration in its constituents. The elastic fibers decrease in concentration and become more erratic, whereas collagen fibers increase in density and become more dense and fibrotic in the deep layer of the lamina propria.[100,101] These alterations are secondary to aging of the fibroblasts and reduction in their productivity.[102–104] The aforementioned anatomical and histologic alterations lead to changes in the viscoelastic properties of the vocal folds with subsequent subjective and objective changes often referred to as presbyphonia.

Given that lung cancer prevails in elderly persons and that age impacts voice negatively, it is fair to postulate that aging is a contributing factor to dysphonia in patients with lung cancer since it causes physiologic changes that make the voice more susceptible to dysfunction caused by additional challenges presented by lung cancer. There are no studies in the current literature comparing the prevalence of dysphonia in elderly versus nonelderly patients with lung cancer. Future studies looking at the prevalence of dysphonia in patients with lung cancer of different age groups are needed to elucidate the cause-effect relationship between aging and dysphonia in these patients.

Metastatic Laryngeal Tumors

Metastatic laryngeal tumors in patients with lung cancer are rare. These are usually either epidermoid carcinoma or adenocarcinoma.

Less common metastatic laryngeal neoplasms include anaplastic carcinoma, oat cell carcinoma, or nonspecific tumors. Based on a review by Ferlito et al in 1988, only 120 cases of secondary laryngeal neoplasms were reported in the literature. The most common primary sites were cutaneous melanoma followed by renal cell carcinoma accounting for 39.1% and 13.3% of the cases, respectively. In that review, only 9 cases of primary lung tumors metastasizing to the larynx were described.[105] Following the review by Ferlito et al, only a few additional cases of secondary laryngeal neoplasms have been reported in patients with lung cancer. Ogata et al in 1993 described a 59-year-old women diagnosed with lung adenocarcinoma who presented with change in voice quality a year after lung resection. The laryngeal exam showed a submucosal hemangioma-like lesion underneath the anterior commissure that resulted in a breathy voice. Tissue biopsy showed papillary adenocarcinoma similar to the pulmonary primary tumor.[106] In 1994, Bernaldez et al described a 56-year-old man diagnosed with lung cancer who presented with dysphonia and dysphagia 1 year following left pneumonectomy. Laryngeal examination showed a left aryepiglottic polypoidal mass that was associated with cervical lymphadenopathy. Histopathologic examination revealed poorly differentiated epidermoid carcinoma consistent with the primary lung malignancy.[107] In 1996, Nicolai et al reported a 69-year-old man who presented with dysphonia secondary to a transglottic mass, and right vocal fold paralysis. Computed tomography of the chest showed an apical lung mass. Histologic examination of both lesions was similar and consistent with poorly differentiated adenocarcinoma.[108]

In all the aforementioned cases, the clinical presentation of metastatic laryngeal neoplasms with lung cancer as a primary was misleading. The laryngeal symptoms can be similar to those reported by patients with primary laryngeal tumors, and laryngeal endoscopic findings are almost always nonspecific. The supraglottis is more commonly affected than the subglottis, and the laryngeal lesion is usually submucosal with intact overlying mucosa.[105] Immunohistochemical studies with special stains are needed to confirm the diagnosis. In cases of pulmonary adenocarcinoma, for instance, the expression of surfactant apoprotein is a "good marker of pulmonary adenocarcinoma" as reported by Ogata et al.[106] The mode of metastasis from the lungs to the larynx is either hematogenous or lymphogenous.[109] The hematogenous route follows the pulmonary circulation and aorta into the laryngeal circulation. A less common mode of spread is retrograde flow via the vertebral venous plexus, as described by Batson.[110] The management strategy of metastatic laryngeal neoplasia depends on the presence or absence of other metastatic lesions. Once the diagnosis of metastatic laryngeal tumor is made, similar to secondary laryngeal tumors with renal or cutaneous primary malignancies, an attempt to treat it should be considered.[111-114] The laryngeal lesion can be managed either surgically or by radiation, depending on the extent of the lesion and the overall medical condition of the patient.

Treatment-Related Dysphonia

Dysphonia in patients with lung cancer may be an adverse event caused by treatment including surgical resection with or without adjuvant therapy such as chemotherapy and/or radiotherapy. Physicians should understand treatment-related dysphonia in patients with lung cancer, particularly with emphasis on surgery and radiation-induced dysphonia.

Surgery-Related Dysphonia

Surgical procedures performed in patients with lung cancer can be diagnostic or therapeutic. The most common diagnostic procedure is mediastinoscopy with or without video assistance. It is frequently performed for tissue sampling and staging, following which surgical resection may be offered as treatment. Various surgical procedures such as pneumonectomy, lobectomy, sublobar resection, or segmentectomy are advocated depending on the stage of the disease, its local growth, and the patient's pulmonary function.[115,116] Both diagnostic and therapeutic surgical procedures performed in patients with lung cancer may lead to dysphonia.

Injury to the Vagus or Recurrent Laryngeal Nerves

Mediastinoscopy and dysphonia. Mediastinoscopy is an alternative or adjunct procedure to noninvasive radiologic studies for staging patients with lung cancer. Despite its high diagnostic yield, it confers certain risks and complications, most common of which is vocal fold paralysis. In a retrospective review of the complications of cervical mediastinoscopy performed on 1459 cases of lung cancer, Lemaire et al noted a morbidity of 1.07% and vocal fold dysfunction in 12 cases.[117] Other complications in that study included hemorrhage, tracheal injury, and pneumothorax. Similarly, Chabowski et al reported transient recurrent laryngeal nerve palsy in 5.5% of patients undergoing mediastinoscopy for staging of lung cancer and diagnosis of mediastinal tumors.[118] Zielinski described transcervical extended mediastinal lymphadenectomy as a variant of conventional mediastinoscopy and reported

temporary or permanent laryngeal palsy in 8 out of 256 patients.[119] Gonfioti et al reported recurrent laryngeal nerve palsy in 0.8% of patients undergoing video-assisted thoracic surgery without video-assisted mediastinoscopy. The authors elaborated on the added value of this technique in reducing the risk of vocal fold paralysis in patients undergoing video-assisted thoracic surgery.[120] Yandamuri et al in their study on the utility of transcervical extended mediastinal lymphadenectomy reported recurrent laryngeal nerve injury in 6.7% of the cases in a group of 157 patients with NSCLC.[121] Similarly, Kara et al reported close to 1% (5 cases) of unilateral vocal fold paralysis in 525 patients with NSCLC who underwent video-assisted mediastinal lymphadenectomy. The affected patients had aspiration and decreased cough effectiveness with an elevated VHI-10 score.[122]

The exact mechanism behind injury to the recurrent laryngeal nerve during mediastinoscopy remains uncertain. What is known, however, is that the proximity of the recurrent laryngeal nerves to the tracheoesophageal groove makes these nerves susceptible to injury during mediastinal lymph node dissection. Based on the study by Benouaich et al, there are two anatomical areas associated with substantial risk to the left recurrent laryngeal nerve during dissection. One is the area between the aorta and the anteroinferior part of the trachea, and the second is the lower part of the trachea on the left side.[123] Roberts and Wadsworth conducted a study on 15 patients who underwent mediastinoscopy while the recurrent laryngeal nerves were monitored using sensing electrodes positioned on laryngeal masks.[124] The authors attributed injury to the recurrent laryngeal nerves to traction in the anterior mediastinum during dissection. In view of the associated morbidity of mediastinoscopy and the need for general anesthesia to perform the procedure, less invasive diagnostic and staging modalities have recently gained popularity. These include thorascopic biopsy and fine needle aspiration under ultrasound guidance using the endobronchial or thoracic approach.[125] Studies are needed to investigate the impact of these procedures on phonation.

Lung resection and dysphonia. A significant cause of vocal fold paralysis in patients with lung cancer undergoing lung resection is injury to the recurrent laryngeal nerve (Figure 4–6). In a review by Mitas et al on complications following oncologic resection in patients with lung cancer, the authors reported high body mass index (BMI above 25), the presence of COPD, and left-sided lesions as the main risk factors.[126] In a study on postoperative complications following pneumonectomy ($n = 50$) and lobectomy ($n = 49$) in patients with lung cancer, Filaire et al reported vocal fold dysfunction in 31% of the cases. The group with vocal fold dysfunction had significantly higher rates of pulmonary complications, reintubation, and pneumonia.[127] The authors advocated early postoperative laryngeal examination in symptomatic patients in order to initiate early treatment. Similarly, in the study by Fourdain et al on the added value of laryngeal endoscopic evaluation postoperatively in patients undergoing surgery for lung cancer, the authors reported vocal fold paralysis in 5.2% of the cases. Right-sided surgeries accounted for 55.6% of the total cases, with lobectomy and pneumonectomy being the most commonly performed procedures (82.8% and 10.4% of the cases, respectively). Given the reduced quality of life associated with vocal fold paralysis, the authors also concurred with the need for routine postoperative laryngeal examination in order to reduce the associated morbidities of aspiration, pneumonia, and

reintubation.[128] In addition to the emphasis on vocal fold paralysis as a common complication of lung resection, it is important to note the large variation in the onset time of dysphonia following surgery. In cases in which the recurrent laryngeal nerve is transected during surgery, dysphonia is noted immediately postoperatively. However, in cases of traction or manipulation of the recurrent laryngeal nerves, the onset of vocal fold dysfunction may be delayed. In a survey by Mitas et al looking at the risk factors and complications of 189 cases who underwent pulmonary oncologic procedures, the authors reported the occurrence of dysphonia between the 8th and 30th days postoperatively.[126] Similar to the disparity in the onset of dysphonia following surgery, the recovery period is also variable. In a review of 69 patients with unilateral vocal fold paralysis secondary to mediastinal lymph node dissection and lung resection, the recovery period of vocal fold motion reached 9 months following surgery, with a rate that varied between 2.8% and 23.5% of the cases.[129] In another review on hoarseness following radical surgery for lung cancer, Sano et al

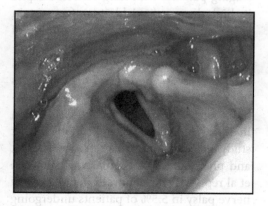

Figure 4–6. Surgery-induced dysphonia. A 70-year-old man diagnosed with lung adenocarcinoma, presented with history of dysphonia and aspiration following left upper lobectomy. On laryngeal exam he had left vocal fold paralysis in the paramedian position.

reported recovery of vocal fold movement in 61.1% and improvement in voice quality in 72.7% over the course of 28 months postoperatively.[130] The study was conducted on 365 patients, 22 of whom had dysphonia and 15 had left recurrent laryngeal nerve injury. In conclusion, both rate and duration of recovery vary markedly depending on the degree of neural injury.

Given the morbidity of unilateral vocal fold paralysis following lung resection, particularly aspiration, pneumonia, and the need for reintubation, early intervention is highly recommended. Mom et al advocated concomitant laryngeal framework surgery with thoracic operations that include vagus or recurrent laryngeal nerve transection.[131] In their review of 25 cases who underwent thyroplasty type I during thoracic surgery, no aspiration or swallowing dysfunction was reported postoperatively.[131] Similarly, in a review by Abraham et al on the outcome of laryngeal framework surgery following intrathoracic surgery, the authors reported improvement in dyspnea, dysphagia, and dysphonia in addition to improvement in pulmonary function.[132] Reconstruction of the injured or severed recurrent laryngeal nerve either by direct anastomosis or using the phrenic nerve also has been reported with rewarding results. In a review by Li et al of 4 cases of vagus or recurrent laryngeal nerve injury who underwent surgical neural repair, the authors reported almost complete recovery with good voice quality and approximation of the vocal folds 2 days postoperatively.[133] This report is not consistent with the timeline expected by laryngologists who perform this procedure, since neural regrowth takes many months. An alternative to these surgical procedures is injection laryngoplasty using different filling materials[134,135] (Figure 4–7). Office-based or bedside injection laryngoplasty for patients with unilateral vocal fold paralysis

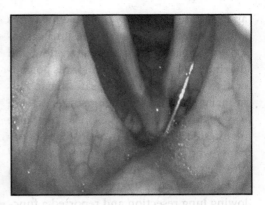

Figure 4–7. A 65-year-old man diagnosed with left vocal fold paralysis secondary to lung adenocarcinoma undergoing percutaneous injection laryngoplasty using hyaluronic acid.

following surgical resection of lung cancer provides immediate relief of aspiration, with improvement in swallowing and phonation. Moreover, early injection laryngoplasty has been reported to obviate the need for permanent medialization in some patients.[136] Further studies are needed to substantiate this conclusion.

Pulmonary Complications of Lung Resection. The respiratory function of patients with lung cancer undergoing surgery is always a major concern.[137] Despite lung resection being the best treatment option for a large percentage of patients with lung cancer, the morbidity of the surgery and its impact on breathing is substantial. In a systematic review on health-related quality of life of patients following resection of NSCLC, Poghosyan et al reported worsening in physical function with the main symptoms being cough, dyspnea, and fatigue.[138] These symptoms were mainly attributed to the surgically induced decline in respiratory function. Similarly, Bolliger et al investigated the impact of lung resection on pulmonary function in 68 lung cancer patients using pulmonary function tests and exercise capacity as outcome measures and reported a decrease in total lung capacity, vital capacity (VC), expiratory flow, and maximum oxygen uptake 3 months postoperatively. In parallel with the decline in pulmonary function following surgery, there was an adverse effect on exercise tolerance manifested by dyspnea in almost 50% of patients who underwent pneumonectomy.[139] Nezu et al examined pulmonary function and exercise capacity 3 and 6 months following lung resection and reported a functional loss of 11.2% to 36.1% for FEV1 and 11.6% to 40.1% for VC. Moreover, there was a decline in maximum oxygen consumption that reached 28.1% in the pneumonectomy group.[140] Keenan et al reported a decrease in FVC, FEV1, and maximum voluntary ventilation up to 81.1%, 66.7%, and 65.2%, respectively, in patients with NSCLC who underwent lobectomy.[141] In a longitudinal study on the long-term effect of lung resection on respiratory function and exercise capacity, Nagamatsu et al reported a significant decrease in maximum oxygen uptake per square meter of surface area 2 weeks after surgery in 18 patients who underwent lobectomy. Notable were the 95% recovery in exercise capacity and the total restoration of the anaerobic threshold after 1 year.[142] Based on a study by Takazakura on diaphragmatic motion following lung resection, the authors reported a decrease on the operated side and an increase on the unoperated side. These changes were not observed after resection of the right middle lobe. The study was conducted on 44 patients in whom diaphragmatic motion was measured during slow and deep breathing using a "spoiled gradient-recalled echo sequence."[143]

In the aforementioned reports, lobectomy and segmentectomy had less effect on pulmonary function than pneumonectomy. In the study by Bolliger, the decline in maximal oxygen uptake and breathing reserve improved at 6 months in the lobectomy group but remained in the pneumonectomy group which also had a decline in exercise capacity.[139] Similarly, in the study by Nezu et al, patients who underwent pneumonectomy remained with a decrease in breathing reserve on follow-up, unlike the lobectomy group (*n* = 62 cases) who had partial recovery in pulmonary function at 6 months postoperatively.[140] The negative effect of lung resection on pulmonary function is less pronounced in "good-risk" patients undergoing segmentectomy for small peripheral lesions. In a comparative study by Takizawa et al on 80 patients with lung cancer treated surgically, the authors reported a reduction in FVC and FEV1 by 5.1% and 6.7%, respectively, in the segmentectomy group with minimal pulmonary loss 12 months after surgery.[144] These findings were supported by Keenan et al in a retrospective study of 54 cases of early stage, NSCLC who underwent segmentectomy. At 1 year following surgery, there was a significant decrease only in the diffusing capacity.[141]

These studies lead us to conclude that lung resection undermines breathing. Given the importance of breathing in phonation, it is clear that the surgically induced decrease in respiratory function is likely to impair voice functional quality.

Chemotherapy-Related Dysphonia

Adjuvant chemotherapy regimens with or without targeted therapy in the form of monoclonal antibodies or tyrosine kinase inhibitors are used commonly in patients with advanced lung cancer, recurrent or metastatic disease. Several drug combinations are approved for treatment, the most common of which are carboplatin-Taxol and gemcitabine-cisplatin.[145] Monoclonal antibody therapy includes vascular endothelial growth factor inhibitor and epidermal growth factor receptor inhibitor therapy. Tyrosine kinase inhibitors are classified as epidermal growth factor receptor tyrosine kinase inhibitors and kinase inhibitors that affect cells with gene changes.

A review of the literature indicates scarcity of reports on the adverse effect of chemotherapy and its adjuvants on phonation. Thatcher et al investigated the effect of Necitumumab, a second-generation immunoglobulin antibody, in combination with gemcitabine and cisplatin in the treatment of NSCLC and reported hypomagnesemia and grade 3 rash in addition to disease-related adverse events. Dysphonia and dysphagia were not reported as side effects of the treatment.[146] Wu et al examined the response of advanced NSCLC to chemotherapy, cisplatin, and gemcitabine combined with afatinib and described rash, stomatitis or mucositis, and diarrhea in 14.6%, 5.4%, and 5.4%, respectively, with no report on change in voice quality in the treated group.[147] However, stomatitis and mucositis often are associated with laryngeal mucosal changes. So, voice effects are likely. Similarly, Langer et al in their investigation on the addition of pembrolizumab to carboplatin and pemetrexed in the treatment of nonsquamous NSCLC reported anemia, decreased neutrophil count, fatigue, and sepsis and thrombocytopenia as adverse events. There was also no report of hoarseness or change in voice quality in either group, those on chemotherapy alone versus those on the combined regimen.[148] In a multicenter, randomized, open-label study, West et al assessed the efficacy and toxicity of chemotherapy using carboplatin and nab-paclitaxel with or without atezolizumab in the treatment of metastatic nonsquamous NSCLC. This investigation that included 131 centers described anemia and neutropenia as adverse events with no mention of dysphonia.[149] However, Wittgen et al investigated the effect and toxicity of aerosolized sustained-release lipid inhalation targeting (SLIT) cisplatin given in a dose-escalating manner in the treatment of lung carcinoma and reported hoarseness in 47.1% in addition to dyspnea and fatigue in 64.7% as adverse events.[150] Goss et al evaluated the impact of cediranib, a vascular endothelial growth factor inhibitor, in combination with cisplatin 80 mg/m^2 and gemcitabine in the treatment of advanced NSCLC. The study, which was conducted on 15 patients, revealed hoarseness in addition to headache at high doses of cediranib.[151] Similarly, in an investigation on the effect of carboplatin and paclitaxel with and without an inhibitor of vascular endothelial growth factor tyrosine kinases (AZD2171), Laurie et al reported fatigue, headache, and hoarseness as side effects when the dosage of AZD2171 reached 45 mg/d.[152]

Despite the scarcity of reports on dysphonia as an adverse event of chemotherapy, chemotherapy is likely to affect phonation through its adverse systemic effects. In a study by Salhi et al that included 16 patients with respiratory cancer who received radical therapy, defined as surgery or chest radiotherapy with or without chemotherapy, the authors showed marked reduction in muscle force evidenced by a decrease in exercise tolerance, in addition to functional impairment that adversely impacted quality of life. Both functional disability and muscle force improved after rehabilitation therapy.[137] In a review of 82 patients who underwent induction chemoradiation followed by surgical resection and who were subjects for a pulmonary rehabilitation program, Tarumi et al[153] reported reduced pulmonary function, namely, forced vital capacity, forced expiratory volume in 1 second, and alteration in the lung diffusing capacity.

Radiotherapy-Related Dysphonia

Radiation-induced injury to the recurrent laryngeal nerve is thought to be mediated via ischemic changes and/or soft tissue fibrosis as a result of scarring of the nerves.[154,155] However, unlike peripheral nerves, the recurrent laryngeal nerves and cranial nerves in general are resilient to radiotherapy with only a few cases of adverse effects being reported in the literature. Most of these are patients with breast cancer, Hodgkin disease, and head and neck cancer.[154,156–160] In the review by Crawley and Sulica on radiation-induced vocal fold paralysis, the primary tumors were nasopharyngeal, thyroid, and breast. A common finding in those reports is the delayed and subtle occurrence of radiation-induced effect.[161]

In patients with lung cancer, vagus or recurrent laryngeal nerve radiation-induced neuropathy has been described primarily in the context of complications following stereotactic body radiotherapy (SBRT). This is a standard treatment option offered to patients with early lung cancer, namely NSCLC, who are inoperable.[162] Despite its favorable control rate, SBRT carries toxicity to many organs in the body such as the vascular system, to the lung parenchyma, and to the central airway, esophageus, and neural structures. Airway toxicity can lead to atelectasis, bronchial strictures, and stenosis as reported by Song et al and Speiser et al.[163,164] Similarly, esophageal toxicity may manifest as esophagitis that can result in strictures and perforations.[165,166] Shultz et al reported vagus and recurrent laryngeal nerve injury in 17% of patients with lung cancer who received SBRT treatment. Predisposing factors included preexisting autoimmune diseases and previous irradiation.[167]

References

1. World Health Organization. *Cancer Fact Sheet*. Updated September 12, 2018. Accessed July 1, 2019. https://www.who.int/news-room/fact-sheets/detail/cancer
2. Ferlay J, Soerjomataram I, Ervik M, et al. Cancer incidence and mortality worldwide: sources, methods and major patterns in GLOBCAN 2012. *Int J Cancer*. 2015;136(5):E359–386.
3. Torre LA, Siegel RL, Jemal A. Lung cancer statistics. *Adv Exp Med Biol*. 2016;893: 1–19.
4. Ryan BM. Lung cancer health disparities. *Carcinogenesis*. 2018;39(6):741–751.
5. Haiman CA, Stram DO, Wilkens LR, et al. Ethnic and racial differences in the smoking-related risk of lung cancer. *N Engl J Med*. 2006;354(4):333–342.
6. SEER Cancer Statistic Review (CSR)1975-2014. National Cancer Institute. Updated April 2, 2018. Accessed July 1, 2019. https://seer.cancer.gov/csr/1975_2014/
7. Siegel RL, Miller KD, Jemal A. Cancer statistics, 2019. *CA Cancer J Clin*. 2019;69 (1):7–34.
8. Midthun DE. Overview of the risk factors, pathology, and clinical manifestations of lung cancer. UpToDate. Updated March 5, 2019. Accessed May 20, 2019. https://www.uptodate.com/contents/overview-of-the-risk-factors-pathology-and-clinical-manifestations-of-lung-cancer
9. Lorenzo-González M, Torres-Durán M, Barbosa-Lorenzo R, Provencio-Pulla M, Barros-Dios JM, Ruano-Ravina A. Radon exposure: a major cause of lung cancer. *Expert Rev Respir Med*. 2019;13(9):839–850.
10. Kocher F, Hilbe W, Seeber A, et al. Longitudinal analysis of 2293 NSCLC patients: a comprehensive study from the TYROL registry. *Lung Cancer*. 2015;87(2):193–200.

11. Chute CG, Greenberg ER, Baron J, Korson R, Baker J, Yates J. Presenting conditions of 1539 population-based lung cancer patients by cell type and stage in New Hampshire and Vermont. *Cancer.* 1985;56 (8):2107–2111.

12. Patel AM, Peters SG. Clinical manifestations of lung cancer. *Mayo Clin Proc.* 993;68(3):273–277.

13. Sahn SA. Malignant pleural effusions. *Clin Chest Med.* 1985;6(1):113–125.

14. Chernow B, Sahn SA. Carcinomatous involvement of the pleura: an analysis of 96 patients. *Am J Med.* 1977;63(5):695–702.

15. Strauss BL, Matthews MJ, Cohen MH, Simon R, Tejada F. Cardiac metastases in lung cancer. *Chest.* 1977;71(5):607–611.

16. Adenle AD, Edwards JE. Clinical and pathologic features of metastatic neoplasms of the pericardium. *Chest.* 1982;81(2):166–169.

17. Hinton J, Cerra-Franco A, Shiue K, et al. Superior vena cava syndrome in a patient with locally advanced lung cancer with good response to definitive chemoradiation: a case report. *J Med Case Rep.* 2018;12(1):301–306.

18. Stenbygaard LE, Soreson JB, Olsen JE. Metastatic pattern at autopsy in nonresectable adenocarcinoma of the lung—a study from a cohort of 259 consecutive patients treated with chemotherapy. *Acta Oncol.* 1997;36(3):301–306.

19. Pagani JJ. Normal adrenal glands in small cell lung carcinoma: CT-guided biopsy. *AJR AM J Roentgenol.* 1983;140(5):949–951.

20. Toloza EM, Harpole L, McCrory DC. Noninvasive staging of non-small cell lung cancer: a review of the current evidence. *Chest.* 2003;123(1 Suppl):137S–146S.

21. Schumacher T, Brink I, Mix M, et al. FDG-PET imaging for the staging and follow-up of small cell lung cancer. *Eur J Nucl Med.* 2001;28(4):483–488.

22. Le Roux BT. The presentation of bronchial carcinoma. *Scott Med J.* 1968;13(2):31–37.

23. Hyde L, Hyde C. Clinical manifestations of lung cancer. *Chest.* 1974;65(3):299–306.

24. Maguire PD, Sibley GS, Zhou SM, et al. Clinical and dosimetric predictors of radiation-induced oesophageal toxicity. *Int J Radiat Oncol Biol Phys.* 1999;45(1): 97–103.

25. Stankey RM, Roshe J, Sogocio RM. Carcinoma of the lung and dysphagia. *Dis Chest.* 1969;55(1):13–17.

26. Camidge DR. The causes of dysphagia in carcinoma of the lung. *J R Soc Med.* 2001;94(11):567–572.

27. Roe JW, Leslie P, Drinnan MJ. Oropharyngeal dysphagia: the experience of patients with non-head and neck cancers receiving specialist palliative care. *Palliat Med.* 2007;21(7):567–574.

28. Counsell CE, Collie DA, Grant R. Incidence of intracranial tumours in the Lothian region of Scotland, 1989–90. *J Neurol Neurosurg Psychiatry.* 1996;61(2):143–150.

29. Joffe N. Symptomatic gastrointestinal metastases secondary to bronchogenic carcinoma. *Clin Radiol.* 1978;29(2):217–225.

30. Antler AS, Ough Y, Pitchumoni CS, Davidian M, Thelmo W. Gastrointestinal metastases from malignant tumors of the lung. *Cancer.* 1982;49(1):170–172.

31. Andersen HA, Prakash UBS. Diagnosis of symptomatic lung cancer. *Semin Respir Med.* 1982;3(3):165–175.

32. Grippi MA. Clinical aspects of lung cancer. *Semin Roentgenol.* 1990;25(1):12–24.

33. Knudsen R, Gaunsbaek MQ, Schultz JH, Nilsson AC, Madsen JS, Asgari N. Vocal cord paralysis as primary and secondary results of malignancy. A prospective descriptive study. *Laryngoscope Investig Otolaryngol.* 2019;4(2):241–245.

34. National Institute for Health and Care Excellence. Lung Cancer: diagnosis management. March 2019. Accessed June 1, 2019. https://www.nice.org.uk/guidance/ng122

35. Lee CF, Carding PN, Fletcher M. The nature and severity of voice disorders in lung cancer patients. *Logoped Phoniatr Vocol.* 2008;33(2):93–103.

36. Mancini I, Body JJ. Assessment of dyspnea in advanced cancer. *Support Care Cancer.* 1999;7(4):229–232.

37. Buccheri G, Ferrigno D, Tamburini M. Karnofsky and ECOG performance status

scoring in lung cancer: a prospective, longitudinal study of 536 patients from a single institution. *Eur J Cancer.* 1995;32A (7):1135–1141.

38. Kaasa S, Bjordal K, Aaronson N, et al. The EORTC core quality of life questionnaire (QLQ-C30): validity and reliability when analysed with patients treated with palliative radiotherapy. *Eur J Cancer.* 1995;31A(13–14):2260–2263.

39. Bernhard J, Ganz PA. Psychological issues in lung cancer patients. *Chest.* 1991; 99(1):216–223.

40. Dankbaar JW, Pameijer FA. Vocal cord paralysis: anatomy, imaging and pathology. *Insights Imaging.* 2014;5(6):743–751.

41. Glazer HS, Aronberg DJ, Lee JK, Sagel SS. Extralaryngeal causes of vocal cord paralysis: CT evaluation. *AJR Am J Roentgenol.* 1983;141(3):527–531.

42. Baumann MH, Heffner JE. Bilateral vocal cord paralysis with respiratory failure: a presenting manifestation of bronchogenic carcinoma. *Arch Intern Med.* 1989;149(6):1453–1454.

43. Gauri LA, Agrawal NK, Banerjee S, Misra SN. Neurological manifestations associated with bronchogenic carcinoma. *J Indian Med Assoc.* 1990;88(8):224–226.

44. Terris DJ, Arnstein DP, Nguyen HH. Contemporary evaluation of unilateral vocal cord paralysis. *Otolaryngol Head Neck Surg.* 1992;107(1):84–90.

45. Benninger MS, Gillen JB, Altman JS. Changing etiology of vocal fold immobility. *Laryngoscope.* 1998;108(9):1346–1350.

46. Havas T, Lowinger D, Priestley J. Unilateral vocal fold paralysis: causes, options and outcomes. *Aust N Z J Surg.* 1999;69(7):509–513.

47. Loughran S, Alves C, MacGregor FB. Current aetiology of unilateral vocal fold paralysis in a teaching hospital in the West of Scotland. *J Laryngol Otol.* 2002; 116(11):907–910.

48. Kraus DH, Ali MK, Ginsberg RJ, et al. Vocal cord medialization for unilateral paralysis associated with intrathoracic malignancies. *J Thorac Cardiovasc Surg.* 1996; 111(2):334–341.

49. Iseli TA, Brown CL, Sizeland AM, Berkowitz RG. Palliative surgery for neoplastic unilateral vocal cord paralysis. *ANZ J Surg.* 2001;71(11):672–674.

50. Koç AO, Turkoglu SB, Erol O, Erbek S. Vocal cord paralysis: What matters between idiopathic and non-idiopathic cases? *Kulak Burun Bogaz Ihtis Derg.* 2016;26(4):228–233.

51. Bilici S, Yildiz M, Yigit O, Misir E. Imaging modalities in the etiologic evaluation of unilateral vocal fold paralysis. *J Voice.* 2019;33(5):813.e1–813.e5.

52. Smith CB, Nelson JE, Berman AR, et al. Lung cancer physicians' referral practices for palliative care consultation. *Ann Oncol.* 2012;23(2):382–387.

53. Cesario A, Ferri L, Galetta D, et al. Preoperative pulmonary rehabilitation and surgery for lung cancer. *Lung Cancer.* 2007; 57(1):118–119.

54. Santoro A, Tomino C, Prinzi G, et al. Tobacco smoking: Risk to develop addiction, chronic obstructive pulmonary disease, and lung cancer. *Recent Pat Anticancer Drug Discov.* 2019;14(1):39–52.

55. Global Strategy for the Diagnosis, Management and Prevention of COPD. Global Initiative for Chronic Obstructive Lung Disease (GOLD). 2018 Report. Accessed June 5, 2019. https://goldcopd.org/wp-content/uploads/2017/11/GOLD-2018-v6.0-FINAL-revised-20-Nov_WMS.pdf

56. Loganathan RS, Stover DE, Shi W, Venkatraman E. Prevalence of COPD in women compared to men around the time of diagnosis of primary lung cancer. *Chest.* 2006; 129(5):1305–1312.

57. Read WL, Tierney RM, Page NC, et al. Differential prognostic impact of comorbidity. *J Clin Oncol.* 2004;22(15):3099–3103.

58. Lin H, Lu Y, Lin L, Meng K, Fan J. Does chronic obstructive pulmonary disease relate to poor prognosis in patients with lung cancer? A meta-analysis. *Medicine* (Baltimore). 2019;98(11):e14837.

59. Rennard SI, Drummond MB. Early chronic obstructive pulmonary disease: definition, assessment, and prevention. *Lancet.* 2015; 385(9979):1778–1788.

60. Houghton AM. Common mechanisms linking chronic obstructive pulmonary disease and lung cancer. *Ann Am Thorac Soc.* 2018;15(4):S273–S277. doi:10.1513/AnnalsATS.201808-537MG

61. Young RP, Duan F, Chiles C, et al. Airflow limitation and histology shift in the National Lung Screening Trial: the NLST-ACRIN cohort substudy. *Am J Respir Crit Care Med.* 2015;192(9):1060–1067.

62. Bosken CH, Wei Q, Amos CI, Spitz MR. An analysis of DNA repair as a determinant of survival in patients with non-small-cell lung cancer. *J Natl Cancer Inst.* 2002;94(14):1091–1099.

63. Anderson GP, Bozinovski S. Acquired somatic mutations in the molecular pathogenesis of COPD. *Trends Pharmacol Sci.* 2003;24(2):71–76.

64. Demedts IK, Demoor T, Bracke KR, Joos GF, Brusselle GG. Role of apoptosis in the pathogenesis of COPD and pulmonary emphysema. *Respir Res.* 2006;7:53.

65. Liloglou T, Bediaga NG, Brown BR, Field JK, Davies MP. Epigenetic biomarkers in lung cancer. *Cancer Lett.* 2014;342(2):200–212.

66. Qiu W, Baccarelli A, Carey VJ, et al. Variable DNA methylation is associated with chronic obstructive pulmonary disease and lung function. *Am J Respir Crit Care Med.* 2012;185(4):373–381.

67. Zhu HX, Shi L, Zhang Y, et al. Myocyte enhancer factor 2D provides a cross-talk between chronic inflammation and lung cancer. *J Transl Med.* 2017;15(1):65–75.

68. Welham NV, Maclagan MA. Vocal fatigue: current knowledge and future directions. *J Voice.* 2003;17(1):21–30.

69. Sataloff RT. Cohn JR, Hawshkaw M. Respiratory dysfunction. In: Sataloff RT. *Professional Voice: The Science and Art of Clinical Care.* 4th ed. San Diego, CA: Plural Publishing; 2017:751–764.

70. Titze IR. Vocal fatigue: some biomechanical considerations. In: Lawrence VL, ed. *Transcripts of the Twelfth Symposium: Care of the Professional Voice. Part One: Scientific Papers.* New York, NY: The Voice Foundation; 1984:97–104.

71. Ryu CH, Han S, Lee MS, et al. Voice changes in elderly adults: prevalence and the effect of social, behavioral, and health status on voice quality. *J Am Geriatr Soc.* 2015;63(8):1608–1614.

72. Kozak E, Maniecka-Aleksandrowicz B, Frank-Piskorska A, Witman D. Evaluation of the effect of chronic steroid inhalation therapy on the state of the upper airway in patients with chronic obstructive pulmonary disease. *Pneumonol Alergol Pol.* 1991;59(9–10):33–37.

73. Hamdan AL. Laryngeal manifestations of respiratory disorders. In Hamdan AL, Sataloff RT, Hawkshaw M. *Laryngeal Manifestations of Systemic Diseases.* San Diego, CA: Plural Publishing; 2018:159–182.

74. Bobbio A, Chetta A, Ampollini L, et al. Preoperative pulmonary rehabilitation in patients undergoing lung resection for non-small cell lung cancer. *Eur J Cardiothorac Surg.* 2008;33(1):95–98.

75. Quist M, Rørth M, Langer S, et al. Safety and feasibility of a combined exercise intervention for inoperable lung cancer patients undergoing chemotherapy: a pilot study. *Lung Cancer.* 2012;75(2):203–208.

76. Ozalevli S, Ilgin D, Kul Karaali H, Bulac S, Akkoclu A. The effect of in-patient chest physiotherapy in lung cancer patients. *Support Care Cancer.* 2010;18(3):351–358.

77. Cheville AL, Kollasch J, Vandenberg J, et al. A home-based exercise program to improve function, fatigue, and sleep quality in patients with Stage IV lung and colorectal cancer: a randomized controlled trial. *J Pain Symptom Manage.* 2013;45(5):811–821.

78. Hamdan AL, Sataloff RT. Sleep, body fatigue, and voice. In Hamdan AL, Sataloff RT, Hawkshaw M. *Laryngeal Manifestations of Systemic Diseases.* San Diego, CA: Plural Publishing; 2018:83–86.

79. Hill KM, Amir Z, Muers MF, Connolly CK, Round CE. Do newly diagnosed lung cancer patients feel their concerns are being met? *Eur J Cancer Care.* 2003;12(1):35–45.

80. Tishelman C, Petersson LM, Degner LF, Sprangers MA. Symptom prevalence,

intensity, and distress in patients with inoperable lung cancer in relation to time of death. *J Clin Oncol.* 2007;25(34):5381–5389.

81. Zabora J, Brintzenhofe-Szoc K, Curbow B, Hooker C, Piantadosi S. The prevalence of psychological distress by cancer site. *Psychooncology.* 2001;10(1):19–28.

82. Hughes JE. Depressive illness and lung cancer. II. Follow-up of inoperable patients. *Eur J Surg Oncol.* 1985;11(1):21–24.

83. McGeough A, Edwards J, Chamberlain RM, Nogeire C. Social isolation in lung cancer patients. *Soc Work Health Care.* 1980;5(4): 433–436.

84. Yates P, Schofield P, Zhao I, Currow D. Supportive and palliative care for lung cancer patients. *J Thorac Dis.* 2013;5(Suppl 5): S623–S628.

85. Cosci F, Fava GA, Sonino N. Mood and anxiety disorders as early manifestations of medical illness: a systematic review. *Psychother Psychosom.* 2015;84(1):22–29.

86. World Health Organization. Depression: let's talk says WHO, as depression tops list of causes of ill health. Updated March 30, 2017. Accessed June 1, 2019. https://www.who.int/en/news-room/detail/30-03-2017-depression-let-s-talk-says-who-as-depression-tops-list-of-causes-of-ill-health

87. Hughes JE. Depressive illness and lung cancer. I. Depression before diagnosis. *Eur J Surg Oncol.* 1985;11(1):15–20.

88. Montazeri A, Milroy R, Hole D, McEwen J, Gillis CR. Anxiety and depression in patients with lung cancer before and after diagnosis: findings from a population in Glasgow, Scotland. *J Epidemiol Community Health.* 1998;52(3):203–204.

89. Brintzenhofe-Szoc KM, Levin TT, Li Y, Kissane DW, Zabora JR. Mixed anxiety/depression symptoms in a large cancer cohort: prevalence by cancer type. *Psychosomatics.* 2009;50(4):383–391.

90. Arrieta Ó, Angulo LP, Núñez-Valencia C, et al. Association of depression and anxiety on quality of life, treatment adherence, and prognosis in patients with advanced non-small cell lung cancer. *Ann Surg Oncol.* 2013;20(6):1941–1948.

91. Mendoza E, Carballo G. Acoustic analysis of induced vocal stress by means of cognitive workload tasks. *J Voice.* 1998;12(3):263–273.

92. Van Lierde K, Van Heule S, De Ley S, Mertens E, Claeys S. Effect of psychological stress on female vocal quality. *Folia Phoniatr Logop.* 2009;61(2):105–111.

93. Giddens CL, Barron KW, Byrd-Craven J, Clark KF, Winter AS. Vocal indices of stress: A review. *J Voice.* 2013;27(3):390.e21–e29.

94. Gomes VE, Batista DDC, Lopes LW, Aquino R, Almeida AA. Symptoms and vocal risk factors in individuals with high and low anxiety. *Folia Phoniatr Logop.* 2019;71(1): 7–15.

95. Schulkes KJ, Hamaker ME, van den Bos F, van Elden LJ. Relevance of a geriatric assessment for elderly patients with lung cancer—a systematic review. *Clin Lung Cancer.* 2016;17(5):341–349.

96. Owonikoko TK, Ragin CC, Belani CP, et al. Lung cancer in elderly patients: an analysis of the surveillance, epidemiology, and end results database. *J Clinical Oncol.* 2007;25(35):5570–5577.

97. Sataloff RT. The effects of age on the voice. In: Sataloff RT. *Professional Voice: The Science and Art of Clinical Care.* 4th ed. San Diego, CA: Plural Publishing; 2017: 585–604.

98. Xue SA, Hao GJ. Changes in the human vocal tract due to aging and the acoustic correlates of speech production: a pilot study. *J Speech Lang Hear Res.* 2003;46(3): 689–701.

99. Linville SE, Rens J. Vocal tract resonance analysis of aging voice using long-term average spectra. *J Voice.* 2001;15(3):323–330.

100. Gonçalves TM, dos Santos DC, Pessin AB, Martins RH. Scanning electron microscopy of the presbylarynx. *Otolaryngol Head Neck Surg.* 2016;154(6):1073–1078.

101. Hirano M, Kurita S, Sakaguchi S. Ageing of the vibratory tissue of human vocal folds. *Acta Otolaryngol.* 1989;107(5–6):428–433.

102. Sato K, Hirano M. Age-related changes of the macula flava of the human vocal fold.

Ann Otol Rhinol Laryngol. 1995;104(11): 839–844.

103. Ximenes Filho JA, Tsuji DH, do Nascimento PH, Sennes LU. Histologic changes in human vocal folds correlated with aging: a histomorphometric study. *Ann Otol Rhinol Laryngol.* 2003;112(10):894–898.

104. Chan RW, Titze IR. Viscoelastic shear properties of human vocal fold mucosa: measurement methodology and empirical results. *J Acoust Soc Am.* 1999;106(4 Pt 1): 2008–2021.

105. Ferlito A, Caruso G, Recher G. Secondary laryngeal tumors. Report of seven cases with review of the literature. *Arch Otolaryngol Head Neck Surg.* 1988;114(6):635–639.

106. Ogata H, Ebihara S, Mukai K, et al. Laryngeal metastasis from a pulmonary papillary adenocarcinoma: a case report. *Jpn J Clin Oncol.* 1993;23(3):199–203.

107. Bernáldez R, Toledano A, Alvarez J, Gavilán J. Pulmonary carcinoma metastatic to the larynx. *J Laryngol Otol.* 1994;108(10): 898–901.

108. Nicolai P, Puxeddu R, Cappiello J, et al. Metastatic neoplasms to the larynx: report of three cases. *Laryngoscope.* 1996;106(7):851–855.

109. Freeland AP, van Nostrand AW, Jahn AF. Metastases to the larynx. *J Otolaryngol.* 1979;8(5):448–456.

110. Batson OV. The Function of the vertebral veins and their role in the spread of metastases. *Ann Surg.* 1940;112(1):138–149.

111. Chamberlain D. Malignant melanoma metastatic to the larynx. *Arch Otolaryngol.* 1966;83(3):231–232.

112. Shaheen OH. A case of metastatic amelanotic melanoma of the larynx. *J Laryngol Otol.* 1960;74:182–187.

113. Maug R, Burke RC, Hwang WS. Metastatic renal carcinoma to larynx. *J Otolaryngol.* 1987;16:16–18.

114. Demir L, Erten C, Somali I, et al. Metastases of renal cell carcinoma to the larynx and thyroid: two case reports on metastasis developing years after nephrectomy. *Can Urol Assoc J.* 2012;6:E209–E212.

115. Abbas AE. Surgical management of lung cancer: history, evolution, and modern advances. Curr Oncol Rep. 2018;20(12):98–104.

116. Roman M, Labbouz S, Valtzoglou V, et al. Lobectomy vs. segmentectomy. A propensity score matched comparison of outcomes. *Eur J Surg Oncol.* 2019;45(5):845–850.

117. Lemaire A, Nikolic I, Petersen T, et al. Nine-year single center experience with cervical mediastinoscopy: complications and false negative rate. *Ann Thorac Surg.* 2006;82(4):1185–1190.

118. Chabowski M, Szymanska-Chabowska A, Skotarczak J, Janczak D, Pawlowski L, Janczak D. The role of mediastinoscopy in the diagnosis of thoracic disease: one-year single center experience. *Adv Exp Med Biol.* 2015;852:1–4.

119. Zieliński M. Transcervical extended mediastinal lymphadenectomy: results of staging in two hundred fifty-six patients with non-small cell lung cancer. *J Thorac Oncol.* 2007;2(4):370–372.

120. Gonfiotti A, Bongiolatti S, Viggiano D, et al. Does videomediastinoscopy with frozen sections improve mediastinal staging during video-assisted thoracic surgery pulmonary resections? *J Thorac Dis.* 2016;8(12):3496–3504.

121. Yandamuri S, Battoo A, Dy G, et al. Transcervical extended mediastinal lymphadenectomy: experience from a North American cancer center. *Ann Thorac Surg.* 2017;104(5):1644–1649.

122. Kara HV, Karaaltin AB, Ersen E, Alaskarov E, Kilic B, Turna A. Minimally invasive injection laryngoplasty in the management of unilateral vocal cord paralysis after video-assisted mediastinal lymph adenectomy. *Wideochir Inn Tech Maloinwazyjne.* 2018;13(3):388–393.

123. Benouaich V, Marcheix B, Carfagna L, Brouchet L, Guitard J. Anatomical bases of left recurrent nerve lesions during mediastinoscopy. *Surg Radiol Anat.* 2009;31(4):295–299.

124. Roberts JR, Wadsworth J. Recurrent laryngeal nerve monitoring during mediastinoscopy: predictors of injury. *Ann Thorac Surg.* 2007;83(2):388–392.

125. Hammoud ZT, Anderson RC, Meyers BF, et al. The current role of mediastinoscopy in the evaluation of thoracic disease. *J Thorac Cardiovasc Surg.* 1999;118(5):894–899.

126. Mitas L, Horvath T, Sobotka M, et al. Complications in patients undergoing pulmonary oncological surgery. *Rozhl Chir.* 2010;89(2):113–117.

127. Filaire M, Mom T, Laurent S, et al. Vocal cord dysfunction after left lung resection for cancer. *Eur J Cardiothorac Surg.* 2001;20(4):705–711.

128. Fourdain A, De Dominicis F, Iquille J, et al. Usefulness of a routine endoscopic assessment of laryngeal lesions after lung cancer surgery. *Respirology.* 2018;23(1):107–110.

129. Laccourreye O, Malinvaud D, Delas B, et al. Early unilateral laryngeal paralysis after pulmonary resection with mediastinal dissection for cancer. *Ann Thorac Surg.* 2010;90(4):1075–1078.

130. Sano Y, Shigematsu H, Okazaki M, et al. Hoarseness after radical surgery with systematic lymph node dissection for primary lung cancer. *Eur J Cardiothorac Surg.* 2019; 55(2):280–285.

131. Mom T, Filaire M, Advenier D, et al. Concomitant type I thyroplasty and thoracic operations for lung cancer: preventing respiratory complications associated with vagus or recurrent laryngeal nerve injury. *J Thorac Cardiovasc Surg.* 2001;121(4): 642–648.

132. Abraham MT, Bains MS, Downey RJ, Korst RJ, Kraus DH. Type I thyroplasty for acute unilateral vocal fold paralysis following intrathoracic surgery. *Ann Otol Rhinol Laryngol.* 2002;111(8):667–671.

133. Li H, Hu Y, Huang J, Yang Y, Xing K, Luo Q. Attempt of peripheral nerve reconstruction during lung cancer surgery. *Thorac Cancer.* 2018;9(5):580–583.

134. Kwon TK, Buckmire R. Injection laryngoplasty for management of unilateral vocal fold paralysis. *Curr Opin Otolaryngol Head Neck Surg.* 2004;12(6):538–542.

135. Lisi C, Hawkshaw MJ, Sataloff RT. Viscosity of materials for laryngeal injection: a review of current knowledge and clinical implications. *J Voice.* 2013;27(1):119–123.

136. Yung KC, Likhterov I, Courey MS. Effect of temporary vocal fold injection medialization on the rate of permanent medialization laryngoplasty in unilateral vocal fold paralysis patients. *Laryngoscope.* 2011; 121(10):2191–2194.

137. Salhi B, Demedts I, Simpelaere A, et al. Endurance and resistance training in radically treated respiratory cancer patients: A pilot study. *Rehabil Res Pract.* 2010;2010:481546. doi:10.1155/2010/481546

138. Poghosyan H, Sheldon LK, Leveille SG, Cooley ME. Health-related quality of life after surgical treatment in patients with non-small cell lung cancer: a systematic review. *Lung Cancer.* 2013;81(1):11–26.

139. Bolliger CT, Jordan P, Soler M, et al. Pulmonary function and exercise capacity after lung resection. *Eur Respir J.* 1996;9(3):415–421.

140. Nezu K, Kushibe K, Tojo T, Takahama M, Kitamura S. Recovery and limitation of exercise capacity after lung resection for lung cancer. *Chest.* 1998;113(6):1511–1516.

141. Keenan RJ, Landreneau RJ, Maley Jr RH, et al. Segmental resection spares pulmonary function in patients with stage I lung cancer. *Ann Thorac Surg.* 2004;78(1):228–233.

142. Nagamatsu Y, Maeshiro K, Kimura NY, et al. Long-term recovery of exercise capacity and pulmonary function after lobectomy. *J Thoracic Cardiovasc Surg.* 2007;134(5): 1273–1278.

143. Takazakura R, Takahashi M, Nitta N, et al. Assessment of diaphragmatic motion after lung resection using magnetic resonance imaging. *Radiat Med.* 2007;25(4):155–163.

144. Takizawa T, Haga M, Yagi N, et al. Pulmonary function after segmentectomy for small peripheral carcinoma of the lung. *J Thorac Cardiovasc Surg.* 1999;118(3): 536–541.

145. National Cancer Institute. Drugs approved for lung cancer. Updated June 18, 2019. Accessed July 1, 2019. https://www.cancer.gov/about-cancer/treatment/drugs/lung

146. Thatcher N, Hirsch FR, Luft AV, et al. Necitumumab plus gemcitabine and cisplatin versus gemcitabine and cisplatin alone as first-line therapy in patients with stage IV squamous non-small-cell lung cancer (SQUIRE): an open-label, randomised, controlled phase 3 trial. *Lancet Oncol.* 2015;16(7):763–774.

147. Wu YL, Zhou C, Hu CP, et al. Afatinib versus cisplatin plus gemcitabine for first-line treatment of Asian patients with advanced non-small-cell lung cancer harbouring EGFR mutations (LUX-Lung 6): an open-label, randomised phase 3 trial. *Lancet Oncol.* 2014;15(2):213–222.

148. Langer CJ, Gadgeel SM, Borghaei H, et al. Carboplatin and pemetrexed with or without pembrolizumab for advanced, non-squamous non-small-cell lung cancer: a randomised, phase 2 cohort of the open-label KEYNOTE-021 study. *Lancet Oncol.* 2016;17(11):1497–1508.

149. West H, McCleod M, Hussein M, et al. Atezolizumab in combination with carboplatin plus nab-paclitaxel chemotherapy compared with chemotherapy alone as first-line treatment for metastatic non-squamous non-small-cell lung cancer (IMpower130): a multicentre, randomised, open-label, phase 3 trial. *Lancet Oncol.* 2019;20(7):924–937.

150. Wittgen BP, Kunst PW, van der Born K, et al. Phase I study of aerosolized SLIT cisplatin in the treatment of patients with carcinoma of the lung. *Clin Cancer Res.* 2007;13(8):2414–2421.

151. Goss G, Shepherd FA, Laurie S, et al. A phase I and pharmacokinetic study of daily oral cediranib, an inhibitor of vascular endothelial growth factor tyrosine kinases, in combination with cisplatin and gemcitabine in patients with advanced non-small cell lung cancer: a study of the National Cancer Institute of Canada Clinical Trials Group. *Eur J Cancer.* 2009;45(5):782–788.

152. Laurie SA, Gauthier I, Arnold A, et al. Phase I and pharmacokinetic study of daily oral AZD2171, an inhibitor of vascular endothelial growth factor tyrosine kinases, in combination with carboplatin and paclitaxel in patients with advanced non-small-cell lung cancer: The National Cancer Institute of Canada clinical trials group. *J Clin Oncol.* 2008;26(11):1871–1878.

153. Tarumi S, Yokomise H, Gotoh M, et al. Pulmonary rehabilitation during induction chemoradiotherapy for lung cancer improves pulmonary function. *J Thorac Cardiovasc Surg.* 2015;149:569–573.

154. Westbrook KC, Ballantyne AJ, Eckler NE, Brown GR. Breast cancer and vocal cord paralysis. *South Med J.* 1974;67(7):805–807.

155. Delanian S, Lefaix JL. The radiation-induced fibroatrophic process: therapeutic perspective via the antioxidant pathway. *Radiother Oncol.* 2004;73(2):119–131.

156. Rosanowski F, Tigges M, Eysholdt U. Esophagomediastinal fistula and recurrent laryngeal nerve paralysis after radiotherapy of Hodgkin's disease. *Laryngorhinootologie.* 1995;74(8):516–517.

157. Chaudhry MR, Akhtar S. Bilateral vocal cord paralysis following radiation therapy for nasopharyngeal carcinoma. *ORL J Otorhinolaryngol Relat Spec.* 1995;57(1):48–49.

158. Cheng VST, Schultz MD. Unilateral hypoglossal nerve atrophy as a late complication of radiation therapy of head and neck carcinoma: a report of four cases and a review of the literature on peripheral and cranial nerve damages after radiation therapy. *Cancer.* 1975;35(6):1537–1544.

159. Stern Y, Marshak G, Shpitzer T, Segal K, Feinmesser R. Vocal cord palsy: possible late complication of radiotherapy for head and neck cancer. *Ann Otol Rhino Laryngol.* 1995;104(4 Pt 1):294–296.

160. Takimoto T, Saito Y, Suzuki M, Nishimura T. Radiation-induced cranial nerve palsy: hypoglossal nerve and vocal cord palsies. *J Laryngol Otol.* 1991;105(1):44–45.

161. Crawley BK, Sulica L. Vocal fold paralysis as a delayed consequence of neck and chest radiotherapy. *Otolaryngol Head Neck Surg.* 2015;153(2):239–243.

162. Kang K, Okoye C, Patel R, et al. Complications from stereotactic body radiotherapy

for lung cancer. *Cancers*. 2015;7(2):981–1004.

163. Song SY, Choi W, Shin SS et al. Fractionated stereotactic body radiation therapy for medically inoperable stage I lung cancer adjacent to central large bronchus. *Lung Cancer*. 2009;66(1):89–93.

164. Speiser BL, Spratling L. Radiation bronchitis and stenosis secondary to high dose rate endobronchial irradiation. *Int J Radiat Oncol Biol Phys*. 1993;25(4):589–597.

165. Timmerman R. Papiez L, McGarry R et al. Extracranial stereotactic radioablation: results of a phase I study in medically inoperable stage I non-small cell lung cancer. *Chest*. 2003;124(5):1946–1955.

166. Wu AJ, Williams E, Modh A et al. Dosimetric predictors of esophageal toxicity after stereotactic body radiotherapy for central lung tumors. *Radiother Oncol*. 2014;112(2):267–271.

167. Shultz DB, Trakul N, Maxim PG, Diehn M, Loo BW Jr. Vagal and recurrent laryngeal neuropathy following stereotactic ablative radiation therapy in the chest. *Pract Radiat Oncol*. 2014;4(4):272–278.

5

Breast Cancer and Voice

Abdul-Latif Hamdan, Robert Thayer Sataloff, Mary J. Hawkshaw, and Dahlia M. Sataloff

Epidemiology and Clinical Presentation

Breast cancer is the most common malignancy encountered in women and the second most common cancer globally.[1] In 2018, it accounted for more than 2 million new cases.[2] Despite the decrease in mortality rate over the last years, it is still the second cause of cancer-related death in women in their fifth and sixth decades.[3,4] Based on the Global Cancer Statistics, it accounts for one-fourth of cancer diagnoses in women and 14% of cancer deaths annually.[5] The prevalence of breast cancer varies with ethnicity and race. In the United States, African American women are less affected than Caucasian women. However, the morbidity and mortality have been reported as higher in the former group.[6]

The incidence of breast cancer is still on the rise despite the increase in health awareness. Based on the Group for Epidemiology and Cancer Registry in Latin Language Countries (GRELL), the increase in the mean rate between 1999 and 2008 was estimated as 1.19% yearly.[7] Important factors that may have a potential role in the etiology and prevention of breast cancer are lifestyle and dietary habits. A meta-analysis

conducted by Fowler and Akinyemiju showed a positive and strong correlation between dietary inflammatory index (DII) and cancer. Subjects with high DII have 25% higher risk of cancer development and 67% increased risk of dying from cancer.[8] With the alarming epidemic of obesity worldwide, there is also circumstantial evidence to suggest that obesity and physical activity are linked strongly to breast cancer.[9,10] As reported by the American Cancer Society, increased adiposity after menopause, more so at the waist area, increases the risk of breast cancer.[10] Given that adipose tissue is a major source of estrogen, the strong intertwining between mammary gland development and exposure to estrogen supports the possible etiologic role of obesity in breast cancer. Based on the study by Jerry et al, hypersensitivity to estrogen exposure, be it endogenous or exogenous, is also a predisposing factor.[11] The prolonged intake of oral contraceptives at a young age and the use of hormone therapy for more than 5 years have been reported as risk factors. The combination of progesterone with estrogen is thought to increase the risk of breast cancer in comparison to intake of estrogen alone.[12] Other environmental chemicals incriminated in the etiology of breast cancer include dichlorodiphenyltrichloroethane, dioxins, and gasoline components.[13]

Family history affects the prevalence of breast cancer, as well. Positive family history doubles the risk of breast cancer if 1 first-degree relative is affected and triples the risk if 2 first-degree relatives are affected.[10] In a study by Armstrong et al on the risk of breast cancer, the authors reported that risk increases up to 13.6% when a first-degree relative is affected.[14] Some women have genetic mutations that increase the risk of breast cancer as well.[15] Deleterious mutations confer a 60% to 80% lifetime risk in *BRCA1* carriers and 40% to 60% in *BRCA2* carriers. There are other gene mutations that increase risk, including *PALB2*, *CHEK2*, and others. Genetic testing and consultation with a genetic counselor are important in selected patients. Risk-reducing strategies include lifestyle modifications, like regular exercise, diet, and weight reduction, and moderation in alcohol intake. Risk-reducing medications, like tamoxifen, can also be recommended. Risk-reducing surgeries, like bilateral salpingo-oophorectomy or bilateral mastectomy, are also options.[16] Other significant risk factors include prior history of breast cancer, atypical hyperplasia and lobular neoplasia, or prior breast biopsy.[16] The risk of developing a second breast cancer is higher in patients with a history of breast cancer in comparison to those with no history of breast cancer.[17] Age also is an important predictive and risk factor in affected patients. The median age at the time of diagnosis of breast cancer is 62 years with less than 3% of patients being diagnosed below the age of 40 years.[5] Women who have had mantle irradiation during adolescence and young adulthood are also at higher risk for developing breast cancer.

Breast cancer is a disease with myriad clinical presentation. In addition to locoregional spread, breast cancer can metastasize systematically to various organs resulting in symptoms and signs that may precede or follow the diagnosis of the primary lesion. In the head and neck region, the sites most commonly affected are the supraclavicular lymph nodes and bony structures.[18,19] In a review by Hirshberg and Buchner, 2 out of 5 patients with metastatic disease to the maxilla or mandible had breast cancer as the primary malignancy.[20] Nahum and Bailey described a patient of poorly differentiated epidermoid carcinoma of the breast who presented with facial pain and opacification of the left maxillary sinus. Histologic examination of the mass filling the maxillary antrum revealed the same pathology as that of the primary tumor. A review of the literature in that report identified 8 cases of breast carcinoma metastasizing to the sinuses.[21] Similarly, in a review by Tracy et al on breast cancer metastasis to the head and neck, the authors reported a case of maxillary sinus adenocarcinoma with evidence of bony erosion on computed tomography (CT).[19] The temporal bone is affected less commonly. Feinmesser et al reported a case of breast adenocarcinoma that metastasized to the temporal bone and highlighted the importance of high-resolution CT in diagnosing metastatic lesions.[22]

Given the diverse clinical presentation of breast cancer, it is important for clinicians to be familiar with the association between breast cancer and voice. A thorough discussion on treatment-induced dysphonia also is presented in view of the morbidity of adjuvant therapy. This information is essential to provide optimal treatment to patients with breast cancer presenting with change in voice quality.

Disease-Induced Dysphonia

Dysphonia in patients with breast cancer is usually the result of recurrent laryngeal nerve palsy, disease invasion of the larynx and its contiguous structures, and/or to laryngeal metastasis.

Recurrent Laryngeal Nerve Palsy

In the absence of metastasis to the larynx or its contiguous structures, dysphonia in patients with breast cancer is usually the result of mass compression or metastatic infiltration of the recurrent laryngeal nerve.[23–27] This is not surprising given that 30% of patients with breast cancer develop metastasis during the course of the disease, which may extend for many years.[23] The lymphatic channels most commonly affected are the internal mammary, supraclavicular, and mediastinal. Metastatic mediastinal lymphadenopathy is common in 8% of patients with breast cancer undergoing surgery and in 25% of those presenting with recurrence of the disease.[24] Given the proximity of these lymph nodes to the course of the recurrent laryngeal nerves, it is not surprising that some patients with breast cancer develop vocal fold paralysis. In a review of unusual complications of metastatic breast cancer, Conklin reported 3 patients with dysphagia; 2 of those patients had recurrent laryngeal nerve palsy. The authors alluded to vocal fold paralysis as an alarming sign of mediastinal invasion in patients with advanced breast cancer.[26] Westbrook et al reported 37 patients with vocal fold paralysis in a group of 3000 patients with breast cancer suspected of having metastasis. All 37 patients referred for laryngeal examination had either dysphonia, dyspnea, or cough. The most common etiology for vocal fold paralysis was disease metastasis, present in 86% of the cases. The paralysis was mostly attributed to compression of the recurrent laryngeal nerve secondary to disease metastasis to the neck and mediastinum. It was unilateral in most patients and more common on the left side in patients with mediastinal disease. The average time between the start of treatment and the onset of paralysis was almost 5 years.[24] However, it is important to note that with advances in technology and the early diagnosis of vocal fold paralysis, treatment is more likely to be initiated early. More current studies are needed to elucidate the true prevalence of vocal fold paralysis in affected patients and the lapse of time between diagnosis and treatment. Vocal fold paralysis can also be bilateral. Khater et al reported a patient with breast cancer who presented with stridor secondary to supraclavicular nodal metastasis and bilateral vocal fold paralysis[28] (Figure 5–1).

Vocal fold paralysis in patients with breast cancer also may be secondary to disease metastasis to the base of the skull. In 1983, Hall et al described 8 patients with metastatic breast cancer who presented with multiple cranial neuropathies secondary to base of skull involvement in the absence of intracranial disease. The fifth and seventh cranial nerves were affected most commonly, and the vagus nerve was involved in 2 patients. Treatment with radiotherapy

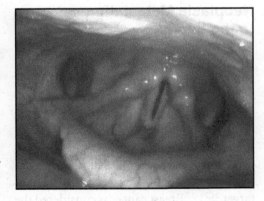

Figure 5–1. A 78-year-old female patient with breast cancer presented to the voice clinic with history of stridor. In-office laryngoscopy revealed bilateral vocal fold paralysis.

improved the palsies in 50% of the cases.[23] In 1987, Saab et al reported a case of adenocarcinoma of the breast who had metastasis to the jugulodigastric lymph nodes and nasopharynx with invasion to the pituitary gland and base of skull. Though the authors did not report any phonatory symptoms in that case, they emphasized the need for a thorough examination of the head and neck region in patients with breast metastasis, keeping in mind the skipping pattern of cervical lymph node metastasis.[29] In 2017, Tracy et al described a case of adenocarcinoma of the breast who presented with dysphonia and right vocal fold paralysis. CT of the head and neck showed a mass at the jugular foramen, the pathology of which was consistent with metastatic adenocarcinoma.[19]

In summary, the presence of dysphonia and vocal fold paralysis in patients with breast cancer should alert the physician to the possibility of recurrent laryngeal nerve compression or invasion. A thorough and diligent workup is mandatory to exclude lymph node metastasis along the course of this nerve in the chest and neck. Disease metastasis to the base of the skull also should be ruled out.

Neoplasia Metastatic to the Larynx

Another cause of dysphonia or change in voice quality in patients with breast cancer is laryngeal metastasis. Breast cancer can metastasize to many organs in the body, the most common of which are bones, lymph nodes, lungs, and liver. Metastasis to the head and neck region is well-described in the literature, with the larynx being a rare target.[24,29–37] Breast cancer is considered the fourth most common metastatic disease to the larynx following cutaneous melanomas, which account for the majority of laryngeal metastatic malignancies.[37] There have been a few cases of laryngeal metastasis reported in patients with primary breast cancer. In 1965, Mazzarella et al described a case of metastatic breast carcinoma to the larynx with cartilaginous involvement of the laryngeal structures. Based on the authors' discussion, the laryngeal perichondrium acted as a barrier to the spread of the disease to endolaryngeal structures.[38] In 1983, Abemayor et al described metastatic cancer to the larynx in a patient with breast and colon cancer. The patient presented with dysphonia and sore throat months following successful treatment of the neoplastic primary lesions. On laryngeal examination, the patient had a large supraglottic mass with fixation of the right vocal fold. The pathology of the laryngeal specimen was consistent with well-differentiated adenocarcinoma identical to that of the colon. The authors highlighted the need for laryngeal examination and imaging in patients with dysphonia and suspected metastatic disease.[39] Batsakis et al, in 1985, reported 11 cases of laryngeal metastasis, with breast cancer being the primary neoplasm in 2. The laryngeal symptoms in all patients were nonspecific, and the supraglottis was the main site for metastasis in 40% of the cases.[37] In a study on secondary laryngeal tumors, Ferlito et al described 7 cases that the authors had encountered over the course of 21 years. In their review of the literature through 1988, they reported 11 cases of metastatic breast cancer to the larynx out of 120 laryngeal tumors.[34] Wanamaker et al described a 77-year-old woman, diagnosed with stage II breast adenocarcinoma, who presented with hoarseness and dyspnea 16 months after left modified radical mastectomy. CT examination showed a laryngeal mass, biopsy of which revealed poorly differentiated carcinoma consistent with breast metastasis.[40] In 2007, Grasso et al reported a 66-year-old woman, diagnosed with infiltrative ductal carcinoma, who presented 8 years after treatment with dysphonia. She had a laryngeal mass that involved the left true vocal fold and aryepiglottic fold. Tissue examination using immunohistochemistry showed atypical cells consistent with metastatic breast cancer. The authors speculated a lymphatic spread in view of the positive involvement of the paratracheal lymph nodes and the deep jugular lymphatic channel.[41] In 2019, Kumar et al reported a 63-year-old patient with breast carcinoma who presented with dysphonia and shortness of breath secondary to a transglottic lesion and impaired mobility of the left true vocal fold. The patient had successful surgical treatment of her primary carcinoma which was followed by hormone therapy 5 years before she presented with laryngeal symptoms.[42] In view of the diffuse metastasis to the larynx, lungs, and skeletal structures, the patient received palliative chemotherapy and radiation therapy.

In many of the patients reported, the clinical presentation of laryngeal metastasis from breast carcinoma could have been misleading. The reported symptoms may be similar to those described by patients with primary laryngeal carcinoma.[39,43] These can include dysphonia, cough, sore throat, shortness of breath, and dyspnea.[39] Laryngeal examination also may be nonspecific. The laryngeal endoscopic findings can be ill-defined with the presence of subtle submucosal lesions.[42,44] The laryngeal sites most commonly affected are the supraglottis in 40% followed by the subglottis in 12%.[37] The mode of metastasis can be either hematogenous or lymphogenous. Hematogenous spread may occur with tumor emboli reaching the ossified cartilages of the larynx via "vena cava-right heart-left heart-aorta-external carotid-upper thyroid artery-laryngeal artery."[37(p459)] In cases of ossification of the laryngeal cartilaginous structures, the thyroid cartilage and hyoid bone were reported as early as 1954 as hosts for metastatic spread in 22% of the laryngeal metastatic cases.[45] Kusama et al reported a 69-year-old woman who developed a painless neck mass 10 years after being diagnosed and treated for breast carcinoma. On positron emission tomography (PET)-CT, the patient was found to have bony metastasis to multiple sites including the hyoid bone.[46] A less common route of metastasis is lymph-borne emboli that can reach the larynx either in an orderly fashion or in a skip pattern.[47]

In summary, a high index of suspicion is needed in order to make the proper diagnosis of breast carcinoma metastasizing to the larynx. Multiple deep laryngeal biopsies must be taken, and special histochemical staining, in addition to electron microscopic examination, are often needed to confirm disease metastasis to the larynx.

Metastasis to Laryngeal Contiguous Structures

Another cause of dysphonia in patients with breast carcinoma is tumor metastasis to laryngeal contiguous structures. Conklin, in 1964, described 2 patients with breast cancer who developed esophageal obstruction and recurrent laryngeal nerve palsy secondary to supraclavicular metastasis.[26] In 1982, Biller et al reported 2 patients with breast cancer who presented with dysphagia and inability to swallow. The symptoms were attributed to esophageal obstruction with circumferential strictures at the level of the upper esophageal sphincter due to neoplastic compression. Both patients had vocal fold paralysis, one unilateral and the other bilateral.[35] Another common metastatic target for breast cancer that can adversely impact phonation is the thyroid gland. Thyroid metastasis occurs in almost 1 out of 4 patients with widespread malignancy.[48] The most common primary carcinomas metastasizing to the thyroid gland are malignant melanoma, lung carcinoma, renal cell carcinoma, and breast carcinoma.[48-51] In 1984, Ivy reported 30 women with thyroid metastatic lesions, 6 of whom had breast cancer as a primary malignancy. Kidney, lung, and lymphoid tissue malignancies were the predominant source of malignancy in the remaining group.[36] In all of the described cases, the presenting sign was a thyroid mass, and the diagnosis of metastatic breast carcinoma was challenging. Although the authors did not elaborate on the laryngeal findings, dysphonia in affected patients is hypothetically due either to impaired mobility of the vocal folds secondary to compression of the recurrent laryngeal nerve, or to tumor invasion to the nerve or laryngeal structures. Similarly, Molina Garrido et al, in 2006, reported a 43-year-old woman with breast carcinoma who presented with metastatic thyroid disease following successful surgical treatment and chemoradiation.[52] The patient had multinodular enlargement of the thyroid gland which impinged on the laryngopharyngeal complex resulting in dysphonia and dysphagia. The authors emphasized the importance of thyroidectomy to acquire the entire thyroid gland as a specimen for diligent tissue examination in patients with suspected thyroid metastasis.[52] In 2012, Slipac described a 42-year-old woman who developed a nodule in the right thyroid gland with enlargement of paratracheal lymph nodes following successful treatment of her breast carcinoma. Histologic examination of the thyroid specimen and immunohistochemistry analysis confirmed metastatic breast carcinoma despite the diagnosis of medullary thyroid carcinoma on fine needle aspiration.[49] In 2017, Plonczak et al reported a 62-year-old woman with bilateral breast cancer who presented with a neck mass and thyroid enlargement 12 years after treatment. Histopathologic examination of the thyroid gland and cervical lymph nodes revealed metastatic breast cancer.[50] All the aforementioned reports lead us to conclude that a high index of suspicion is needed in the workup of thyroid metastasis in patients with a history of breast cancer. Moreover, examination of the entire thyroid gland as a specimen may be essential to confirm the diagnosis.

Anxiety, Stress, and Dysphonia in Breast Cancer

Cancer patients are prone to experience psychological disorders and affective mood alterations. The most commonly reported ones that often require psychological intervention are anxiety and depression.[53,54] When present, these can lead to disruptive behavior such as social isolation and to somatic symptoms related to autonomic overactivity.[54] In patients with breast cancer, the reported prevalence of anxiety and depression ranges between 1.7% and 23%.[55,56] In 2005, Burgess et al investigated anxiety and depression within 5 years following the diagnosis of breast cancer in 170 women. Using validated questionnaires, the authors reported that 1 out of 2 patients with breast cancer experience depression and anxiety within the first year following diagnosis. The prevalence seems to taper with time except in patients with stressful life experiences, prior history of psychological disorders, and no confiding relationship.[57] Fafouti et al examined the psychopathologic profile of 109 patients with breast cancer versus 71 healthy controls. Using the Montgomery-Åsberg Depression Rating Scale (MADRS) and the

Spielberger State-Trait Anxiety Inventory (STAI), the authors reported higher scores in the cancer group and a positive association between breast cancer and the different psychological measures used.[58] In a study by Jacob et al on the prevalence of depression and anxiety in patients with breast cancer, the authors reported a figure of 8.8 per 100 person-years. The main factors associated with a higher risk of depression and anxiety included younger age at the time of diagnosis and presence of metastasis.[59] The same authors reported depression in 36.9% and anxiety in 35.1% of patients with breast cancer who were diagnosed by general practitioners and gynecological practices. Again, prior history of depression and presence of metastasis were considered significant risk factors for depression and anxiety.[60] Similarly, in a study by Kostev et al that included 4842 patients, the risk of depression and anxiety within 3 years of diagnosis following treatment was higher in those with suspected breast cancer or genital organ cancer in comparison with those with no cancer (14.1% versus 10.5%).[61] In all the previously discussed reports, the prevalence of abnormal affective mood disorders and psychopathologic profile has been linked to older age, prior history of psychiatric or psychological disturbances, and lack of confiding relationships.

Given the reported high prevalence of anxiety and depression in patients with breast cancer, and given the strong association between anxiety, depression, and voice,[62] it is imperative to recognize that patients with breast cancer suffering from affective mood disorders are more likely to experience phonatory disturbances. Although there are no studies in the literature on the prevalence of dysphonia in patients with breast cancer with and without anxiety and depression, the association between these conditions and dysphonia warrants future investigation. Intervention using either medications or other psychological treatments should be considered in affected patients.

Cluster of Body Fatigue, Pain, and Insomnia in Patients With Breast Cancer

Other significant risks for dysphonia in patients with breast cancer include history of fibromyalgia, body fatigue, and/or pain. Chronic musculoskeletal pain, be it widespread or local, is common in the general population. Its overall prevalence is in the range of 11%,[63] and its pattern is markedly influenced by many factors.[64-67] Significant triggers reported in the literature include low socioeconomic status, unemployment, exposure to traumatic events, and low level of education.[64,68] Cancer per se also has been described as a pain trigger, with patients with cancer being at an increased risk of having pain in comparison to the normal population. In a study by Schrier et al in 2012, conducted on 40 patients with breast cancer versus 40 healthy controls matched to age, the authors reported 4 times higher rates of widespread pain. In addition, 3 patients in the cancer group met the American College of Rheumatology criteria for fibromyalgia in comparison with only 1 in the control group, which was not statistically significant.[69] Affected subjects are impacted not only by the threat imposed by the disease itself but also by treatment-induced physical and mental adverse events.

An equally important somatic and physical impairment in patients with breast cancer is sleep disturbance. In the review by Schrier et al, 60% of patients with breast cancer were affected by disturbed sleep and insomnia in comparison with only 35% in the control group.[69] Based on the study by Palesh et al, the disturbed nocturnal sleep in patients with metastatic breast cancer is also associated with reduced respiratory sinus arrhythmia and diurnal cortisol rhythm variations.[70] The presence of insomnia has been shown to exacerbate the frequency and severity of psychological symptoms and body fatigue leading to poor quality of life.[71-73] Based on a systematic review on the prevalence and risk factors for sleep disturbances in patients diagnosed and treated for breast cancer, Leysen et al described depressive symptoms and fatigue as significant risk factors with odds ratios of 3.20 and 2.82, respectively.[73]

Given the high level of body fatigue, pain, and sleep deprivation in patients with breast cancer, and given the known association between these impairments and voice,[74] we can extrapolate that patients with breast cancer suffering from body pain and/or insomnia are at a higher risk to develop vocal disorders in comparison to normal subjects.

Treatment-Induced Dysphonia in Patients With Breast Cancer

Breast tissue resection (total or partial mastectomy) is one of the key components of breast cancer management.[75] Surgery is often followed by adjuvant therapy, which can include radiotherapy, chemotherapy, and/or hormone therapy. In selected cases, chemotherapy or endocrine therapy may precede surgery (neoadjuvant). Each of these adjuvant or neoadjuvant therapies may affect the voice.

Radiation-Induced Dysphonia

Radiation therapy to the breast is standard after partial mastectomy. In women over 70

to 75 years of age with favorable, hormone-receptor positive lesions, radiation therapy may be omitted. When given, it may be delivered externally to the whole breast or partially to the lumpectomy site (partial breast irradiation, PBI). PBI can be given externally or via a catheter placed at the lumpectomy site. Radiation therapy is also recommended in some patients postmastectomy. Indications for radiotherapy include large lesions (more than 5 cm), positive posterior margin, 4 or more lymph nodes involvement, and unfavorable tumor phenotypes with lymph node metastasis.[76] It is also considered in patients with 1 to 3 positive lymph nodes if there are other unfavorable risk factors. Despite its well-documented added value, radiation therapy has many adverse effects among which is damage to the recurrent laryngeal nerve along its course in the chest. Depending on several factors such as dose of irradiation, source, and field application, irradiation may lead to injury to the neural axons, myelin sheath, and the adjacent connective tissue structures resulting in perineural fibrosis and scarring.[77] Irradiation-induced recurrent laryngeal neuropathy can be progressive and may occur years after therapy, with the left recurrent laryngeal nerve being more affected than the right one.[78,79] In a study by Pradat and Delanian on the late effect of radiation on peripheral nerves, the authors described multiple phases of injury leading to fibrogenesis and atrophic changes with subsequent apoptosis.[80] Stern et al described 3 cases of head and neck cancer patients who developed late vocal fold palsy postirradiation. The paralysis was bilateral in 2 out of the 3 cases and occurred between 21 and 34 years after treatment. The authors highlighted the need to dissociate recurrence of the disease from irradiation-induced damage.[81] Crawley and Sulica reported 10 cases of delayed vocal fold paralysis postradiotherapy to the neck and chest. The mean time elapsed between completion of therapy and development of vocal fold paralysis was 21 years.[78] In another study by Johansson et al on late complication of mediastinal irradiation, 12 out of 150 patients diagnosed with breast cancer and treated by irradiation developed delayed vocal fold paralysis.[79] The authors attributed the recurrent laryngeal nerve palsy to an overlap in the field of irradiation at the trachea-esophageal groove. The areas of fibrosis and scarring in the vicinity of the affected nerves were referred to as hotspots.

In cases of extensive nodal positivity, radiation is also delivered regionally to the supraclavicular nodes. The purpose of radiotherapy to the neck in addition to chest is to control the microscopic spread of the disease. As a result, radiation-induced inflammatory changes in the laryngeal and pharyngeal mucosa may occur. Animal studies have shown that the laryngeal mucosa can be affected negatively by 20 Gy radiotherapy or more.[82,83] The exposure of the laryngeal mucosa to ionizing radiation results in inflammatory changes and vascular congestion with subsequent edema. Irradiation may also adversely affect glandular mucosal secretions. Sato et al investigated the adverse effect of radiation on laryngeal mucosal glands and described a decrease in the size and function of these glands with subsequent mucosal dehydration[84]; the effect of dehydration on phonation is well known.[85-89]

Mucosal alterations, edema, and dehydration can lead to phonatory changes. In a study by Sagiroglu et al on 29 patients with breast cancer who underwent supraclavicular radiotherapy for locally advanced disease, the authors reported an increase in cycle-to-cycle variation in intensity from 1.94 to 2.45, and in the Acoustic Voice Quality Index (AVQI) from 3.36 to 3.91 at 1 month posttreatment. These acoustic changes reverted to normal at 6 months following surgery. The AVQI decreased to 3.33 at 6 months, and the shimmer decreased to 1.57. In parallel with these acoustic changes were signs of inflammatory changes in the laryngeal mucosa on stroboscopic evaluation which also reverted back to normal.[90] In another report by Fiets et al on the acute toxicity of whole breast irradiation and regional therapy in cases of infraclavicular, supraclavicular, or parasternal lymph node metastasis, the authors described various degrees of laryngopharyngeal symptoms such as dysphagia, cough, and dyspnea.[91] These symptoms, in addition to the findings reported by Sagiroglu et al,[90] are in accordance with the results of numerous studies on the adverse effect of neck irradiation on voice in the management of non-laryngeal carcinoma.[85,92,93] In a study by Hamdan et al on the vocal changes following radiotherapy to the neck while sparing the vocal folds, 15% of the irradiated subjects described their voice as poor and 85% as fair. This self-perceived evaluation was substantiated by an increase in all the perceptual parameters posttreatment. The study was performed on 15 patients with nasopharyngeal or tongue tumors.[85] Similarly, Fung et al reported overall increased supraglottic activity and a high voice handicap in 27% of patients who received radiotherapy for non-laryngeal malignancies.[92]

In conclusion, radiation therapy to the chest and neck in patients with breast cancer can result in voice symptoms. These symptoms may be attributed either to radiation-induced recurrent laryngeal neuropathy along its course in the chest and neck or to inflammatory changes in the laryngeal mucosa. A thorough investigation of the cause of dysphonia in patients with breast cancer is warranted, as are additional studies.

Endocrine Therapy-Induced Dysphonia

Endocrine therapy has been proven beneficial in patients with breast cancer with steroid receptor expression. It is used commonly either as an adjuvant or neoadjuvant therapy in patients with estrogen receptor (ER)-positive and progesterone receptor (PR)-positive tumors. Two-thirds of patients with breast cancer are hormone receptor positive. Endocrine therapy aims at either blocking the proliferative effect of estrogen on breast tissue or lowering the rate of estrogen production at various sites.[94] The former is achieved primarily using selective estrogen receptor modulators such as tamoxifen and toremifene or selective estrogen receptor degraders such as fulvestrant (AstraZeneca, Cambridge, United Kingdom). Aromatase inhibitors (AIs) such as anastrozole and letrozole are prescribed commonly to reduce estrogen production in postmenopausal women.[95,96] These medications act primarily by inhibiting the peripheral conversion of androstenedione and testosterone available in adipose tissue to estrogen.[94]

Given the well-known systemic effect of estrogen depletion or suppression on the phonatory apparatus and its impact on voice, one would speculate that endocrine therapy in patients with breast cancer must lead to vocal symptoms similar to those reported in postmenopausal women. These include throat clearing, deepening of the voice, loss of the high notes, and voice fatigue.[97] These symptoms occur in up to two-thirds of postmenopausal women who do not use hormone replacement therapy and are attributed to vocal fold atrophic changes and to decrease in laryngeal glandular secretions. Current literature is scarce on the effect of estrogen depletion on voice in women with breast cancer following hormonal therapy. There is only 1 report by Hersxheimer et al on tamoxifen and the singing voice highlighting the irreversible change in voice quality that can be induced by estrogen receptor modulators.[98] Patients with breast cancer treated with estrogen receptor modulators should be informed about dysphonia as a possible side effect of treatment. More research on the impact of hormone therapy on voice is needed.

Aromatase inhibitors may also impact phonation indirectly through their adverse effect on the musculoskeletal system. Despite the favorable effect of AI on the rate of recurrence in patients with breast cancer,[99] their benefit comes with a cost. Aromatase-induced arthralgia (AIA) is a broad term used to describe a heterogeneous cluster of symptoms related to both muscles and joints. Its adverse effect on patients' quality of life leads to discontinuation of therapy in up to 31% of patients within a year.[100] Significant predictors include a low body mass index, prior hormonal treatment, and the stage of the disease with stage I patients being more affected than stage III patients.[101-103] Given the known impact of body fatigue and pain on phonation,[74] physicians should be aware that breast cancer patients treated with AI and suffering from muscle pain may complain of change in voice quality. Professional voice users are at an increased risk given the high susceptibility of their phonatory apparatus to voice symptoms associated with body fatigue and pain.

Chemotherapy and Voice in Patients With Breast Cancer

Chemotherapy is one of the many therapeutic options given to patients with breast cancer. It is used either preoperatively or postoperatively in combination with other adjuvant therapies such as radiotherapy, immuno-therapy, targeted therapy, and endocrine therapy. Several combinations of drugs for the treatment of breast carcinoma are commonly used including AC (doxorubicin hydrochloride and cyclophosphamide) with or without paclitaxel, CAF (cyclophosphamide with doxorubicin hydrochloride and fluorouracil), and FEC (fluorouracil, epirubicin hydrochloride, and cyclophosphamide).[104] There are no published studies on dysphonia as an adverse effect of chemotherapy in patients with breast cancer, though there are a few in patients treated for lung cancer.[105,106] Nevertheless, a review of the many side effects of chemotherapy led us to conclude that the phonatory apparatus is at jeopardy during treatment,[107] as reviewed by Mattioni et al in a chapter entitled "Cancer Chemotherapy: An Overview and Voice Implications."[108] Cough, in addition to dehydration secondary to diarrhea and vomiting, may well lead to dysphonia given the known adverse effect of phonotrauma and dehydration on voice.[88,89,109] Increased awareness of vocal symptoms and diligent workup of dysphonia in patients with breast cancer undergoing chemotherapy is warranted.

Additional information on the impact of breast cancer on voice, and on voice professionals, can be found in other literature.[16]

Surgical Treatment of Breast Cancer and Dysphonia

The surgical treatment of breast cancer consists primarily of either lumpectomy or mastectomy. The choice of surgical procedure depends on the local extent of the disease, the presence of more than one affected site within the breast, soft tissue or skin changes adjacent to the tumor site, and the stage of the disease.[17] With either surgery, staging of the axilla is often included. For the majority of patients, this involves a sentinel biopsy, a procedure that removes the main draining nodes (average 1 to 3 nodes removed). For more advanced disease, an axillary lymph node dissection may be required. Morbidity, including rates of lymphedema and arm stiffness, is higher with an axillary lymph node dissection.

The shoulder pain and stiffness that may occur as a result of dissection of axillary lymph nodes may affect phonation, particularly in professional voice users who are vulnerable to body pain and fatigue.[74] Another challenge to the phonatory apparatus following surgical treatment is reconstruction. Reconstruction postmastectomy may be performed with implant-based techniques, autologous techniques, or a combination of both. Most reconstructions utilize the implant-based procedures. Autologous techniques include pedicled transverse rectus abdominus myocutaneous (TRAM) flaps, latissimus dorsi flaps, which also require an implant, and free flaps such as the deep inferior epigastric perforator (DIEP), superficial inferior epigastric perforator (SIEP), gluteal flaps, and so on. Very advanced disease requiring removal of large amounts of local structures may be treated with thoracoepigastric or thoracoabdominal flaps, or musculocutaneous flaps from the abdomen.[110]

The use of these flaps and the resultant surgical defects may jeopardize abdominal support in breathing and phonation. Following these procedures, singers are advised not to sing before regaining adequate abdominal muscle strength to allow optimal support (power source) for phonation.[17]

References

1. Bonilla JM, Tabanera MT, Mendoza LR. Breast cancer in the 21st century: from

early detection to new therapies. *Radiología* (English Edition). 2017;59(5):368–379.

2. World Cancer Research Fund. Breast cancer statistics. Accessed August 23, 2019. https://www.wcrf.org/dietandcancer/cancer-trends/breast-cancer-statistics

3. CancerNet. Breast cancer: statistics. Cancer Net Editorial Board. Updated January 2019. Accessed July 1, 2019. http://www.cancer.net/cancer-types/breast-cancer/statistics

4. Yedjou CG, Tchounwou PB, Payton M, et al. Assessing the racial and ethnic disparities in breast cancer mortality in the United States. *Int J Environ Res Public Health*. 2017; 14(5). doi:10.3390lijerph14050486

5. Rediq A, McAllister S. Breast cancer as a systemic disease: a view of metastasis. *J Intern Med*. 2013;274(2):113–126.

6. Radecka B, Litwiniuk M. Breast cancer in young women. *Ginekologia polska*. 2016;87(9): 659–663.

7. Leclere B, Molinie F, Tretarre B, et al. Trends in incidence of breast cancer among women under 40 in seven European countries: a GRELL cooperative study. *Cancer Epidemiol*. 2013;37(5):544–549.

8. Fowler ME, Akinyemiju TF. Meta-analysis of the association between dietary inflammatory index (DII) and cancer outcomes. *Int J Cancer*. 2017;141(11):2215–2227.

9. Taha Z, Eltom SE. The role of diet and lifestyle in women with breast cancer: an update review of related research in the Middle East. *Biores Open Access*. 2018;7(1):73–80.

10. American Cancer Society medical and editorial content team. Lifestyle-related Breast Cancer Risk Factors. Updated September 6, 2017. Accessed July 1, 2019. https://www.cancer.org/cancer/breast-cancer/risk-and-prevention/lifestyle-related-breast-cancer-risk-factors.html

11. Jerry DJ, Shull JD, Hadsell DL, et al. Genetic variation in sensitivity to estrogens and breast cancer risk. *Mamm Genome*. 2018; 29(1-2):24–37.

12. Chlebowski RT, Kuller LH, Prentice RL, et al. Breast cancer after use of estrogen plus progestin in post-menopausal women. *NEJM*. 2009;360(6):573–587.

13. Rodgers KM, Udesky JO, Rudel RA, Brody JG. Environmental chemicals and breast cancer: an updated review of epidemiological literature informed by biological mechanisms. *Environ Res*. 2018;160:152–182.

14. Armstrong K, Eisen A, Weber B. Assessing the risk of breast cancer. *NEJM*. 2000;342(8):564–571.

15. Anders CK, Johnson RH, Litton J, Phillips M, Bleyer A. Breast cancer before age 40 years. *Semin Oncol*. 2009;36(3):237–249.

16. Gail, MH, Constantino, JP, Byant J, et al. Weighing the risks and benefits of tamoxifen treatment for preventing breast cancer. *J Natl Cancer Inst*. 1999;91(21):1829–1846.

17. Sataloff DM, Sataloff RT. Breast cancer in professional voice users. In: Sataloff RT. *Professional Voice: The Science and Art of Clinical Care*. 4th ed. San Diego, CA: Plural Publishing; 2017:689–694.

18. Kiricuta IC, Willner J, Kolbl O, Bohndorf W. The prognostic significance of the supraclavicular lymph node metastases in breast cancer patients. *Int J Radiat Oncol Biol Phys*. 1994;28(2):387–393.

19. Tracy JC, Mildenhall NR, Wein RO, O'Leary MA. Breast cancer metastases to the head and neck: case series and literature review. *Ear, Nose, Throat J*. 2017;96(3):E21–E24.

20. Hirshberg A, Buchner A. Metastatic tumors to the oral region. An overview. *Eur J Cancer B Oral Oncol*. 1995;31B(6):355–360.

21. Nahum AM, Bailey BJ. Malignant tumors metastatic to the paranasal sinuses: case report and review of the literature. *Laryngoscope*. 1963;73(7):942–953.

22. Feinmesser R, Libson Y, Uziely B, Gay I. Metastatic carcinoma to the temporal bone. *Am J Otol*. 1986;7(2):119–120.

23. O'Shaughnessy J. Extending survival with chemotherapy in metastatic breast cancer. *Oncologist*. 2005;10(Suppl 3):20–29.

24. Westbrook KC, Ballantyne AJ, Eckles NE, Brown GR. Breast cancer and vocal cord paralysis. *South Med J*. 1974;67(7):805–807.

25. Morrissey AT, O'Connell DA, Allegretto M. Medialization thyroplasty for unilateral vocal cord paralysis secondary to advanced

extralaryngeal malignant disease: review of operative morbidity and patient life expectancy. *J Otolaryngol Head Neck Surg.* 2012;41(1);41–45.

26. Conklin EF. Some unusual complications of metastatic carcinoma of the breast. *Ann Surg.* 1964;159(4):489–495.

27. Handforth A, Nag S, Robertson DM. Polyneuropathy with vagus and phrenic nerve involvement in breast cancer. Report of a case with spontaneous remission. *Arch Neurol.* 1984;41(6):666–668.

28. Khater A, El-Badrawy A, Ebrahem MA. Stridor as the first presentation of metastatic breast cancer that was managed with chemotherapy: a case report. *Indian J Surg Oncol.* 2018;9(3):336–339.

29. Saab GA, Abdul-Karim FW, Samara M. Breast carcinoma metastatic to the nasopharynx. *J Laryngol Otol.* 1987;101(7):723–725.

30. Saldanha CB, Bennett JD, Evans JN, Pambakian H. Metastasis to the temporal bone, secondary to carcinoma of the bladder. *J Laryngol Otol.* 1989;103(6):599–601.

31. Batsakis JG, Bautina E. Metastases to major salivary glands. *Ann Otol Rhinol Laryngol.* 1990;99(6 Pt 1):501–503.

32. Bernstein JM, Montgomery WW, Balogh K Jr. Metastatic tumors to the maxilla, nose, and paranasal sinuses. *Laryngoscope.* 1966;76(4):621–650.

33. Zachariades N. Neoplasms metastatic to the mouth, jaws and surrounding tissues. *J Craniomaxillofac Surg.* 1989;17(6):283–290.

34. Ferlito A, Caruso G, Recher G. Secondary laryngeal tumors: report of seven cases with review of the literature. *Arch Otolaryngol Head Neck Surg.* 1988;114(6):635–639.

35. Biller HF, Diktaban T, Fink W, Lawson W. Breast carcinoma metastasizing to the cervical esophagus. *Laryngoscope.* 1982;92(9 Pt 1):999–1000.

36. Ivy HK. Cancer metastatic to the thyroid: a diagnostic problem. *Mayo Clin Proc.* 1984;59(12):856–859.

37. Batsakis JG, Luna MA, Byers RM. Metastases to the larynx. *Head Neck Surg.* 1985;7(6):458–460.

38. Mazzarella LA, Pina LH, Wolff D. Asymptomatic metastasis to the larynx. *Laryngoscope.* 1966;76(9):1547–1554.

39. Abemayor E, Cochran AJ, Calcaterra TC. Metastatic cancer to the larynx. Diagnosis and management. *Cancer.* 1983;52(10):1944–1948.

40. Wanamaker JR, Kraus DH, Eliachar I, Lavertu P. Manifestations of metastatic breast carcinoma to the head and neck. *Head Neck.* 1993;15(3):257–262.

41. Grasso RF, Quattrocchi CC, Piciucchi S, et al. Vocal cord metastasis from breast cancer. *J Clin Oncol.* 2007;25(13):1803–1805.

42. Kumar R, Kumar S, Gogia A, Kakkar A, Mathur SR. Laryngeal metastases from breast cancer: a rare clinical entity. *Curr Probl Cancer.* 2019;43(2):130–134.

43. Freeland AP, van Nostrand AW, Jahn AF. Metastases to the larynx. *J Otolaryngol.* 1979;8(5):448–456.

44. Barnes L. Metastases to the head and neck: an overview. *Head Neck Pathol.* 2009;3(3):217–224.

45. Ehrlich A. Tumor involving the laryngeal cartilages. *AMA Arch Otolaryngol.* 1954;59(2):178–185.

46. Kusama H, Okishiro M, Ishida T, et al. A case of hyoid bone metastasis from breast cancer. *Gan To Kagaku Ryoho.* 2014;41(12):1915–1917.

47. Ritchie WW, Messmer JM, Whitley DP, Gopelrud DR. Uterine carcinoma metastatic to the larynx. *Laryngoscope.* 1985;95(1):97–98.

48. Lam KY, Lo CY. Metastatic tumors of the thyroid gland: a study of 79 cases in Chinese patients. *Arch Pathol Lab Med.* 1998;122(1):37–41.

49. Slipac J, Janjanin S, Liepava D, Hutinec Z, Bence-Zigman Z. Thyroid metastasis from breast carcinoma resembling medullary thyroid carcinoma. *Coll Antropol.* 2012;36(2):63–66.

50. Plonczak AM, DiMarco AN, Dina R, Gujral DM, Palazzo FF. Breast cancer metastases to the thyroid gland—an uncommon sentinel for diffuse metastatic disease: a case

report and review of the literature. *J Med Case Rep.* 2017;11(1):269.

51. Wood K, Vini L, Harmer C. Metastases to the thyroid gland: the Royal Marsden experience. *Eur J Surg Oncol,* 2004;30(6): 583–588.

52. Molina Garrido MJ, Guillen Ponce C, Macia Escalante S, Martinez y Sevila C, Carrato Mena A. Dysphagia and dysphonia in a woman with a previous breast cancer. *Clin Transl Oncol.* 2006;8(7):533–535.

53. Maass SW, Roorda C, Berendsen AJ, Verhaak PF, de Bock GH. The prevalence of long-term symptoms of depression and anxiety after breast cancer treatment: a systematic review. *Maturitas.* 2015;82(1):100–108.

54. Jassim GA, Whitford DL, Hickey A, Carter B. Psychological interventions for women with non-metastatic breast cancer. *Cochrane Database of Syst Rev.* 2015;(5):CD008729.

55. Lee MS, Love SB, Mitchell JB, et al. Mastectomy or conservation for early breast cancer: psychological morbidity. *Eur J Cancer.* 1992;28(8–9):1340–1344.

56. Fallowfield LJ, Hall A, Maguire P, Baum M, A'Hern RP. Psychological effects of being offered choice of surgery for breast cancer. *BMJ.* 1994;309(6952):448.

57. Burgess C, Cornelius V, Love S, Graham J, Richards M, Ramirez A. Depression and anxiety in women with early breast cancer: five year observational cohort study. *BMJ.* 2005;330(7493):702.

58. Fafouti M, Paparrigopoulos T, Zervas Y, et al. Depression, anxiety and general psychopathology in breast cancer patients: a cross-sectional control study. *In Vivo.* 2010; 24(5):803–810.

59. Jacob L, Kalder M, Kostev K. Incidence of depression and anxiety among women newly diagnosed with breast or genital organ cancer in Germany. *Psycho-Oncol.* 2017; 26(10):1535–1540.

60. Jacob L, Bleicher L, Kostev K, Kalder M. Prevalence of depression, anxiety and their risk factors in German women with breast cancer in general and gynecological prac-

tices. *J Cancer Res Clin Oncol.* 2016;142(2): 447–452.

61. Kostev K, Jacob L, Kalder M. Risk of depression, anxiety, and adjustment disorders in women with a suspected but unconfirmed diagnosis of breast or genital organ cancer in Germany. *Cancer Causes Control.* 2017;28(10):1021–1026.

62. Rosen DC, Heuer RJ, Sasso DA, Sataloff RT. Psychological aspects of voice disorders. In: Hamdan AL, Sataloff RT, Hawkshaw M. *Laryngeal Manifestations of Systemic Diseases.* San Diego, CA: Plural Publishing; 2018:119–150.

63. Croft P, Rigby AS, Boswell R, Schollum J, Silman A. The prevalence of chronic widespread pain in the general population. *J Rheumatol.* 1993;20(4):710–713.

64. Bergman S, Herrstrom P, Hogstrom K, Petersson IF, Svensson B, Jacobsson LT. Chronic musculoskeletal pain prevalence rates, and sociodemographic associations in a Swedish population study. *J Rheumatol.* 2001;28(6):1369–1377.

65. Bergman S, Herrstrom P, Jacobsson LT, Petersson IF. Chronic widespread pain: a three year follow-up of pain distribution and risk factors. *J Rheumatol.* 2002;29(4):818–825.

66. Nguyen M, Ugarte C, Fuller I, Haas G, Portenoy RK. Access to care for chronic pain: racial and ethnic differences. *J Pain.* 2005;6(5):301–314.

67. Portenoy RK, Ugarte C, Fuller I, Haas G. Population-based survey of pain in the United States: differences among white African American, and Hispanic subjects. *J Pain.* 2004;5(6):317–328.

68. Roth RS, Punch MR, Bachman JE. Educational achievement and pain disability among women with chronic pelvic pain. *J Psychosom Res.* 2001;51(4):563–569.

69. Schrier M, Amital D, Arnson Y, et al. Association of fibromyalgia characteristics in patients with non-metastatic breast cancer and the protective role of resilience. *Rheumatol Int.* 2012;32(10):3017–3023.

70. Palesh O, Zeitzer JM, Conrad A, et al. Vagal regulation, cortisol, and sleep disruption

in women with metastatic breast cancer. *J Clin Sleep Med.* 2008;4(5):441–449.

71. Fiorentino L, Rissling M, Liu L, Ancoli-Israel S. The symptom cluster of sleep, fatigue and depressive symptoms in breast cancer patients: severity of the problem and treatment options. *Drug Discov Today Dis Models.* 2011;8(4):167–173.

72. Reinsel RA, Starr TD, O'Sullivan B, Passik SD, Kavey NB. Polysomnographic study of sleep in survivors of breast cancer. *J Clin Sleep Med.* 2015;11(12):1361–1370.

73. Leysen L, Lahousse A, Nijs J, et al. Prevalence and risk factors of sleep disturbances in breast cancer survivors: systematic review and meta-analyses. *Support Care Cancer.* 2019;27(12):4401–4433.

74. Hamdan AL, Sataloff RT, Hawkshaw MJ. Sleep, body fatigue, and voice. In: Hamdan AL, Sataloff RT, Hawkshaw M. eds. *Laryngeal Manifestations of Systemic Diseases.* San Diego, CA: Plural Publishing; 2018:83–86.

75. Gabriel CA, Domchek SM. Breast cancer in young women. *Breast Cancer Res.* 2010;12(5):212.

76. Partridge AH, Pagani O, Abulkhair O, et al. First international consensus guidelines for breast cancer in young women (BCY1). *Breast.* 2014;23(3):209–220.

77. Delanian S, Lefaix JL, Pradat PF. Radiation-induced neuropathy in cancer survivors. *Radiother Oncol.* 2012;105(3):273–282.

78. Crawley BK, Sulica L. Vocal fold paralysis as a delayed consequence of neck and chest radiotherapy. *Otolaryngol Head Neck Surg.* 2015;153(2):239–243.

79. Johansson S, Lofroth PO, Denekamp J. Left sided vocal cord paralysis: a newly recognized late complication of mediastinal irradiation. *Radiother Oncol.* 2001;58(3):287–294.

80. Pradat PF, Delanian S. Late radiation injury to peripheral nerves. *Handb Clin Neurol.* 2013;115:743–758.

81. Stern Y, Marshak G, Segal K, Shpitzer T, Feinmesser R. Vocal cord palsy: possible late complication of radiotherapy for head and neck cancer. *Ann Otol Rhinol Laryngol.* 1995;104(4 Pt 1):294–296.

82. Oyan S, Tatlipinar A, Atasoy BM, et al. Early effects of irradiation on laryngeal mucosa in a gastroesophageal reflux model: an experimental study. *Eur Arch Otorhinolaryngol.* 2018;275(8):2089–2094.

83. Lidegran M, Forsgren S, Dahlqvist A, Franzen L, Domeij S. Short and long term irradiation effects of on laryngeal mucosa of the rat. *Acta Oncol.* 1999;38(8):1081–1091.

84. Sato K, Nakashima T. Effect of irradiation on the human laryngeal glands. *Ann Otol Rhinol Laryngol.* 2008;117(10):734–739.

85. Hamdan AL, Geara F, Rameh C, Husseini ST, Eid T, Fuleihan N. Vocal changes following radiotherapy to the head and neck for non-laryngeal tumors. *Eur Arch Otorhinolaryngol.* 2009;266(9):1435–1439.

86. Solomon NP, DiMattia MS. Effects of a vocally fatiguing task and systemic hydration on phonation threshold pressure. *J Voice.* 2000;14:341–362.

87. Hamdan AL, Siabi A, Rameh C. Effect of fasting on voice in women. *J Voice.* 2007; 21(4):495–501.

88. Hamdan AL, Ashkar J, Sibai A, Oubari D, Husseini ST. Effect of fasting on voice in males. *Am J Otolaryngol.* 2011;32(2):124–129.

89. Solomon NP, Glaze LE, Arnold RR, van Mersbergen M. Effects of a vocally fatiguing task and systemic hydration on men's voices. *J Voice.* 2003;17(1):31–46.

90. Sagiroglu S, Kurtul N. The effect of supraclavicular radiotherapy on Acoustic Voice Quality Index (AVQI), spectral amplitude and perturbation values. *J Voice.* 2019. doi:10.1016/j.jvoice.2019.01.003

91. Fiets WE, Van Helvoirt RP, Nortier JW, Van der Tweel I, Struikmans H. Acute toxicity of concurrent adjuvant radiotherapy and chemotherapy (CMF or AC) in breast cancer patients: a prospective, comparative, non-randomised study. *Eur J Cancer.* 2003;39(8):1081–1088.

92. Fung K, Yoo J, Leeper HA, et al. Effects of head and neck radiation therapy on

vocal function. *J Otolaryngol.* 2001;30(3): 133–139.

93. Colton RH, Sagerman RH, Chung CT, Yu YW, Reed GF. Voice change after radiotherapy: some preliminary results. *Radiology.* 1978;127(3):821–824.

94. Deslypere JP, Verdonck L, Vermeulen A. Fat tissue: a steroid reservoir and site of steroid metabolism. *J Clin Endocrinol Metab.* 1985;61(3):564–570.

95. Davies C, Pan H, Godwin J, et al. Long-term effects of continuing adjuvant tamoxifen to 10 years versus stopping at 5 years after diagnosis of oestrogen receptor-positive breast cancer: ATLAS, a randomised trial. *Lancet.* 2013;381:805–816.

96. Gray RG, Rea D, Handley K, et al. Long-term effects of continuing adjuvant tamoxifen to 10 years versus stopping at 5 years in 6,953 women with early breast cancer. *J Clin Oncol* (Meeting Abstracts). 2013;31 (18 Suppl 5).

97. Abitbol J, Abitbol P, Abitbol B. Sex hormones and the female voice. *J Voice.* 1999; 13(3):424–446.

98. Herxheimer A. Tamoxifen and the singing voice. *PloS Med.* 2005;2(9):e311–e326.

99. Petrelli F, Coinu A, Cabiddu M, Ghilardi M, Lonati V, Barni S. Five or more years of adjuvant endocrine therapy in breast cancer: a meta-analysis of published randomized trials. *Breast Cancer Res Treat.* 2013;140: 233–240.

100. Ziller V, Kalder M, Albert US, et al. Adhere to adjuvant endocrine therapy in post-menopausal women with breast cancer. *Ann Oncol.* 2009;20:431–436.

101. Beckwée D, Leysen L, Meuwis K, Adriaenssens N. Prevalence of aromatase inhibitor-induced arthralgia in breast cancer: a systematic review and meta-analysis. *Support Care Cancer.* 2017;25(5):1673–1686.

102. Crew KD, Greenlee H, Capodice J, et al. Prevalence of joint symptoms in postmeno-pausal women taking aromatase inhibitors for early-stage breast cancer. *J Clin Oncol.* 2007;25:3877–3883.

103. Horimoto Y, Saito M, Kasumi F. Arthralgia in 329 patients taking aromatase inhibitors. *Breast Care.* 2009;4:319–323.

104. American Cancer Society. Chemotherapy for breast cancer. Accessed July 1, 2019. https:// www.cancer.org/cancer/breast-cancer/treat ment/chemotherapy-for-breast-cancer.html

105. Wittgen BP, Kunst PW, van der Born K, et al. Phase I study of aerosolized SLIT cisplatin in the treatment of patients with carcinoma of the lung. *Clin Cancer Res.* 2007;13(8): 2414–2421.

106. Laurie SA, Gauthier I, Arnold A, et al. Phase I and pharmacokinetic study of daily oral AZD2171, an inhibitor of vascular endothelial growth factor tyrosine kinases, in combination with carboplatin and paclitaxel in patients with advanced non–small-cell lung cancer: The National Cancer Institute of Canada clinical trials group. *J Clin Oncol.* 2008;26(11):1871–1878.

107. Given CW, Sikorskii A, Tamkus D, et al. Managing symptoms among patients with breast cancer during chemotherapy: results of a two-arm behavioral trial. *J Clin Oncol.* 2008;26(36):5855–5862.

108. Mattioni J, Opperman DA, Solimando DA, Sataloff RT. Cancer chemotherapy: An overview and voice implications: In: Sataloff RT. *Professional Voice: The Science and Art of Clinical Care.* 4th ed. San Diego, CA: Plural Publishing; 2017:1137–1140.

109. Hamdan AL, Ashkar J, Sibai A, Oubari D, Husseini ST. Effect of fasting on voice in males. *Am J Otolaryngol.* 2011;32(2): 124–129.

110. Bllington A, Dayicioglu D, Smith P, Kiluk J. Review of procedures for reconstruction of soft tissue chest wall defects following advanced breast malignancies. *Cancer Control.* 2019;26:1–7.

6

Colorectal Cancer and Voice

Abdul-Latif Hamdan, Robert Thayer Sataloff, and Mary J. Hawkshaw

Epidemiology and Clinical Presentation of Colonic Cancer

Colorectal cancer (CRC) is the third most common cancer in the world, accounting for 1.8 million new cases in 2018.[1] It ranks third to lung and prostate cancers in men, and second to breast cancer in women.[2] The highest incidences have been reported in Northern Europe, Australia, and Northern America.[3] The risk of being diagnosed with CRC increases with age, particularly in the fifth decade.[4,5] In a review by Amersi et al, less than 10% of diagnosed CRC cases occur in patients younger than 50 years.[5] However, recent studies indicate that the incidence in subjects above the age of 50 years has decreased, while that of younger subjects has increased.[6,7] In a study by Bailey et al on age-related disparity in the incidence of CRC, the authors estimated an increase in colon and rectal cancer of 27.7% and 46%, respectively, in subjects in their fourth and fifth decades.[6] Colorectal cancer affects both genders with a higher risk reported in men compared to women.[8-11] Based on a study by Hirai et al that included 6218 subjects, male gender was a risk factor for colorectal neoplasia with an odds ratio of

1.95 irrespective of the anatomical location of the lesion.[8] Similarly, in a meta-analysis by Nguyen et al on gender as a risk factor for CRC, the pooled risk estimate for neoplasia in men was 1.83 in comparison to women.[9] It is noteworthy that the 5-year survival rate is lower in women compared to men, partially due to gender-related differences in screening tool specificity.[10]

According to the World Health Organization, CRC accounted for 861 000 mortalities a year in 2018.[12] This figure has dropped over the last decades secondary to improvement in screening, early diagnosis, and treatment.[13,14] Based on Colorectal Cancer Statistics 2017, the mortality rate of CRC witnessed a drop by almost one-third between 1999 and 2007.[15] This drop is commensurate with a yearly decrease of 2% as reported by Cronin et al.[13] CRC mortality remains considerably higher in countries with low economic status, such as Eastern Europe and parts of Latin America, in comparison with countries with high economic status, such as the United States and Western Europe.[16] In a review on CRC mortality rates in Europe by Bosetti et al, the authors highlighted the disparities in these rates among different countries. The approximate decline of 2% per year for men and women was more sustained in Northern Europe in comparison to Eastern countries such as the Czech Republic and Slovakia.[16] The differences in the rates across geographic areas can be attributed partially to Western behavior and lifestyle.[17] This is in alignment with the association between CRC incidence and the Human Development Index (HDI). In an ecological study by Khazaei et al looking at the geographic disparity of CRC across 172 countries, the authors reported a positive correlation between HDI and CRC incidence and mortality.[18]

The development of colorectal carcinoma starts with an abnormal proliferation of the gastrointestinal epithelium. This leads to the formation of a polyp that later evolves or transforms into carcinoma in patients with genetic mutations and or epigenetic abnormalities.[19-21] The site most commonly affected is the proximal colon in 41% of the cases, followed by the rectum and the distal colon in 28% and 22%, respectively.[22] There are various types of CRC, the most common of which is adenocarcinoma accounting for 95% of all cases.[23] Less common cancers include carcinoid tumors, gastrointestinal stromal tumors, lymphomas, and sarcomas.[23-24] Several risk factors for CRC have been identified in the literature. These include diet, alcohol consumption, smoking, caffeine, obesity, physical activity, and intake of nonsteroidal anti-inflammatory drugs.[25-36] He et al in 2019 reported a lower risk of CRC in subjects who consume a diet rich in cereal fibers and whole grains. The hazard ratios reported were 0.75 and 0.72, respectively.[25] This concurs with the review by Thanikachalam and Khan that supported the protective role of nutrition in the prevalence of CRC.[26] Excessive meat and saturated fat consumption has been shown to increase the risk of CRC.[27] Suggested mechanisms include increased formation of deoxycholic acid and lithocholic acid.[28] Excessive alcohol consumption has

also been linked strongly to the increased risk of colorectal polyps and cancer.[29,30] Based on a study by Pelucchi et al, consuming 4 alcoholic drinks or more a day increases the predisposition to develop cancer by 50%. The authors examined the relation between various cancers in the body and the extent of alcohol consumption.[31] This review agreed with the review of the World Cancer Research Fund and the report of the International Agency for Research of Cancer, both of which confirmed the link between alcohol intake and CRC in men.[32] Nicotine and its carcinogenic metabolic derivatives may also increase the odds of developing colorectal cancer.[33] In a meta-analysis looking at the association between cigarette smoking and CRC, Botteri et al reported a dose-dependent association and an absolute increase in risk of 10.8% cases per 100 000 person-years.[33] These findings agree with the review of Fedewa et al on the major risk factors for cancer in the United States, which highlights the high prevalence of cigarette smoking (17.8%) in adults nationally.[34] Obesity and increased body mass index (BMI) have also been shown to increase the chance of developing CRC.[35] The increase has been attributed to the inflammatory state induced by excess adipose tissue in obese subjects with unhealthy eating habits. Physical activity has been shown to reduce the prevalence of colorectal cancer and its mortality. In a large review by Shaw et al, the pooled association of CRC with physical activity ranged between 0.65 and 0.74 depending on BMI.[36]

In addition to the aforementioned risk factors, past medical history of diabetes, inflammatory bowel diseases, and positive family history of CRC have been associated with a higher incidence of CRC. A meta-analysis in 2016 by Luo et al showed that diabetes mellitus (DM) increases the risk of colorectal neoplasia with a relative risk of 1.35.[37] This is in agreement with a large cohort study on 7598 cases, which also demonstrated an association between DM and risk of CRC.[38] Similarly, inflammatory bowel diseases such as ulcerative colitis increase the cumulative incidence of CRC by almost 10% at 40 years in comparison to normal controls.[39] Last but not least, a positive family history of CRC is an important risk factor. Based on a review of the literature on familial risks of colorectal cancer, Butterworth et al reported an increase in the pooled risk estimate for CRC to 2.24 when a first-degree relative was affected, and to 3.97 when 2 relatives were affected.[40] In another systematic review by Mehraban that included 906 981 patients, the authors reported a relative risk of CRC of 1.87 when a first-degree relative was affected and emphasized the importance of screening patients with positive family history.[41]

Patients diagnosed with colorectal cancer suffer marked reduction in quality of life. This is secondary either to symptoms confined to the locoregional growth of the tumor, such as hematochezia, tenesmus, and bleeding, or to distant metastasis. These symptoms may include incremental pain, neuropathies, difficulty sleeping, decreased physical functioning, stress, and depression.[42–45] Janseen et al reported worsening quality of life in CRC patients in comparison to the general population,[43] and Denlinger et al emphasized the role of health care providers in addressing this condition.[42] This problem is not only disease induced but also treatment induced, as numerous adverse events have been reported following chemoradiation therapy in the treatment of CRC.[46–48] These are not limited to physical symptoms such as changes in bowel habits but also to emotional symptoms and social impediments.[46] It is worth noting that treatment-induced adverse events are more pronounced in long-term survivors, the number of whom has increased markedly due to early detection.[49,50]

Given the diverse clinical presentation of CRC with its potentially indolent course, and the strong link of voice to systemic diseases, this chapter reviews the different mechanisms by which patients with colorectal cancer may suffer from change in voice quality throughout the course of the disease and its management. A review of the literature on this topic is included. This information is invaluable to otolaryngologists who encounter patients with dysphonia and history of colorectal carcinoma.

Disease-Induced Dysphonia

Disease-induced dysphonia in patients with colorectal carcinoma can be the result of disease metastasis to the larynx and its contiguous structures, or disease metastasis to intrathoracic structures along the course of the recurrent laryngeal nerve. Other possible causes include body fatigue and the psychopathologic profile of affected patients.

Disease Metastasis to Laryngeal Structures

Dysphonia in patients with CRC can be the result of disease metastasis to the larynx. The occurrence of laryngeal metastasis is rare; but when present, it invariably denotes lung metastasis, which is typically the route to the larynx.[50–52] A review of the literature shows numerous cases of CRC metastasizing to the larynx. In 1972, Whicker et al described a patient with sigmoid carcinoma who presented with hoarseness and stridor 2 years after surgical treatment. On laryngeal examination, the patient had a reddish subglottic mass. Biopsy and histologic examination of that mass revealed adeno-carcinoma consistent with the primary neoplastic lesion. The patient was treated successfully by irradiation with complete regression of the tumor.[53] In 1976, Levine and Applebaum reported a patient with ad-enocarcinoma of the ascending colon who presented initially with history of cough, choking, and globus sensation. On laryngeal examination, he had a large, pedunculated, hemorrhagic laryngeal mass arising from the right arytenoid.[54] Pathologic examina-tion of the lesion revealed adenocarcinoma. Further metastatic workup led to the diag-nosis of a lesion at the right hepatic flexure. In 1983, Abemayor et al described a patient with breast carcinoma and adenocarcinoma of the transverse colon who presented with hoarseness and throat pain in addition to neck swelling. On laryngeal examination, the patient had a large supraglottic mass obliterating the pyriform sinus and fixing the right vocal fold. The patient had a bi-opsy of that mass followed by a tracheotomy to secure the airway. The microscopic ap-pearance of the lesion was similar to that of the colon, namely, mucin-secreting ad-enocarcinoma.[55] In 1985, Batsakis reported 11 patients with laryngeal metastasis at necropsy, one of whom had colorectal ad-enocarcinoma as a primary neoplasia. The age and clinical presentation of that patient were not described.[56] In 1990, Cavicchi et al reported a 59-year-old woman who pre-sented with dysphonia and dyspnea a year after having undergone surgery for a well-differentiated adenocarcinoma of the colon with metastasis to the lungs. On laryngeal examination, she had a sessile subglottic polypoidal lesion, the histology of which was consistent with metastatic colonic ad-enocarcinoma. Conservative excision of the laryngeal lesion was performed while sparing the larynx.[57] In 1996, Nicolai et al reviewed 1442 cases of laryngeal malig-nancies and reported 2 cases of metastatic laryngeal tumors with colonic cancer as a primary neoplasia. The first patient was a 53-year-old woman diagnosed with well-differentiated adenocarcinoma of the colon who presented with shortness of breath secondary to a large subglottic mass. The biopsy of the laryngeal lesion was consis-tent with the primary neoplasia. The sec-ond patient was a 58-year-old woman with moderately differentiated colon adenocarci-noma who also had dyspnea secondary to 2 sessile subglottic lesions. The pathology of the laryngeal lesions was similar to that of the primary tumor.[58] In 1997, Puxeddu de-scribed a 65-year-old man who developed symptoms of airway distress and dysphonia 2 years after being diagnosed and treated for colonic adenocarcinoma. On examina-tion, the patient had a left transglottic le-sion with partial erosion of the thyroid and cricoid cartilages and fixation of the left true vocal fold. Histologic examination of the laryngeal lesion also showed moderately differentiated adenocarcinoma similar to the primary colon tumor.[59] In 1998, Hilger described a patient with rectal adenocarci-noma who presented with airway obstruc-tive symptoms and dysphonia 3 years after treatment. On laryngeal examination, the patient had narrowing of the glottis with extrinsic mass compression. Neck and la-ryngeal biopsies showed a nonthyroid ad-enocarcinoma with features comparable to the rectal neoplastic lesion. Further histo-logic examination of the laryngeal speci-men confirmed metastatic infiltration of the larynx.[60] In 2005, Sano et al, reported a patient with dyspnea and dysphonia 10 years after having undergone colectomy and lobectomy for a colon adenocarcinoma with lung metastasis. On laryngeal exami-nation, the patient had a large mass almost occluding the subglottic space and neces-sitating a tracheotomy to secure the airway.

The histopathologic examination of that mass confirmed that the lesion was metastatic adenocarcinoma.[61] In 2006, Marioni et al, described a 78-year-old patient who presented with a transglottic mass that involved both vocal folds 5 years after being diagnosed and treated for colon adenocarcinoma. Computed tomography (CT) of the larynx showed invasion of the thyroid cartilage with narrowing of the airway. The patient had total laryngectomy and thyroidectomy, and the laryngeal pathology was consistent with metastatic CRC adenocarcinoma.[62] In 2007, Ramanathan et al reported a 51-year-old man who presented with a neck mass and change in voice quality. Laryngeal examination revealed an immobile right vocal fold, and CT showed a mass eroding the thyroid cartilage and hyoid bone. Histopathologic examination of that lesion was consistent with moderately differentiated adenocarcinoma. Further radiologic evaluation looking for a primary mass revealed a rectal mass, the pathology of which was similar to the laryngeal lesion.[63] In 2011, Ta and Kim described a 60-year-old man who presented with dyspnea and dysphonia 4 years after being diagnosed and treated for rectal adenocarcinoma and lung metastasis. The laryngeal symptoms were due to subglottic narrowing with tattered appearance of the cricoid cartilage and upper tracheal rings. The lesion was resected submucosally, and the pathology was consistent with adenocarcinoma of rectal origin, positively staining for CK20.[52] The patient had left supraclavicular lymphadenopathy that substantiated a lymphogenous metastatic route. In 2014, Terashima et al reported a 54-year-old woman who developed laryngeal metastasis 3 years after being diagnosed with moderately differentiated adenocarcinoma of the colon. The patient presented with hoarseness and a right subglottic nodular mass on laryngeal

endoscopy. The pathology examination of the laryngeal tissue was similar to that of the primary lesion.[51]

Laryngeal metastasis should be considered in the differential diagnosis of patients presenting with a laryngeal mass and history of CRC. Both genders are affected, and the mean age at the time of diagnosis usually is between the sixth and ninth decades.[52,56] The diagnosis of laryngeal metastasis can be challenging, given the large lapse of time between the onset of CRC and laryngeal symptoms. The clinical picture of affected patients may be similar to that observed in those with primary laryngeal tumors. Patients may be asymptomatic or complain of symptoms related to airway compromise and/or change in voice quality. Based on the review by Ta and Kim, dyspnea and dysphonia are the presenting complaints in patients with CRC and laryngeal metastasis in 60% and 20% of the cases, respectively. Other rare symptoms that may precede or follow the diagnosis include referred otalgia and globus sensation.[52] The laryngeal examination may be nonspecific. The most common pathology seen on laryngeal endoscopy is a submucosal nodular or fungating lesion with intact overlying mucosa. The laryngeal sites most commonly affected are the supraglottis and subglottis.[64,65] Transglottic lesions are seen in only 21% of the cases, and the glottis is rarely affected (7%).[52] In cases of transglottic lesions with erosion of the laryngeal framework, patients also may present with a neck mass or swelling. The diagnosis of laryngeal metastasis in patients with CRC requires adequate tissue sampling and immunohistochemistry evaluation using specific tumor markers. It is important to note that by the time the diagnosis of laryngeal metastasis is made, patients are usually in the terminal stage of the disease. The treatment strategy should be individualized, taking into consideration the overall health of the patient, the biological behavior of the tumor, the symptoms, and the extent of the laryngeal pathology. Commonly adopted treatment modalities of laryngeal metastasis include endoscopic resection, partial or total laryngectomy, and tracheotomy to alleviate airway obstruction. Nevertheless, it should be kept in mind that the overall prognosis is usually poor. The longest survival of 4½ years has been reported by Terashima et al following a laryngectomy for a laryngeal metastatic adenocarcinoma.[51]

Disease Metastasis to Structures Contiguous With the Larynx

Dysphonia in patients with CRC can be secondary to metastasis to structures contiguous with the larynx.[66] This is not surprising given that 1 out of 3 patients with CRC has metastasis at the time of diagnosis.[67] Among the contiguous structures, the thyroid gland is a common metastatic target. Although this latter is affected more frequently by renal and pulmonary malignancies, it also can be affected by CRC.[68,69] The metastasis is thought to be hematogenous given the high rate of concomitant lung and liver metastasis in affected patients.[70] A less common route for metastasis that may explain solitary thyroid metastatic nodules in the absence of liver metastasis is the vertebral circulation. The tumor cells may drain through the vertebral vessels to the inferior vena cava.[71] However, the fast blood flow and high oxygen and iodine environment are considered by some authors as impediments to hematogenous implantation of metastatic cells.[72,73]

The prevalence of thyroid metastasis in patients with CRC varies in the literature

between autopsy series and clinical series, with higher figures being reported in the former. In 2006, Lievre et al reported a prevalence of 0.1% in their review of the medical records of 5862 patients with CRC.[66] In 2013, Froylich et al reviewed the literature and reported 34 cases of CRC metastasizing to the thyroid gland. Tumors arising from the rectum and sigmoid accounted for the majority of the cases, with concomitant involvement of other organs in almost 85% of patients.[74] In 2015, Onorati et al reviewed the literature on CRC metastasis to the thyroid gland and reported 52 cases, of which 3 were solitary thyroid lesions. The authors reported the fourth case and emphasized the importance of cytologic examination of asymptomatic thyroid nodules in patients with suspected metastatic lesions.[75] In a review of 1295 patients with thyroid carcinoma that included 10 metastatic cases, CRC was the primary tumor in 3 patients.[68] Intrathyroid metastasis was highlighted in the differential diagnosis of thyroid carcinoma. In another study on nonthyroid cancer by Chung et al in 2012, CRC accounted for 10.4% of metastatic thyroid cases, while renal carcinoma was the predominant primary, accounting for 48.1% of the cases.[69] In the multi-institutional review by HooKim et al in 2015, colorectal cancer accounted for only 3.6% of secondary thyroid neoplasms. The majority of patients had renal cell carcinoma as a primary metastatic tumor (50%).[76] Similarly, in 2016, Surov et al reported CRC in 12% of 33 patients with thyroid metastasis. Again, renal carcinoma was the primary tumor in 79% of the cases.[77]

Despite the ubiquity of reports on thyroid metastasis in CRC,[67,70,75,76,78–91] only a few described dysphonia as a symptom in affected patients.[66,81,84,85,88,92] In 2000, Danikas et al reported a 79-year-old man who presented with dysphagia and dysphonia secondary to an enlarging neck mass. The patient underwent total thyroidectomy and laryngectomy with neck dissection after the diagnosis of thyroid anaplastic carcinoma by needle biopsy had been suggested. Further workup of the patient revealed a rectal mass consistent with poorly differentiated carcinoma.[92] In 2006, Lievre et al reported thyroid metastasis in 6 of 5862 cases of CRC, 3 of whom had dysphonia in addition to dysphagia and cervical adenopathy. The diagnosis was made using radiologic imaging, and treatment consisted primarily of thyroidectomy except in 1 patient who had distant organ metastasis.[66] In the same year, Youn et al reported an 85-year-old woman who developed hoarseness and neck swelling almost 2 years after being diagnosed and treated for colon cancer. On examination, she had an enlarged thyroid gland with elevated serum thyrotropin (TSH). Core biopsy and immune-histochemical staining of the suspected site revealed poorly differentiated adenocarcinoma that stained positive for carcinoembryonic antigen (CEA).[81] In 2014, Alherabi et al described a 40-year-old man with colon adenocarcinoma and diffuse metastasis who presented with dysphonia and dysphagia. On examination, he had a thyroid mass that was consistent with colon metastatic disease on fine needle aspiration and biopsy.[88] The authors emphasized the need to have a low threshold of suspicion in the workup of patients with CRC and a thyroid lesion. In 2016, Minami et al described a 61-year-old woman with a history of colon cancer and metastasis to the lungs and liver who presented with hoarseness, thyroid gland enlargement, and cervical lymphadenopathy. Immunohistochemical staining of the thyroid specimen confirmed the diagnosis of metastatic adenocarcinoma that was treated by chemotherapy following surgery.[85] In 2017, Coehlo

et al reported a 64-year-old woman who had been diagnosed with sigmoid cancer and lung metastasis who presented with goiter and a hypodense thyroid nodule on positron emission tomography (PET) scan several years after treatment. In addition, she developed internal jugular adenopathy, the cytology of which confirmed the diagnosis of metastatic CRC. Hoarseness and dysphagia were reported as symptoms of disease recurrence 10 months after treatment.[84]

In all the reported cases, the diagnosis of thyroid metastasis in patients with CRC was made during the staging process of the disease or on routine follow-up. The time between diagnosis of CRC and thyroid metastasis ranged from 6 months to 20 years.[74,76] This explains the advanced stage of the disease at the time of diagnosis in up to two-thirds of the cases.[74] A high index of suspicion is needed to make the diagnosis of thyroid metastasis given that 50% may be asymptomatic.[66] In the review of Surov et al, the main presenting complaint was a painless neck mass in 85% of the cases.[77] A minority of patients may present with hypothyroidism secondary to the metastasis, or with Hashimoto thyroiditis coexisting with CRC metastasis.[81,93] A rising serum level of CEA usually mandates radiologic investigation using CT and magnetic resonance imaging. The thyroid metastatic lesion usually is described as nonhomogeneous, hypodense, and irregular in shape.[77] Additional radiologic tests in the workup of affected patients include [18F]-fluoro-2-deoxy-D-glucose position emission tomography.[82] In the review by Froylich et al of 34 cases with thyroid disease, PET-CT was helpful in detecting the signs of metastasis prior to histologic examination.[74] It is important to note that not all cases of thyroid metastasis from CRC have radiologic evidence of metastasis to the lungs and liver. Skip patterns with isolated thyroid metastatic nodules have been reported. In 2005, Philips et al described an 81-year-old woman diagnosed with colon adenocarcinoma who presented with thyroid metastasis in the absence of other distant metastasis.[83] Fine needle aspiration and cytology (FNAC) is gaining more popularity as a reliable diagnostic test in differentiating primary thyroid tumors from metastatic lesions. The combination of FNAC with molecular biology investigation in the diagnosis and management of solitary thyroid nodules has been further emphasized by Onorati et al in their review of solitary thyroid metastatic nodules in patients with CRC.[75] Metastatic thyroid gland lesions usually stain negative for CK7, an important marker for primary thyroid tumors, and positive for CK20, a reliable tumor marker for CRC.[85] Once the diagnosis is made, the treatment strategy is based on the overall medical condition of the patient and on the presence or absence of other metastatic sites. If metastasis is confined to the thyroid gland, curative thyroidectomy with or without neck dissection is usually performed. In the presence of invasion of the laryngotracheal framework, cricotracheal resection and anastomosis may be needed.[94] In cases of diffuse metastasis, palliative chemotherapy is recommended.[95]

Mass Compression of the Recurrent Laryngeal Nerve

With advances in radiologic imaging, colorectal cancer has been shown to metastasize to various sites in the body, with the lungs and liver being affected most commonly.[96,97] Metastasis to intrathoracic structures has been described and considered the result of re-metastasis from metastatic lesions to the lungs. There are many reports in the literature of CRC metastasizing to intrathoracic structures in the context of distant metastasis late in the course of the disease.[89,98–106] Yamada et al described a 64-year-old woman with colon cancer who developed an 18-mm inferior mediastinal mass seen on PET-CT, 3½ years after her initial diagnosis. The pathology was consistent with adenocarcinoma similar to the primary neoplasm.[99] Yamamoto et al reported a patient with cecum cancer who was referred for investigation and management of 2 mediastinal masses that appeared 15 months after treatment. Radiologic imaging showed no invasion of adjacent structures with an increase in uptake F-18 on PET. Surgical resection of these lesions revealed rectal cancer metastasis.[89] Lee et al reported a mediastinal metastatic tumor in a patient with colon cancer 4 years after treatment. The patient underwent total thymectomy, and the pathology was consistent with adenocarcinoma suggesting metastasis from the colon.[100] Iwata reported a 75-year-old man who developed a 6-cm mediastinal mass close to 2 years after being treated for his colon cancer. Histopathologic examination confirmed the metastatic nature of the lymphadenopathy.[101] Sano et al described a case of posterior mediastinal metastasis with infiltration of the descending aorta in a 29-year-old man diagnosed with colon adenocarcinoma.[102] The lesion was resected successfully through a posterolateral thoracotomy.[102] Kuba et al reported a 57-year-old woman diagnosed with moderately differentiated adenocarcinoma of the sigmoid colon who presented with an abnormal finding on chest x-ray. Further radiologic evaluation using CT showed a 5-cm mediastinal mass, the aspiration of which using the transbronchial route was suggestive of adenocarcinoma. The lesion was resected, and histopathologic examination was similar to the primary sigmoid neoplasia.[103] Kitami et al described 2 cases of mediastinal metastasis following surgical resection of colon cancer. There was involvement of the para-aortic lymph nodes despite the lack of lung metastasis.[105]

In all of these reports, the diagnosis of mediastinal involvement was made either during the preoperative staging of CRC or late during the posttreatment follow-up with the use of CT, PET, or serum testing for CEA level. In any case, dysphonia was not described as a presenting or delayed symptom of mediastinal lymph node metastasis. Nevertheless, compression of the recurrent laryngeal nerve by an enlarged mediastinal mass remains a potential cause of vocal fold paralysis in patients with CRC. The presence of vocal and swallowing dysfunction in affected subjects should always alert the treating physician to the possibility of mediastinal lymph node metastasis. When suspected, laryngeal examination and radiologic investigation to exclude vocal fold paralysis are warranted. In addition, if lung metastasis impairs lung function or partially obstructs airflow, that will affect the power source of the voice and could lead to dysphonia.

Body Fatigue, Pain, and Vocal Dysfunction in Patients With Colorectal Carcinoma

Patients with CRC suffer from a large array of systemic symptoms aside from those secondary to the local growth of the tumor. Numerous investigators have shown that affected individuals often complain of excessive fatigue, nausea, and dysfunction of many systems in the body leading to a decline in their global health.[107-110] Based on a study by Lashbrook et al, CRC cancer survivors display high scores for fatigability and low scores for physical performance in comparison to healthy individuals.[107] Based

on the analysis by Agasi et al, the systemic complaints are independent of age and are clustered invariably under emotional and pain-related symptoms in addition to dyspnea.[108] Heldens et al, in their study on the association between physical fitness and surgical outcome in patients with CRC undergoing resection, highlighted the high level of perceived fatigability and the preoperative decline in physical activity in affected patients.[109] The results of the study by Thong et al in their survey using the Multidimensional Fatigue Inventory and other validated questionnaires showed that 1 out of 5 patients with cancer (22%) experience high fatigue and moderate distress (class 3 cancer-related fatigue).[110] It is also important to note that cancer-related body fatigue and the decrease in exercise function are associated with body mass index and muscle mass. Vissers et al have shown that patients with high BMI and increased waist circumference are more likely to experience fatigue and a decrease in both physical and emotional function. The study was conducted using a self-assessment questionnaire on health-related quality of life in 1111 patients with CRC, two-thirds of whom (66%) were either overweight or obese.[111] Similarly, Neefjes et al demonstrated the close association between muscle mass and cancer-related fatigue. In their study on 223 cancer patients in which skeletal muscle index (SMI) was computed using CT imaging and fatigue was assessed using a validated assessment questionnaire, the authors demonstrated a negative correlation between cancer-related fatigue and SMI, and alluded to the positive effect of increasing muscle mass as a mitigating factor.[112]

All of these assertions on the increase in body fatigability and the decrease in physical function in patients with CRC lead us to conclude that the vocal apparatus, given its musculoskeletal structure, is in jeopardy.

Phonation is a complex process that mandates adequate health and fitness, more so in professional voice users in whom singing and physical fitness are strongly intertwined, and in whom the importance of good athletic conditioning, especially aerobics, is well established. Disease-induced body fatigue in patients with CRC can inadvertently affect phonation through its impact on the musculoskeletal structure of the phonatory system. A more detailed discussion on the interplay between body fatigue and voice can be found in the chapter entitled "Sleep, body fatigue, and voice" in the book *Laryngeal Manifestations of Systemic Diseases*.[113]

Depression, Anxiety, and Voice in Patients With Colorectal Carcinoma

Patients diagnosed with CRC experience depression and anxiety symptoms more than healthy subjects. Based on an investigation by Bamonti et al, almost 1 out of 5 patients with cancer suffers from depression that may persist over the years. The most important psychosocial predictors of depression are prior history of depression symptoms and/or pain.[114] Other factors associated with anxiety and depression in patients with CRC include having a high educational level and living alone in a rural area.[107] Gonzalez-Saenz de Tejada et al reported an association between social support, functional status, and anxiety in patients with CRC. Improvement in social support leads to a decrease in the level of anxiety with subsequent improvement in quality of life.[115] The impact of high levels of anxiety and depression on quality of life has been emphasized by Trudel-Fitzgerald et al in their investigation on the association between distress and engaging in unhealthy lifestyle behavior.[116] Dhillon et al also reported a correlation between cognitive ability and CRC, which can lead to worsening in quality of life.[117] Similarly, Reese et al conducted a study on 141 patients with colorectal cancer and alluded to the need to address the psychosocial-induced impairment in quality of life that was more significant in women compared to men.[118]

Given that patients with CRC suffer from high levels of anxiety and depression, and given the adverse impact of affective mood disorders on phonation, it is reasonable to suggest that CRC patients are more likely to experience phonatory disturbances. The aforementioned hypothesis is well-supported in the literature on voice and systemic diseases.[119] Numerous studies have demonstrated the etiologic role of depression and anxiety in patients with functional and organic voice disorders. To list a few, in 2008 Dietrich et al showed that patients with vocal fold pathologies had higher scores of stress in comparison to normal subjects. The pathogenic role of stress has been correlated with laryngopharyngeal reflux disease and the higher self-perceived level of stress.[120] Misono et al, in their study on the relationship between distress and impact of dysphonia on quality of life, concurred that there is an association between voice handicap and psychological distress and an inverse relationship between voice handicap and low perceived control.[121]

In summary, long-term survivors of CRC experience emotional disturbances that negatively impact their quality of life. Despite the lack of any investigation on the association between dysphonia and disease-induced depression or anxiety in patients with CRC, affected patients are at higher risk of developing phonatory disturbances. Future investigation looking at the association or causality between these 2 variables is needed.

Treatment-Induced Dysphonia

Surgical Treatment of Colorectal Carcinoma and Dysphonia

Treatment of CRC consists primarily of surgical resection with or without adjuvant chemoradiation. In most cases, the main treatment is local excision or resection of the affected site with anastomosis or colostomy. Complete mesocolic resection or total mesorectal excision is done based on the location and extent of the tumor. These procedures usually are performed using either an open approach or laparoscopically, with excellent disease control and a 5-year survival that can exceed 90% in early stages of the disease.[122] Nevertheless, surgical treatment has been shown to markedly impact quality of life in patients with advanced disease. In a study by Nasvall et al on patients with a permanent stoma following surgical resection of rectal carcinoma, the authors showed a lower quality of life in the study group in comparison to the control group.[123] Kasparek et al also have reported a decrease in quality of life and higher scores for body fatigue and weight loss in patients who underwent abdominoperineal resection in comparison to those who had coloanal anastomosis.[124] Scheneider et al reported fatigue in 23% and limited activity in 15% of long-term CRC survivors. The study was conducted on 474 survivors in whom self-reported symptoms 4 years after diagnosis were analyzed. Most of the health-related symptoms were more prominent in patients who underwent additional radiation therapy.[125] In a study on the impact of different treatment regimens on health-related quality of life, McLachlan et al reported negative adverse effects leading to weight loss and fatigue in patients with CRC.[126]

Given the well-known impact of body fatigue on voice, it is suggested that patients with CRC who experience body fatigue and weight loss following surgical resection are at higher risk for change in voice quality. Future research is needed.

Chemoradiation Therapy of Colorectal Carcinoma and Dysphonia

Similar to surgery, chemoradiation therapy may lead to body fatigue and decreased physical ability. Barreto et al, in 2016, investigated chemotherapy-induced cachexia in an animal study using common chemotherapy regimens such as 5-FU in combination with leucovorin and oxaliplatin.[127] The authors demonstrated that cachexia, defined as "increased fatigability and loss of muscle function,"[127(p1)] is secondary to drug-induced muscle atrophy and depletion in muscle fibers of mitochondrial content. Other significant adverse effects of chemotherapy that may jeopardize phonation are neurotoxicity and pulmonary changes. Chemotherapeutic agents including antimetabolites such as fluorouracil and methotrexate, and alkylating agents such as cyclophosphamide can induce irreversible neural damage to the laryngeal and respiratory system resulting in reduced fine control of vocal pitch and loudness. Similarly, drug-induced pulmonary infiltrates and/or interstitial changes reported with the use of plant alkaloids (taxanes) and endocrine agents (tamoxifen) can decrease the breathing capacity and support.[128] Chemotherapy also may adversely impact voice by causing dehydration secondary to vomiting and diarrhea.[129-131] These may carry potential risks to the professional voice given the paramount importance of hydration in phonation. In a review by Buccafusca G et al, patients with CRC on treatment may suffer from gastrointestinal disorders in addition to sensory neuropathy and sexual dysfunction.[132] Adverse laryngeal events also may arise secondary to chemotherapy-induced blood dyscrasia. This may jeopardize the phonatory apparatus by altering laryngeal blood supply and interfering with the normal repair mechanisms.[128] Dysphonia also may be the result of targeted therapy. Caruso et al described a patient with metastatic colon carcinoma who presented with dysphonia following therapy with antivascular endothelial growth factor monoclonal antibody. On laryngeal examination, she had bilateral, whitish vocal fold lesions with disruption of the mucosal waves. These lesions were attributed to vascular supply inhibition with secondary necrosis.[133] Similar drug-induced complications have been reported in patients receiving bevacizumab, an angiogenesis inhibitor, in combination with other chemotherapeutic agents in the management of various cancers.[134,135] Finally, an important side effect to consider, especially with the use of alkylating agents, is ototoxicity. Hearing is crucial, especially in professional voice users in whom auditory feedback is essential for optimal vocal performance.[136]

The short- and long-term side effects of chemoradiation therapy may adversely affect phonation given the strong link between voice and well-being. More research is needed to establish the cause/effect relationships between the various chemotherapeutic agents used in the treatment of CRC and voice.

References

1. World Cancer Research Fund. Colorectal cancer statistics. Published 2019. Accessed September 2, 2019. https://www.wcrf.org/dietandcancer/cancer-trends/colorectal-cancer-statistics

2. National Cancer Institute. Common cancer types. Updated February 21, 2019. Accessed September 2, 2019. https://www.cancer.gov/types/common-cancers

3. Meyer B, Are C. Current status and future directions in colorectal cancer. *Indian J Surg Oncol.* 2017;8(4):455–456.

4. Siegel RL, Miller KD, Jemal A. Cancer statistics, 2018. *CA Cancer J Clin.* 2018;68(1): 7–30.

5. Amersi F, Agustin M, Ko CY. Colorectal cancer: Epidemiology, risk factors, and health services. *Clin Colon Rectal Surg.* 2005;18(3): 133–140.

6. Bailey CE, Hu CY, You YN, et al. Increasing disparities in the age-related incidences of colon and rectal cancers in the United States, 1975–2010. *JAMA Surg.* 2015;150(1):17–22.

7. Kim NH, Jung YS, Yang HJ, et al. Prevalence of and risk factors for colorectal neoplasia in asymptomatic young adults (20–39 Years Old). *Clin Gastroenterol Hepatol.* 2019;17(1): 115–122.

8. Hirai HW, Ching JY, Wu JC, Sung JJ, Chan FK, Ng SC. Risk factors for advanced colorectal neoplasms in the proximal colon in 6218 subjects undergoing complete colonoscopy. *J Gastroenterol Hepatol.* 2019;34(1):113–119.

9. Nguyen SP, Bent S, Chen YH, Terdiman JP. Gender as a risk factor for advanced neoplasia and colorectal cancer: a systematic review and meta-analysis. *Clin Gastroenterol Hepatol.* 2009;7(6):676–681.

10. Kim SE, Paik HY, Yoon H, Lee JE, Kim N, Sung MK. Sex-and gender-specific disparities in colorectal cancer risk. *World J Gastroenterol.* 2015;21(17):5167–5175.

11. Kolligs FT. Diagnostics and epidemiology of colorectal cancer. *Visc Med.* 2016; 32(3):158–164.

12. Macrae FA. Colorectal cancer: epidemiology, risk factors and protective factors. World Health Organization GLOBOCAN. 2019. Updated August 6, 2019. Accessed

September 2, 2019. https://www.uptodate .com/contents/colorectal-cancer-epidemi ology-risk-factors-and-protective-factors

13. Cronin KA, Lake AJ, Scott S, et al. Annual report to the nation on the status of cancer, part I: national cancer statistics. *Cancer.* 2018; 124(13):2785–2800.

14. Siegel RL, Miller KD, Jemal A. Cancer statistics, 2019. *CA Cancer J Clin.* 2019;69 (1):7.

15. Siegel RL, Miller KD, Fedewa SA et al. Colorectal cancer statistics, 2017. *CA Cancer J Clin.* 2017;67(3):177–193.

16. Bosetti C, Levi F, Rosato V, et al. Recent trends in colorectal cancer mortality in Europe. *Int J Cancer.* 2011;129(1):180–191.

17. Favoriti P, Carbone G, Greco M, Pirozzi F, Pirozzi RE, Corcione F. Worldwide burden of colorectal cancer: A review. *Updates Surg.* 2016;68(1):7–11.

18. Khazaei S, Rezaeian S, Khazaei S et al. Effects of human development index and its components on colorectal cancer incidence and mortality: a global ecological study. *Asian Pac J Cancer Prev.* 2015;17(S3):253–256.

19. Pancione M, Remo A, Colantuoni V. Genetic and epigenetic events generate multiple pathways in colorectal cancer progression. *Patholog Res Int.* 2012;2012:509348.

20. Ewing I, Hurley JJ, Josephides E, Millar A. The molecular genetics of colorectal cancer. *Frontline Gastroenterol.* 2014;5(1):26–30.

21. Valastyan S, Weinberg RA. Tumor metastasis: molecular insights and evolving paradigms. *Cell.* 2011;147(2):275–292.

22. Cheng L, Eng C, Nieman LZ, Kapadia AS, Du XL. Trends in colorectal cancer incidence by anatomic site and disease stage in the United States from 1976 to 2005. *Am J Clin Oncol.* 2011;34(6):573–580.

23. American Cancer Society. What is colorectal cancer? Updated February 21, 2018. Accessed August 29, 2019. https://www.can cer.org/cancer/colon-rectal-cancer/about /what-is-colorectal-cancer.html

24. American Society of Clinical Oncology. Colorectal cancer: introduction. Updated November 2018. Accessed August 29, 2019. https://www.cancer.net/cancer-types/colo rectal-cancer/introduction

25. He X, Wu K, Zhang X, et al. Dietary intake of fiber, whole grains and risk of colorectal cancer: An updated analysis according to food sources, tumor location and molecular subtypes in two large US cohorts. *Int J Cancer.* 2019;145(11):3040–3051.

26. Thanikachalam K, Khan G. Colorectal cancer and nutrition. *Nutrients.* 2019;11(1): 164.

27. Gerhardsson de Verdier M, Hagman U, Peters RK, Steineck G, Övervik E. Meat, cooking methods and colorectal cancer: a case referent-study in Stockholm. *Int J Cancer.* 1991;49(4):520–525.

28. Marley AR, Nan H. Epidemiology of colorectal cancer. *Int J Mol Epidemiol Genet.* 2016;7(3):105–114.

29. Cho E, Smith-Warner SA, Ritz J, et al. Alcohol intake and colorectal cancer: A pooled analysis of 8 cohort studies. *Ann Intern Med.* 2004;140(8):603–613.

30. Shrubsole MJ, Wu H, Ness RM, Shyr Y, Smalley WE, Zheng W. Alcohol drinking, cigarette smoking, and risk of colorectal adenomatous and hyperplastic polyps. *Am J Epidemiol.* 2008;167(9):1050–1058.

31. Pelucchi C, Tramacere I, Boffetta P, Negri E, La Vecchia C. Alcohol consumption and cancer risk. *Nutr Cancer.* 2011;63(7):983–990.

32. Roswall N, Weirderpass E. Alcohol as a risk factor for cancer: existing evidence in a global perspective. *J Prev Med Public Health.* 2015;48(1):1–9.

33. Botteri E, Iodice S, Bagnardi V, Raimondi S, Lowenfels AB, Maisonneuve P. Smoking and colorectal cancer: A meta-analysis. *JAMA.* 2008;300:2765–2778.

34. Fedewa SA, Sauer AG, Siegel RL, Jemal A. Prevalence of major risk factors and use of screening tests for cancer in the United States. *Cancer Epidemiol Biomarkers Prev.* 2015;24(4):637–652.

35. Stone TW, McPherson M, Gail Darlington L. Obesity and cancer: Existing and new

hypotheses for a causal connection. *EBio-Medicine*. 2018;30;14–28.

36. Shaw E, Farris MS, Stone CR, et al. Effects of physical activity on colorectal cancer risk among family history and body mass index subgroups: a systematic review and meta-analysis. *BMC Cancer*. 2018;18(1):71.

37. Luo S, Li JY, Zhao LN, et al. Diabetes mellitus increases the risk of colorectal neoplasia: an updated a meta-analysis. *Clin Res Hepatol Gastroenterol*. 2016;40(1):110–123.

38. Jarvandi S, Davidson NO, Schootman M. Increased risk of colorectal cancer in type 2 diabetes is independent of diet quality. *PLoS One*. 2013;8(9):e74616.

39. Rutter MD, Saunders BP, Wilkinson KH, et al. Thirty-year analysis of a colonoscopic surveillance program for neoplasia in ulcerative colitis. *Gastroenterology*. 2006;130(4):1030–1038.

40. Butterworth AS, Higgins JP, Pharoah P. Relative and absolute risk of colorectal cancer for individuals with a family history: A meta-analysis. *Eur J Cancer*. 2006;42(2):216–227.

41. Mehraban Far P, Alsahrani A, Yaghoobi M. Quantitative risk of positive family history in developing colorectal cancer: A meta-analysis. *World J Gastroenterol*. 2019;25(30):4278–4291.

42. Denlinger CS, Barsevick AM. The challenges of colorectal cancer survivorship. *J Natl Compr Canc Netw*. 2009;7(8):883–893.

43. Jansen L, Koch L, Brenner H, Arndt V. Quality of life among long-term (≥5 years) colorectal cancer survivors—systematic review. *Eur J Cancer*. 2010;46(16):2879–2888.

44. Floriani I, Torri V, Rulli E, et al. Performance of imaging modalities in diagnosis of liver metastases from colorectal cancer: a systematic review and meta-analysis. *J Magn Reson Imaging*. 2010;31(1):19–31.

45. Niekel MC, Bipat S, Stoker J. Diagnostic imaging of colorectal liver metastases with CT, MR imaging, FDG PET, and/or FDG PET/CT: a meta-analysis of prospective studies including patients who have not previously undergone treatment. *Radiology*. 2010;257(3):674–684.

46. Arndt V, Merx H, Stegmaier C, Ziegler H, Brenner H. Restrictions in quality of life in colorectal cancer patients over three years after diagnosis: a population based study. *Eur J Cancer*. 2006;42(12):1848–1857.

47. Ramsey SD, Berry K, Moinpour C, Giedzinska A, Andersen MR. Quality of life in long term survivors of colorectal cancer. *Am J Gastroenterol*. 2002;97(5):1228–1234.

48. Jansen L, Harrmann A, Stegmaier C, Singer S, Brenner H, Arndt V. Health-related quality of life during the 10 years after diagnosis of colorectal cancer: a population-based study. *J Clin Oncol*. 2011;29(24):3263–3269.

49. Glowacka-Mrotek I, Tarkowska M, Nowikiewicz T, et al. Prospective evaluation of the quality of life of patients undergoing surgery for colorectal cancer depending on the surgical technique. *Int J Colorectal Dis*. 2019;34(9):1601–1610.

50. Mols F, Vingerhoets AJ, Coebergh JW, van de Poll-Franse LV. Quality of life among long-term breast cancer survivors: a systematic review. *Eur J Cancer*. 2005;41(17):2613–2619.

51. Terashima S, Watanabe S, Shoji M. Long-term survival after resection of metastases in the lungs and larynx originating from sigmoid colon cancer: report of a case. *Fukushima J Med Sci*. 2014;60(1):82–85.

52. Ta JQ, Kim JY. Rectal adenocarcinoma metastatic to the larynx. *ENT*. 2011;90(4):E28–31.

53. Whicker JH, Carder GA, Devine KD. Metastasis to the larynx. Report of a case and review of the literature. *Arch Otolaryngol*. 1972;96:182–184.

54. Levine HL, Applebaum EL. Metastatic adenocarcinoma to the larynx: report of a case. *Trans Sect Am Otolaryngol Am Acad Ophthalmol Otolaryngol*. 1976;82(5):536–541.

55. Abemayor E, Cochran AJ, Calcaterra TC. Metastatic cancer to the larynx: Diagnosis and management. *Cancer*. 1983;52:1944–1948.

56. Batsakis JG, Luna MA, Byers RM. Metastases to the larynx. *Head Neck Surg*. 1985;7:458–460.

57. Cavicchi O, Farneti G, Occhiuzzi L, Sorrenti G. Laryngeal metastasis from colonic adenocarcinoma. *J Laryngol Otol.* 1990;104:730–732.

58. Nicolai P, Puxeddu R, Cappiello J, et al. Metastatic neoplasms to the larynx: report of three cases. *Laryngoscope.* 1996;106(7):851–855.

59. Puxeddu R, Pelagatti CL, Ambu R. Colon adenocarcinoma metastatic to the larynx. *Eur Arch Otorhinolaryngol.* 1997;254(7):353–355.

60. Hilger AW, Prichard AJ, Jones T. Adenocarcinoma of the larynx—a distant metastasis from a rectal primary. *J Laryngol Otol.* 1998;112(2):199–201.

61. Sano D, Matsuda H, Yoshida T, et al. A case of metastatic colon adenocarcinoma in the larynx. *Acta Oto-Laryngologica.* 2005;125(2):220–222.

62. Marioni G, De Filippis C, Ottaviano G, et al. Laryngeal metastasis from sigmoid colon adenocarcinoma followed by peristomal recurrence. *Acta Oto-Laryngologica.* 2006;126(6):661–663.

63. Ramanathan Y, Rajagopalan R, Abdul Rahman N. Laryngeal metastasis from a rectal carcinoma. *ENT.* 2007;86(11):685–686.

64. Glanz H, Kleinsasser O. Metastases to the larynx. *HNO.* 1978;26(5):163–167.

65. Ferlito A, Caruso G, Recher G. Secondary laryngeal tumors: Report of seven cases with review of the literature. *Arch Otolaryngol Head Neck Surg.* 1988;114:635–639.

66. Lièvre A, Leboulleux S, Boige V, et al. Thyroid metastases from colorectal cancer: the Institut Gustave Roussy experience. *Eur J Cancer.* 2006;42(12):1756–1759.

67. Jemal A, Tiwari RC, Murray T, et al. Cancer statistics, 2004. *CA Cancer J Clin.* 2004;54(1):8–29.

68. Moghaddam PA, Cornejo KM, Khan A. Metastatic carcinoma to the thyroid gland: A single institution 20-year experience and review of the literature. *Endocr Pathol.* 2013;24(3):116–124.

69. Chung AY, Tran TB, Brumund KT, Weisman RA, Bouvet M. Metastases to the thyroid: a review of the literature from the last decade. *Thyroid.* 2012;22(3):258–268.

70. Nakamura K, Nozawa K, Aoyagi Y, et al. A case report of thyroid gland metastasis associated with lung metastasis from colon cancer. *Tumori.* 2011;97(2):229–232.

71. Batson OV. The function of the vertebral veins and their role in the spread of metastases. *Ann Surg.* 1940;112(1):138–149.

72. Willis RA. Metastatic tumours in the thyroid gland. *Am J Pathol.* 1931;7(3):187–208.

73. Nixon IJ, Whitcher M, Glick J, et al. Surgical management of metastases to the thyroid gland. *Ann Surg Oncol.* 2011;18:800–804.

74. Froylich D, Shiloni E, Hazzan D. Metachronous colon metastasis to the thyroid: a case report and literature review. *Case Rep Surg.* 2013;2013:241678. doi:10.1155/2013/241678

75. Onorati M, Uboldi P, Bianchi CL, et al. Solitary thyroid metastasis from colon cancer: fine-needle aspiration cytology and molecular biology approach. *Pathologica.* 2015;107(3–4):192–196.

76. HooKim K, Gaitor J, Lin O, Reid MD. Secondary tumors involving the thyroid gland: A multi-institutional analysis of 28 cases diagnosed on fine-needle aspiration. *Diagn Cytopathol.* 2015;43(11):904–911.

77. Surov A, Machens A, Holzhausen HJ, Spielmann RP, Dralle H. Radiological features of metastases to the thyroid. *Acta Radiol.* 2016;57(4):444–450.

78. Kumamoto K, Utsumi Y, Sugano K, Hoshino M, Suzuki S, Takenoshita S. Colon carcinoma metastasis to the thyroid gland: report of a case with a review of the literature. *Tumori.* 2006;92(3):252–256.

79. Cherk MH, Moore M, Serpell J, Swain S, Topliss DJ. Metastatic colorectal cancer to a primary thyroid cancer. *World J Surg Oncol.* 2008;6:122.

80. Mesko TW, Friedman J, Sendzischew H, Nixon DD. Rectal carcinoma metastatic to the thyroid gland. *J Laryngol Otol.* 1996;110(2):192–195.

81. Youn JC, Rhee Y, Park SY, et al. Severe hypothyroidism induced by thyroid metastasis of colon adenocarcinoma: a case

report and review of the literature. *Endocr J.* 2006;53(3):339–343.

82. Malani AK, Gupta C, Rangineni S, Gupta V. Thyroid metastasis from colorectal cancer: role of [18F]-fluoro-2-deoxy-D-glucose positron emission tomography. *Clin Colorectal Cancer.* 2005;5(4):287–291.

83. Phillips JS, Lishman S, Jani P. Colonic carcinoma metastasis to the thyroid: a case of skip metastasis. *J Laryngol Otol.* 2005;119 (10):834–836.

84. Coelho MI, Albano MN, Costa Almeida CE, Reis LS, Moreira N, Almeida CM. Colon cancer metastasis to the thyroid gland: a case report. *Int J Surg Case Rep.* 2017;37: 221–224.

85. Minami S, Inoue K, Irie J, et al. Metastasis of colon cancer to the thyroid and cervical lymph nodes: a case report. *Surg Case Rep.* 2016;2(1):108–111.

86. Roloff GW, Yang Z, Wood LV, Neychev VK. Colon cancer metastasis to the thyroid gland: report of a case with unique molecular profile. *Clin Case Rep.* 2016;4(6): 549–553.

87. Yeo SJ, Kim KJ, Kim BY, et al. Metastasis of colon cancer to medullary thyroid carcinoma: a case report. *J Korean Med Sci.* 2014;29(10):1432–1435.

88. Alherabi AZ, Marglani OA, Gazzaz MJ, Abbas MM. Colon cancer metastasis to the thyroid gland. *Saudi Med J.* 2014;35(8): 868–871.

89. Yamamoto Y, Kodama K, Ide Y, Takeda M. Thymic and mediastinal lymph node metastasis of colon cancer. *Ann Thorac Surg.* 2017;103(1):e13–e15.

90. Ishikawa M, Hirano S, Tsuji T, Ito J. Management of metastasis to the thyroid gland. *Auris Nasus Larynx.* 2011;38(3):426–430.

91. Cozzolino I, Malapelle U, Carlomagno C, Palombini L, Troncone G. Metastasis of colon cancer to the thyroid gland: A case diagnosed on fine-needle aspirate by a combined cytological, immunocytochemical, and molecular approach. *Diagn Cytopathol.* 2010;38(12):932–935.

92. Danikas D, Theodorou SJ, Matthews WE, Rienzo AA. Unusually aggressive rectal carcinoid metastasizing to larynx, pancreas, adrenal glands, and brain. *Am Surg.* 2000;66(12):1179–1180.

93. Takashima S, Takayama F, Wang Q, Kobayashi S, Sone S. Thyroid metastasis from rectal carcinoma coexisting with Hashimoto's thyroiditis: gray-scale and power Doppler sonographic findings. *J Clin Ultrasound.* 1998;26(7):361–365.

94. Piazza C, Bolzoni A, Peretti G, Antonelli AR. Thyroid metastasis from rectal adenocarcinoma involving the airway treated by crico-tracheal resection and anastomosis: the role of palliative surgery. *Eur Arch Otorhinolaryngol.* 2004;261(9):469–472.

95. Hacker U, Lenz G, Brehm G, Müller-Höcker J, Schalhorn A, Hiddemann W. Metastasis of a rectal adenocarcinoma to the thyroid gland: diagnostic and therapeutic implications. *Anticancer Res.* 2003;23(6D): 4973–4976.

96. Kekelidze M, D'Errico L, Pansini M, Tyndall A, Hohmann J. Colorectal cancer: current imaging methods and future perspectives for the diagnosis, staging and therapeutic response evaluation. *World J Gastroenterol.* 2013;19(46):8502–8514.

97. Leufkens AM, van den Bosch MA, van Leeuwen MS, Siersema PD. Diagnostic accuracy of computed tomography for colon cancer staging: a systematic review. *Scand J Gastroenterol.* 2011;46(7-8):887–894.

98. Martins C, Sousa P, Araujo T, Castro-Pocas F. Mediastinal mass in a patient with colorectal cancer: a diagnostic challenge. *GE Port J Gastroenterol.* 2017;24:193–197.

99. Yamada K, Uchiyama T, Uchisako H, Adachi A, Yamashita Y. A case of mediastinal lymph node metastasis from liver metastasis of colon cancer. *Gan To Kagaku Ryoho.* 2017;44(7):603–606.

100. Lee M, Choi SJ, Yoon YH, Kim JT, Baek WK, Kim YS. Metastatic thymic adenocarcinoma from colorectal cancer. *Korean J Thorac Cardiovasc Surg.* 2015;48(6):447–451.

101. Iwata T, Chung K, Hanada S, et al. Solitary bulky mediastinal lymph node metastasis from colon cancer. *Ann Thorac Cardiovasc Surg.* 2013;19(4):313–315.

102. Sano A, Murakawa T, Morota T, Nakajima J. Resection of a posterior mediastinal metastasis of colon cancer. *Ann Thorac Surg.* 2011;92(1):353–354.

103. Kuba H, Sato N, Uchiyama A, et al. Mediastinal lymph node metastasis of colon cancer: report of a case. *Surg Today.* 1999;29(4): 375–377.

104. Kurosaki I, Hatakeyama K, Nihei K, et al. Mediastinal lymph node recurrence without pulmonary metastasis of hepatic metastatic of colon cancer a case report. *Jpn J Cancer Clin.* 1999;45:1220–1223.

105. Kitami A, Suzuki T, Suzuki S, Hori G. Two cases of postoperative mediastinal lymph nodes metastasis of colonic cancer. *J Jpn Surg Assoc.* 1995;56:2595–2598.

106. Musallam KM, Taher AT, Tawil AN, Chakhachiro ZI, Habbal MZ, Shamseddine AI. Solitary mediastinal lymph node metastasis in rectosigmoid carcinoma: a case report. *Cases J.* 2008;1(1):69.

107. Lashbrook M, Bernardes CM, Kirshbaum MN, Valery PC. Physical functioning and psychological morbidity among regional and rural cancer survivors: A report from a regional cancer centre. *Aust J Rural Health.* 2018;26(3):211–219.

108. Agasi-Idenburg SC, Thong MS, Punt CJ, Stuiver MM, Aaronson NK. Comparison of symptom clusters associated with fatigue in older and younger survivors of colorectal cancer. *Support Care Cancer.* 2017; 25(2):625–632.

109. Heldens AF, Bongers BC, Lenssen AF, Stassen LP, Buhre WF, van Meeteren NL. The association between performance parameters of physical fitness and postoperative outcomes in patients undergoing colorectal surgery: An evaluation of care data. *Eur J Surg Oncol.* 2017;43(11):2084–2092.

110. Thong MS, Mols F, van de Poll-Franse LV, et al. Identifying the subtypes of cancer-related fatigue: results from the population-based PROFILES registry. *J Cancer Surv.* 2018;12(1):38–46.

111. Vissers PA, Martucci RB, Mols F, et al. The impact of body mass index and waist circumference on health-related quality of life among colorectal cancer survivors: results from the PROFILES registry. *Nutr Cancer.* 2017;69(8):1177–1184.

112. Neefjes EC, Van Den Hurk RM, Blauwhoff-Buskermolen S, et al. Muscle mass as a target to reduce fatigue in patients with advanced cancer. *J Cachexia Sarcopenia Muscle.* 2017;8(4):623–629.

113. Hamdan AL, Sataloff RT, Hawkshaw MJ. Sleep, body fatigue, and voice. In: Hamdan AL, Sataloff RT, Hawkshaw M. Eds. *Laryngeal Manifestations of Systemic Diseases.* San Diego, CA: Plural Publishing; 2018:83–86.

114. Bamonti PM, Moye J, Naik AD. Pain is associated with continuing depression in cancer survivors. *Psychol Health Med.* 2018;23(10): 1182–1195.

115. Gonzalez-Saenz de Tejada M, Bilbao A, Baré M, et al. Association between social support, functional status, and change in health-related quality of life and changes in anxiety and depression in colorectal cancer patients. *Psychooncology.* 2017;26(9):1263–1269.

116. Trudel-Fitzgerald C, Tworoger SS, Poole EM, et al. Psychological symptoms and subsequent healthy lifestyle after a colorectal cancer diagnosis. *Health Psychol.* 2018;37(3): 207–217.

117. Dhillon HM, Tannock IF, Pond GR, Renton C, Rourke SB, Vardy JL. Perceived cognitive impairment in people with colorectal cancer who do and do not receive chemotherapy. *J Cancer Surviv.* 2018;12(2):178–185.

118. Reese JB, Handorf E, Haythornthwaite JA. Sexual quality of life, body image distress, and psychosocial outcomes in colorectal cancer: A longitudinal study. *Support Care Cancer.* 2018;26(10):3431–3440.

119. Rosen DC, Heuer RJ, Sasso DA, Sataloff RT. Psychological aspects of voice disorders. In: Sataloff RT. *Professional Voice: The Science and Art of Clinical Care.* 4th ed. San Diego, CA: Plural Publishing; 2017:705–736.

120. Dietrich M, Abbott KV, Gartner-Schmidt J, Rosen CA. The frequency of perceived stress, anxiety, and depression in patients with common pathologies affecting voice. *J Voice.* 2008;22(4):472–488.

121. Misono S, Haut C, Meredith L, et al. Dysphonia, perceived control, and psychosocial distress: a qualitative study. *J Voice*. 2019;33 (5):682–690.

122. Siani LM, Pulica C. Stage I-IIIC right colonic cancer treated with complete mesocolic exicision and central vascular ligation: quality of surgical specimen and long-term oncologic outcome according to the plane of surgery. *Minerva Chir*. 2014;69(4):199–208.

123. Näsvall P, Dahlstrand U, Löwenmark T, Rutegård J, Gunnarsson U, Strigård K. Quality of life in patients with a permanent stoma after rectal cancer surgery. *Qual Life Res*. 2017;26(1):55–64.

124. Kasparek MS, Hassan I, Cima RR, Larson DR, Gullerud RE, Wolff BG. Quality of life after coloanal anastomosis and abdominoperineal resection for distal rectal cancers: sphincter preservation vs quality of life. *Colorectal Dis*. 2011;13(8):872–877.

125. Schneider EC, Malin JL, Kahn KL, Ko CY, Adams J, Epstein AM. Surviving colorectal cancer: patient-reported symptoms 4 years after diagnosis. *Cancer*. 2007;110(9): 2075–2082.

126. McLachlan SA, Fisher RJ, Zalcberg J, et al. The impact on health-related quality of life in the first 12 months: A randomised comparison of preoperative short-course radiation versus long-course chemoradiation for T3 rectal cancer (Trans-Tasman Radiation Oncology Group Trial 01.04). *Eur J Cancer*. 2016;55:15–26.

127. Barreto R, Waning DL, Gao H, Liu Y, Zimmers TA, Bonetto A. Chemotherapy-related cachexia is associated with mitochondrial depletion and the activation of ERK1/2 and p38 MAPKs. *Oncotarget*. 2016;7(28):43442–43460.

128. Mattioni J, Opperman DA, Solimando, Jr. DA, Sataloff RT, ed. Cancer chemotherapy: an overview and voice implications. In: Sataloff RT. *Professional Voice: The Science and Art of Clinical Care*. 4th ed. San Diego, CA: Plural Publishing; 2017:1137–1141.

129. Verdolini K, Min Y, Titze IR, et al. Biological mechanisms underlying voice changes due to dehydration. *J Speech Lang Hear Res*. 2002;45:268–281.

130. Solomon NP, DiMattia MS. Effects of a vocally fatiguing task and systemic hydration on phonation threshold pressure. *J Voice*. 2000;14(3):341–362.

131. Hamdan AL, Siabi A, Rameh C. Effect of fasting on voice. *J Voice*. 2007;21(4):495–501.

132. Buccafusca G, Proserpio I, Tralongo AC, Rametta Giuliano S, Tralongo P. Early colorectal cancer: diagnosis, treatment and survivorship care. *Crit Rev Oncol Hematol*. 2019;136:20–30.

133. Caruso AM, Meyer TK, Allen CT. Hoarseness after metastatic colon cancer treatment. *JAMA Otolaryngol Head Neck Surg*. 2014;140(9):881–882.

134. Hartl DM, Ferté C, Loriot Y, et al. Dysphonia induced by vascular endothelium growth factor/vascular endothelium growth factor receptor inhibitors. *Invest New Drugs*. 2010;28(6):884–886.

135. Hartl DM, Bahleda R, Hollebecque A, Bosq J, Massard C, Soria JC. Bevacizumab-induced laryngeal necrosis. *Ann Oncol*. 2012;23(1):276–278.

136. Hamdan AL, Abouchakra KS, Al-Hazzouri Z, Zeytoun G. Transient-evoked otoacoustic emissions in a group of professional singers who have normal pure-tone hearing thresholds. *Ear Hear*. 2008;29(3):360–377.

7

Prostate Cancer and Voice

Abdul-Latif Hamdan, Robert Thayer Sataloff, and Mary Hawkshaw

Epidemiology and Pathogenesis

Prostate cancer is the second most common malignancy in men. The estimated incidence is 109.5 per 100 000 with 174 650 new cases diagnosed in 2019.[1] Prostate cancer affects mainly men in their seventh decade of life, with less than 10% of those affected being below the age of 45 years.[1,2] There are ethnic/racial differences with a higher prevalence rate being reported in African Americans compared to Caucasians and Asians (233.8 per 100 000 versus 149.5 and 88.3 per 100 000 respectively).[1] Native Americans are the least affected with an estimated prevalence of 75.3 per 100 000.[1] The variation in prevalence rate and disease outcome is linked to exogenous and endogenous factors.[3,4] Genomic studies have identified mutations in *HOXB13* and DNA repair genes (*BRCA2*) in diseased subjects.[5,6] Despite the advances in screening and early diagnosis, prostate cancer is still among the 6 leading causes of cancer-related deaths in the world. The estimated number of mortalities in 2018 was 359 000 with an expected increase to 740 000 deaths in 2040. The increase in mortality rate has been attributed to population growth and aging worldwide.[7]

The true etiology of prostate cancer is still unknown. Several factors have been implicated among which are endogenous hormone balance, smoking, alcohol intake, family history, diet, obesity, and physical activity. The possible etiologic role of endogenous hormone balance is based on the high expression of steroid hormone receptors and the increased level of testosterone in prostate cancer tissue. Both estrogens and androgens are contributors to progression as well as development of prostate cancer.[8] Smoking is also a major risk factor. In a large meta-analysis conducted by Islami et al, the adjusted relative risk of cigarette smoking for prostate cancer was 0.90.[9] Moreover, cigarette smoking has been shown to increase prostate-specific antigen (PSA) and to have detrimental effects on the oncologic outcome of patients diagnosed with prostate cancer.[10] The association between alcohol consumption and prostate cancer is also well established.[11,12] Zhao et al reviewed 27 studies on the association between prostate cancer and alcohol intake and reported a dose-response relationship between them. The adjusted relative risk estimates increased with the increase in amount of alcohol consumed.[12] Positive family history is a significant risk factor, as well. Based on a review by Xu et al which included 2321 patients with prostate cancer, 3.6% had a positive family history. This latter increased the risk of prostate cancer by almost 2-fold.[13] In a prospective study that included 11 654 patients, Thalgott et al demonstrated the adverse impact of family history on disease control and recurrence. Subjects with a family history were more likely to develop advanced local disease at an early age.[14] Diet and obesity are also linked strongly to prostate cancer. In a study by Dickerman et al on the association between fat distribution and prostate cancer, the authors reported a strong link between the 2 and emphasized the adverse effect of visceral fat on disease outcome.[15] Hence, lifestyle factors such as eating well, exercising, and reducing weight, are highly recommended to reduce the risk of prostate cancer.[16-18]

The histopathology of prostate cancer is heterogeneous. It is usually multifocal with an overlap in the presence of benign glandular tissue hypertrophy, neoplastic proliferation of prostatic intraepithelial tissue, and adenocarcinoma.[19] The pathology most frequently encountered is adenocarcinoma. Unspecified histology may be present in one out of five patients, and poorly differentiated carcinoma accounts for 5.2% of the cases.[20] The diagnosis of prostate carcinoma usually entails digital rectal examination and the use of specific immunohistochemistry markers, namely prostatic acid phosphatase.[3] PSA is an effective screening tool with some association with disease-specific mortality rate.[21] Based on a study by Gamble et al on the use of tumor marker hyperreactivity, the specificity of PSA immune-staining can reach up to 98%.[22] Other diagnostic modalities, such as prostate ultrasound and biopsy, are often requested preoperatively in order to confirm diagnosis, estimate disease prognosis, and plan management. The natural course of prostate cancer can be indolent or aggressive depending on the grade and clinical stage of the disease. Four out of 5 patients have localized disease at the time of diagnosis, whereas 20% may present with advanced disease that can be resistant to androgen therapy.[23-25] What is alarming about prostate cancer is the high rate of distant metastasis with more than 1 organ affected. In an autopsy study by Saitoh et al, 2 or more organs were the target of metastasis in up to 67.9% of cases, and only 1 out of 4 patients do not develop metastasis during the course of the disease. Based on that study, the metastatic rate is higher in patients with prostate adenocarcinoma in comparison to with patients with squamous cell carcinoma or poorly differentiated carcinoma.[20] Neoplastic lesions can disseminate either in a 1-step process in which tumor cells spread in a direct fashion to an organ, or in a 2-step process in which tumor cells seed to a distant metastatic site and metastasize further from that site in a cascade fashion.[26,27]

Given the systemic manifestation of prostate cancer and its high rate of spread to distant organs, the phonatory apparatus is undoubtedly in jeopardy. This chapter reviews the literature on the association between prostate cancer and voice, with an emphasis on laryngeal metastasis. A discussion of the adverse effects of treatment and the impact of androgen depletion therapy on voice also is presented. This information is useful to otolaryngologists and voice therapists who encounter patients with dysphonia and history of prostate cancer.

Disease-Induced Dysphonia

Prostate Carcinoma With Metastasis to the Larynx

It is estimated that 10% to 15% of patients with prostate cancer have metastasis at the time of diagnosis. Bones, lungs, and liver are the organs most commonly affected.[27] Laryngeal metastasis from a primary prostate cancer is rare. According to a 1957 report by Quinn and McCabe, the scarcity is attributed to the terminal position of the larynx in relation to the lymphatic and vascular circulation, and to the nonossified nature of the laryngeal framework. This latter acts as an impediment to hematogenous spread that usually targets osseous structures.[28] However, we doubt this is correct since much of the laryngeal framework is ossified by the time men are in their 60s, and this disease presents when they are in their 70s. Nevertheless, blood-borne tumor cells from prostate carcinoma, similar to other primary subdiaphragmatic malignancies, can reach the larynx bypassing the filtering role of the pulmonary and hepatic circulation. The hematogenous route is via the vertebral venous system also known as the Batson plexus, or possibly through the external carotid artery system.[29] An alternative metastatic route is the lymphatic system.[30,31] To that end, Butler et al reported supraclavicular lymphadenopathy as an early sign of metastatic prostate carcinoma,[32] and Welsh and Welsh described the interconnection between the laryngeal lymphatics and the supraclavicular nodes commonly affected in patients with prostate cancer.[33]

The literature documents a substantial number of patients with prostate cancer and laryngeal metastasis. In 1954, Ehrlich described 5 cases of laryngeal metastasis, among whom a 70-year-old man with history of prostate adenocarcinoma. Based on autopsy, metastatic disease affected both the thyroid and cricoid cartilages.[34] In 1957, Quinn and McCabe described 2 cases of metastatic laryngeal adenocarcinoma. The first case was an 83-year-old man with prostate adenocarcinoma who presented with sore throat and referred ear pain. On laryngeal examination, he had an ulcerative arytenoid mass with normal mobility of the vocal folds. Histologic examination of the laryngeal mass showed findings similar to the prostate lesion. The second patient had dysphonia secondary to impaired mobility of the left vocal fold, in addition to thickening of the left true and false vocal folds. The patient underwent suspension microlaryngoscopy and biopsy of the thickened mucosa which showed moderately well-differentiated adenocarcinoma. Metastatic workup revealed elevated acid phosphatase and a hypertrophic nodular prostate indicative of carcinoma.[28] In 1984, Coakley and Ranson reported a 64-year-old man with prostate adenocarcinoma who presented with stridor. On laryngeal examination, the patient had a subglottic mass, the histologic examination of which revealed poorly differentiated malignant cells similar to the primary prostate neoplasm.[35] In 1985, Batsakis et al described a case of prostate laryngeal metastasis in their report of 11 cases of laryngeal metastasis. It is noteworthy that melanoma, renal cell carcinoma, and breast carcinoma were the most common primaries that metastasized to the larynx.[36] In 1986, Hessan et al described a 70-year-old man who complained of hoarseness of 5 months' duration as the presenting symptom of metastatic prostate cancer. Laryngeal examination revealed an erosive lesion arising from the ossified thyroid cartilage and obliterating the laryngeal ventricle. Histochemical staining of the lesion showed adenocarcinoma metastasizing from a primary prostate tumor that was missed on initial evaluation.[37] In 1988, Ferlito reviewed the literature on laryngeal metastatic tumors and reported 120 cases. The most common primaries were melanoma and renal and lung carcinomas. In only 8 cases, the primary was prostate cancer with adenocarcinoma as the main pathology (7 out of the 8 cases).[38] In 1989, McMenamin et al described 4 patients with prostate cancer who presented with neck metastasis but no laryngeal involvement or phonatory symptoms.[39] In 1990, Grignon et al reported a 71-year-old patient who noticed a change in voice quality 6 months after being diagnosed with poorly differentiated carcinoma of the prostate. On laryngeal examination, he had swelling of the right false and true vocal folds. Histopathologic examination of a laryngeal biopsy revealed cells that resembled the primary tumor and was consistent with metastatic carcinoma.[40] In 1993, Park and Park reported a 66-year-old man with prostate adenocarcinoma who presented with dysphonia and left vocal fold paralysis. Computed tomography (CT) of the neck showed a destructive lesion of the thyroid cartilage with obliteration of the pyriform sinus on the side of the paralysis. On immunoperoxidase staining, the tumor was positive for PSA and was consistent with metastatic, moderately differentiated adenocarcinoma.[41] In 2002, Prescher et al performed a postmortem analysis on 6 patients with history of prostate cancer and multiple metastases. Interestingly, there was microscopic tumor cell infiltration of the ossified structures of the laryngeal framework in all 6 cases despite the fact that none of the patients had a history of phonatory or airway symptoms. The authors highlighted the high prevalence of microscopic hematopoietic laryngeal metastasis in patients with prostate cancer and multiple metastasis.[42] A decade later in 2011, Escudero et al described a 49-year-old man who presented with a history of hematuria and cervical mass of 3 months' duration. On examination, the patient had tumor infiltration of the bladder visceral wall suggestive of a malignant process in the prostate. A biopsy of the prostate gland performed using the transrectal approach revealed prostatic adenocarcinoma. CT of the neck requested for further evalu-

ation of the cervical mass showed a lesion in the thyroid lamina. Pathologic examination of the thyroid cartilage following hemilaryngectomy revealed metastatic prostate cancer.[43] A year later in 2012, Oliveira et al described a 73-year-old man who had dysphonia a month after being diagnosed with prostate adenocarcinoma and bone involvement. Laryngeal examination revealed right vocal fold paralysis and signs of mucosal inflammation. Biopsy of the lesion and immunohistochemical analysis using low-weight cytokeratin and PSA confirmed metastatic disease.[44]

All of these reports clearly indicate that the larynx is a metastatic target in patients with prostate carcinoma. Physicians should be on the alert for the possibility of laryngeal metastasis in patients with dysphonia and history of prostate cancer. The index of suspicion should be higher in elderly patients with bone metastasis. Based on the postmortem study by Ehrlich, there was histologic evidence of metastasis to the laryngeal cartilages primarily in patients with prostate cancer who had diffuse bone metastasis and bony metaplasia (ossification) of the laryngeal hyaline cartilages.[34] The diagnosis of laryngeal metastasis in patients with prostate cancer can be very challenging given the diversity in clinical presentation. Laryngeal involvement by metastatic disease is often subtle and misleading, and some patients have no symptoms or nonradiographic signs. A careful medical history and a diligent laryngeal examination are crucial in making the diagnosis. Patients may be asymptomatic or complain of symptoms commonly reported in patients with primary laryngeal neoplasia. Symptoms may include neck pain, dysphonia, sore throat, referred ear pain, or shortness of breath and stridor. Similarly, laryngeal endoscopy may be nonspecific. Patients may have unilateral or bilateral vocal fold paralysis or may present with a submucosal lesion that is hard to delineate. In rare cases, patients may have an ulcerative lesion with erosion of the laryngeal structures. The supraglottis is the site affected most commonly in 40% of the cases, followed by the subglottis in 12% of the cases.[36] The glottis is rarely involved, and the presence of multiple lesions is not uncommon. Radiologic imaging using CT and/or magnetic resonance imaging is useful in delineating the extent of the laryngeal lesion and in assessing the presence or absence of cervical lymph node involvement. A biopsy is nearly always recommended, and special stains often are needed to confirm the diagnosis. Surgical treatment may be either conservative or radical depending on the extent and growth of the laryngeal tumor.

In summary, the larynx should be recognized as a metastatic target in patients with dysphonia and history of prostate carcinoma. Elderly subjects with ossified laryngeal cartilages are more likely to be affected, and laryngeal ossification is normal in this age group. A diligent laryngeal examination is mandatory, and biopsy is often needed to make the diagnosis.

Prostate Carcinoma Metastasizing to Structures Contiguous With the Larynx

Metastasis from prostate cancer to structures contiguous with the larynx is not uncommon. The bronchial tree is an important metastatic target that may impact phonation adversely. Endobronchial metastasis from extrathoracic neoplasms has been described thoroughly in the literature. Marchioni et al reported the clinical and pathologic characteristics of 174 patients with extrathoracic neoplasms and endobronchial metastasis, of whom 4.5% had prostate cancer. The mean latency period from diagnosis of the primary

neoplasms to metastasis was 136 months. The most common symptoms were dyspnea in 23% of the cases, followed by cough and hemoptysis in 15% and 12% of the cases, respectively.[45] Lalli et al reported a 55-year-old man who presented with hemoptysis, cough, and dyspnea. Bronchoscopic examination revealed multiple polypoidal lesions, the pathology of which was consistent with well-differentiated adenocarcinoma. Biopsy of the prostate through a transperineal approach revealed the same pathology.[46] Similarly, Shen et al reported a 72-year-old man who presented with a mass in the superior lobar bronchus in addition to multiple pulmonary lesions. Histopathologic examination of that mass using P504S and PSA confirmed the presence of mucinous adenocarcinoma compatible with the pathology retrieved from a prostate biopsy.[47] Similarly, Asghar Nawaz and Shackcloth described an 80-year-old man with history of metastatic stromal cell sarcoma who presented with dyspnea. CT of the chest showed an obstructive lesion of the right main bronchus. Histologic examination of that lesion was similar to that of the prostate. The patient was treated successfully using endoscopic cryotherapy.[48]

In all the earlier reports, dyspnea and cough were the main symptoms of endobronchial metastasis. Given the critical paramount role of breathing in phonation, it is fair to assume that endobronchial metastasis from prostate carcinoma may jeopardize phonation by interfering with the power source of phonation, especially if there is partial obstruction of bronchi. There are no current studies on the prevalence of dysphonia in patients with prostate cancer and endobronchial metastasis. Future research is warranted.

Another structure contiguous with the larynx that may be affected in patients with prostate cancer is the thyroid gland.

This latter is a known metastatic target that may present with clinical signs and symptoms many years after the primary tumor has been diagnosed. Affected individuals are usually in their seventh decade of life, and the incidence of metastasis varies from 1.25% to 24% of cases.[49] The most common primary malignancies that metastasize to the thyroid gland arise from the kidneys, breasts, and gastrointestinal system.[49] Metastasis from prostate neoplasia to the thyroid gland is rare, with only 6 cases reported in the literature. In 1994, Ro et al reported a case of thyroid gland metastasis in a 71-year-old man with prostate adenocarcinoma. The patient presented with an enlarging goiter and evidence of a multicystic thyroid mass on CT. Fine-needle aspiration and biopsy of that mass confirmed the metastatic nature of the lesion. It is noteworthy that the patient developed hoarseness, shortness of breath, and hypoxia only following his thyroid surgery.[50] In 1995, Michelow et al described a 70-year-old man who presented with a thyroid nodule and para-aortic lymphadenopathy. Fine-needle aspiration of the thyroid mass was suspicious for adenocarcinoma. Further investigation looking for a primary led to the diagnosis of prostate adenocarcinoma.[51] In 1998, Momma et al reported a patient with primary adenocarcinoma of the prostate who developed multiple organ metastasis despite hormone therapy. The metastasis to the thyroid gland was confirmed by immunohistochemical staining for CEA and CA19-9.[52] In 2004, Bayram et al reported a 77-year-old man with known prostate adenocarcinoma, who presented with a slowly growing nodular goiter. Fine-needle aspiration and biopsy of the thyroid revealed metastatic prostate adenocarcinoma.[53] In 2007, Selimoglu et al described a 73-year-old patient with prostate cancer who presented with a large thyroid nodule (44 mm × 53 mm) displacing the trachea and internal jugular vein. Fine-needle aspiration and biopsy of the nodule revealed atypical cells that stained positive for PAS.[54] In 2013, Albsoul et al reported a patient with prostate adenocarcinoma who developed multinodular goiter with retrosternal extension that led to compression symptoms. The patient underwent total thyroidectomy, and the pathology was consistent with metastatic prostate adenocarcinoma.[55]

In all these cases, the main presentation of thyroid metastasis was thyroid enlargement and/or mass. Despite the fact that none of the affected subjects had dysphonia, voice change is common in primary thyroid or metastatic cancer, and it is likely to occur in some patients with prostate cancer despite the absence of current reports.

Recurrent Laryngeal Nerve Palsy in Patients With Prostate Cancer

Vocal fold paralysis in patients with prostate cancer is uncommon. In the absence of laryngeal metastasis, it is usually the result of compression or invasion of the recurrent laryngeal nerve along its course in the chest. The most common intrathoracic structures affected are the mediastinal lymph nodes. This is not surprising given that lymph nodes are common metastatic targets in patients with prostate cancer.[20] Metastasis to the mediastinal and paratracheal lymph nodes has been described in the literature.[56] Riquet et al reported on extrathoracic malignancies, among which metastatic prostate carcinoma occurred in 37 out of 565 patients with mediastinal lymphadenopathy. The authors alluded to the favorable role of surgical intervention in the management of these cases.[57] In an analysis of 1435 patients with prostate cancer, Lindell et al in 1982 reported intrathoracic metastatic disease and mediastinal adenopathy with and without pulmonary nodules in 5.2% and 0.83% of the cases, respectively.[58] In 1983, Yam et al described 2 patients who presented with lung and mediastinal disease secondary to metastatic adenocarcinoma of unknown origin. Further investigation using prostatic acid phosphatase (PAP) as a marker led to the diagnosis of prostate cancer. The authors referred to the usefulness and added value of PAP in the investigation of metastatic adenocarcinoma of undetermined origin.[59] In 1987, Cho and Epstein reported mediastinal lymphadenopathy in a patient with prostate cancer.[60] The authors highlighted the need to include prostate cancer in the metastatic workup of patients with supradiaphragmatic lymphadenopathy. In 1999, Old was the first to report a patient with prostate carcinoma who presented years after treatment with left recurrent laryngeal nerve palsy. His symptoms and signs were attributed to massive lymphadenopathy in the mediastinum and neck. Histologic examination of the lymph nodes confirmed the presence of metastatic prostate disease, and the patient was treated successfully by radiation.[61] In 2002, Oyan et al reported a 56-year-old man who presented with weight loss and mediastinal lymphadenopathy as part of generalized lymphadenopathy that affected the neck, chest, abdomen, and inguinal areas. Histologic examination of the cervical lymph nodes revealed metastatic adenocarcinoma. Further investigation led to the diagnosis of a primary prostate carcinoma.[62] In 2003, Ikekubo et al reported an 81-year-old man who presented with painful cervical lymphadenopathy. Using 201T1 and 99mTc-MIBI scans, the patient was found to have evidence of mediastinal disease. Immunohistochemical evaluation of the mediastinal lymph node confirmed the presence of metastatic prostate carcinoma. Supradiaphragmatic lymphade-

nopathy was the presenting sign of prostate cancer in this patient.[63] In 2007, Roca et al reported mediastinal lymphadenopathy, in addition to cutaneous and pulmonary metastasis, 8 years after a patient had been diagnosed with prostate carcinoma. The authors emphasized that late onset of mediastinal metastasis is a sign of aggressive tumor behavior.[64] That same year, Perez et al described a 73-year-old patient with prostate cancer and bone metastasis who developed shortness of breath secondary to paratracheal and hilar lymphadenopathy. Biopsy of those lymph nodes showed metastatic prostate adenocarcinoma.[65] In 2009, Riquet et al described 2 cases of prostate carcinoma among 37 cases of extrathoracic malignancies presenting with mediastinal lymphadenopathies. The authors highlighted the possibility of having isolated hilar or mediastinal lymphadenopathy in patients with extrathoracic carcinoma.[57] In 2016, Soydal et al reported the usefulness of Ga prostate-specific membrane antigen positron emission tomography (PET)/CT in showing pathologic uptake in metastatic mediastinal lymph nodes of affected patients[66]; and Su et al reported the usefulness of ^{18}F-fludeoxyglucose (FDG)-PET/CT in detecting mediastinal and lung nodules despite the negative yield of magnetic resonance imaging.[67] Metastasis to the thymus should be considered as another potential cause of vocal fold paralysis in patients with prostate cancer and mediastinal disease.[68]

In summary, mediastinal lymphadenopathy in patients with prostate cancer rarely leads to recurrent laryngeal nerve palsy. Despite its common presentation with compressive vascular and pulmonary symptoms,[69–74] it is rarely the cause of vocal fold paralysis.

Another site for potential compression of the recurrent laryngeal nerve is the supraclavicular area. Supraclavicular lymphadenopathy has been reported in patients with prostate cancer and is often mistaken for lymphoma.[59,60,75–77] In the study by Yam et al, 7 patients, 2 of whom had known prostate cancer, presented with supraclavicular lymphadenopathy on the left side secondary to metastatic adenocarcinoma.[59] In 1987, Cho and Epstein reported 26 patients with metastatic prostate carcinoma, 23 of whom had either supraclavicular or cervical lymphadenopathy. Only 7 out of the 26 patients had a history of known prostate cancer at the time of presentation, and the majority had inconclusive histological examination. The authors emphasized the importance of *prostate specific acid phosphatase* (PSAP) immunohistochemical staining in patients with suspected metastatic disease.[60] In the case report by Oyan et al, left-sided cervical lymphadenopathy was part of the generalized lymphadenopathy suggestive of a lymphoproliferative disease.[62] Similarly, Tan-Shalaby reported a patient with left bulky cervical adenopathy despite hormone therapy and radiation to his primary prostate cancer. The pathology of the mass was consistent with metastatic prostatic carcinoma.[77]

In summary, cervical lymphadenopathy may be the first sign of metastatic disease in patients with known or unknown prostate cancer. Supraclavicular lymphadenopathy, in addition to bone pain,[78] should alert the physician to the possibility of distant metastasis. These signs should be sought in patients with dysphonia.

Age as a Demographic Variable in Patients With Prostate Cancer and Dysphonia

Dysphonia is common in elderly patients, with marked impact on quality of life.[79–81] The etiology includes a variety of disorders.

Woo et al reported systemic diseases in almost 1 out of 2 elderly patients who present with dysphonia.[80] Neurologic diseases and inflammatory vocal fold lesions accounted for the majority of the causes. Gregory et al reported laryngopharyngeal reflux disease and muscle tension dysphonia in 91% and 73% of cases, respectively. The study included 175 subjects between the ages of 65 and 89 years.[82] In the absence of systemic diseases and vocal fold inflammatory disorders, dysphonia in elderly patients is often the result of physiologic aging. Affected patients complain of change in pitch and loudness and/or vocal fatigue. In professional voice users, additional vocal symptoms such as loss of range, diminished power, and inability to sustain a note are commonly reported. Perceptual evaluation often reveals a breathy, asthenic, and strained voice. Acoustic analysis shows an increase in the perturbation parameters, jitter and shimmer, an increase in noise-to-harmonic ratio, and variations in habitual pitch in men and women. These acoustic changes are secondary to alterations in the histologic structures of the vocal folds.[83–87] There are also variations in the upper airflow measurements. There is a decrease in the mean airway resistance and peak airflow.[88,89] This decrease parallels the decrease in maximal vocal intensity reported by Morris and Brown[90] and the reduced ability to control loudness described by Baker et al.[91]

Given the effects of aging on voice and the fact that prostate cancer is a disease of elderly patients, affected patients are more likely to experience phonatory disturbances. This conclusion remains hypothetical in the absence of any study comparing vocal symptoms in young versus elderly patients with prostate cancer. However, in elderly patients with dysphonia, it seems important to avoid attributing the dysphonia to aging without considering other serious causes such as prostate cancer.

Depression, Anxiety, and Dysphonia in Patients With Prostate Cancer

Prostate cancer has adverse effects on the mental well-being of affected patients and their partners.[92] The most common psychological burdens reported are depression and anxiety.[93] In an investigation on patients with prostate cancer who were on active surveillance, Watts et al in 2015 reported higher rates of depression and anxiety in comparison to the normal population matched according to age.[94] These results agreed with those of a previous study by the same authors who described depression and anxiety in 17.27% and 27.04% of the cases, respectively.[95] The study was a systemic review conducted in 2014, which included 4494 patients with prostate cancer. Similarly, in a retrospective analysis of 5862 patients with prostate cancer, Pompe et al reported abnormal Patient Health Questionnaire-4 (PHQ-4) in 28% of cases. This was used as an outcome measure of depression and anxiety with a score ranging from 0 to 6 indicating the severity of disease. Moreover, there was a negative association between PHQ-4 scores and the surgical and functional outcomes.[96] In another study conducted on 100 patients with prostate cancer, Burnet et al also reported anxiety in 21% of the cases.[97] Important predictive factors to consider in the evaluation of psychological burden in patients with prostate cancer are age and the presence of other morbidities. In a study on the effect of androgen deprivation therapy on the psychological status of affected patients, Chipperfield et al concluded that younger patients and those with multiple morbidities were at higher risk of developing depression and anxiety.[98] Another important predictive factor is the course of treatment. In the study by Watts et al, the prevalence of depression decreased during treatment and increased afterward.[94]

Patients with prostate cancer carry a high risk of psychological burden. The impact of psychological factors on the phonatory system is well known.[99–101] Patients with prostate cancer and suffering from anxiety and depression should be evaluated for voice disorders, and serious diseases including prostate cancer should be considered when evaluating voice patients with anxiety and depression. Future research is warranted.

Treatment-Induced Dysphonia

Hormone Therapy of Prostate Cancer and Voice

In the last 2 decades, a marked improvement has been realized in the management of prostate cancer. Androgen deprivation therapy (ADT) has gained popularity as a viable treatment alternative to surgical castration.[102] It has proven to be very effective in normalizing or markedly decreasing PSA level even in patients with advanced prostate cancer.[103,104] The effect is mediated by the high affinity of prostate cancerous tissue to sex hormones. The gonadotropin-releasing hormone agonists result in a decrease in serum testosterone to almost a castrated level only a few weeks after initiation of therapy. The flare in serum testosterone witnessed during the first week of treatment may be mitigated by the administration of anti-androgens.[105–107]

With this effective treatment modality come significant systemic adverse effects. Patients with prostate cancer who undergo ADT invariably suffer from hypogonadism, a clinical syndrome characterized by symptoms of impotence, gynecomastia, excessive weight, and fatigue.[108–115] In parallel with the change in body composition, there are alterations in lipid and glucose metabolism. There is an increase in cholesterol and triglycerides, a decrease in insulin sensitivity, and an increase in the incidence of diabetes mellitus.[116–119] There is also an increase in arterial stiffness and atherogenic risks.[120,121] With these metabolic alterations, there is bone loss and a decline in bone density leading to a higher incidence of fractures.[122–124]

Given that the larynx is a hormone target, the hypogonadal state that follows ADT poses a substantial risk to phonation.[125,126] The impact of sex hormones on voice is well-recognized at puberty when voice becomes a secondary sexual characteristic and an acoustic cue to the speaker's gender.[127,128] Numerous clinical investigations also have demonstrated the strong association between sex hormones and voice in adults. To list a few, Meuser and Nieschlag reported a correlation between testosterone/estradiol ratios and the different vocal registers in a group of 102 male singers. Tenors had lower ratios in comparison with baritones and basses.[129] Pedersen et al reported a negative correlation between the fundamental frequency and testosterone level. The study included 19 men between the ages of 16 years and 19.5 years.[130] Dabbs et al showed an inverse relationship between testosterone level and vocal pitch in a group of 61 undergraduate male subjects with a mean age of 19.7 years (standard deviation [SD] = 1.5). Testosterone level was measured in saliva using radioimmunoassay, and vocal pitch was assessed while asking the patient to count to 10 and sustain different vowels.[131] Similarly, Evans et al reported a significant negative correlation between fundamental frequency and testosterone levels. The study was conducted on 40 male subjects, and saliva samples were collected at various intervals throughout the day to match the variation in serum circulating testosterone level.[132]

In view of the strong interplay between sex hormones and voice, one would speculate that alterations in androgen level in patients undergoing ADT might adversely impact voice. Yet, there is no consensus in the literature on the impact of androgen deprivation or replacement on voice in adults despite the ubiquity of reports on the role of sex hormones in sexual dimorphism. In 2010, Gugatschka et al reported no significant impact of androgen level on voice in elderly men. The study was conducted on 62 men stratified as hypogonadal (lowered level of sex hormones) versus normal. All subjects had undergone a comprehensive voice evaluation that included subjective and objective voice measurements.[133] In a prospective study on the effect of androgen ablation therapy using gonadotropin-releasing hormone agonists and antiandrogens in a group of patients with prostate cancer, Hamdan et al reported a significant difference in habitual pitch in the study group in comparison to a control group. Moreover, there was a significant increase in the perturbation parameters in patients with prostate cancer on ADT. However, there was no significant difference in the prevalence of phonatory symptoms between the 2 groups.[134] Akcam et al investigated the impact of androgen hormonal therapy on voice in 24 patients with hypogonadotrophic hypogonadism.[135] Following administration of hormone therapy, there was almost normalization of the mean fundamental frequency in the treated group. These results were in alignment with animal studies on the effect of androgen on laryngeal structures. Sassoon et al reported androgen-induced myogenesis and chondrogenesis in juvenile larynges of South African clawed frogs, further corroborating the role of testosterone in sexual dimorphism at puberty.[136]

In summary, the literature on the impact of ADT on voice is scarce. More research to elucidate the impact of hormone therapy on voice is needed. Given the increased survivals of patients with prostate cancer, physicians and voice therapists should be aware of the potential long-term adverse effect of hypogonadism on the phonatory apparatus.

Surgery for Prostate Cancer and Voice

Surgery is a main treatment option for patients with prostate cancer.[137,138] Tumor growth and progression may be suppressed by surgical removal of prostate tissue using various approaches.[138] With surgery come physical impairments that may further lead to mental impairments. In 2019, Jarzemski et al studied the impact of surgery and adjuvant therapy on the mental well-being of 100 patients with prostate cancer. The authors reported an association between the physical symptoms, deferred memory, depression, and anxiety. They alluded to the need for psychiatric assistance in addressing the psychological burden of therapy.[139] Albaugh et al conducted a study using open-ended questions and interviews looking at the sexual experience and quality of life of patients with prostate cancer following treatment. Aside from sexual dysfunction being the main physical impairment, a high percentage of patients suffered from depression and anxiety. The authors emphasized the need to identify these burdens in the management of affected patients.[140] Similarly, in a survey that included 4719 patients with prostate cancer who were followed up for 11.5 years, Meissner et al reported that low global health, psychological status, and younger age are important predictors of anxiety in patients with prostate cancer.[141]

This leads us to conclude that surgical treatment of prostate carcinoma is associated not only with physical impairments but also with psychological ones. These may have a negative effect on voice that needs to be addressed in the management of surgical patients and that also requires research.

Chemotherapy and Voice in Patients With Prostate Cancer

Chemotherapy is one of many treatment options for prostate cancer. Many drugs are in use including docetaxel and cabazitaxel, among others. Associated side effects include anemia, neutropenia, thrombocytopenia, organ-related inflammatory disorders, memory and cognitive disorders, generalized fatigue, and sleep disturbances. Other significant side effects include diarrhea, nausea, and vomiting.[1] Although there are no reports in the literature on dysphonia as an adverse effect of chemotherapy in the treatment of prostate cancer, the phonatory apparatus is in jeopardy given the strong link between body well-being and voice, and the known impact of dehydration on the phonatory system.[142,143] A thorough review of the implications of chemotherapy on voice can be found in the literature.[144]

References

1. National Cancer Institute: Surveillance Epidemiology and End Results (SEER). Cancer stat facts: Prostate cancer. Accessed September 2, 2019. https://seer.cancer.gov/statfacts/html/prost.html
2. Cancer Research UK. Prostate cancer statistics. Accessed September 2, 2019. https://www.cancerresearchuk.org/health-professional/cancer-statistics/statistics-by-cancer-type/prostate-cancer#heading-Three
3. NCCN guidelines and clinical resources. National Comprehensive Cancer Network.

Accessed September 2, 2019. https://www.nccn.org/professionals/physician_gls/default.aspx

4. Breyer JP, Avritt TG, McReynolds KM, Dupont WD, Smith JR. Confirmation of the HOXB13 G84E germline mutation in familial prostate cancer. *Cancer Epidemiol Biomarkers Prev.* 2012;21:1348–1353.

5. Pritchard CC, Mateo J, Walsh MF, et al. Inherited DNA-repair gene mutations in men with metastatic prostate cancer. *N Engl J Med.* 2016;375(5):443–453.

6. Qi X, Wang Y, Hou J, Huang Y. A single nucleotide polymorphism in HPGD gene is associated with prostate cancer risk. *J Cancer.* 2017;8(19):4083–4086.

7. Culp MB, Soerjomataram I, Efstathiou JA, Bray F, Jemal A. Recent global patterns in prostate cancer incidence and mortality rates. *Eur Urol.* 2020;77(1):38–52.

8. Dobbs RW, Malhotra NR, Greenwald DT, Wang AY, Prins GS, Abern MR. Estrogens and prostate cancer. *Prostate Cancer Prostatic Dis.* 2019;22(2):185–194.

9. Islami F, Moreira DM, Boffetta P, Freedland SJ. A systematic review and meta-analysis of tobacco use and prostate cancer mortality and incidence in prospective cohort studies. *Eur Urol.* 2014;66:1054–1064.

10. Shiota M, Ushijima M, Imada K, et al. Cigarette smoking augments androgen receptor activity and promotes resistance to antiandrogen therapy. *Prostate.* 2019;79(10):1147–1155.

11. Kawada T. Lifestyles, health habits, and prostate cancer. *J Cancer Res Clin Oncol.* 2019 Feb 21. doi:10.1007/s00432-019-02871-w

12. Zhao J, Stockwell T, Roemer A, Chikritzhs T. Is alcohol consumption a risk factor for prostate cancer? A systematic review and meta-analysis. *BMC Cancer.* 2016;16(1):845.

13. Xu Y, Huang D, Wu Y, et al. Family history is significantly associated with prostate cancer and its early onset in Chinese population. *Prostate.* 2019;79(15):1762–1766.

14. Thalgott M, Kron M, Brath JM, et al. Men with family history of prostate cancer have a higher risk of disease recurrence after radical prostatectomy. *World J Urol.* 2018;36(2):177–185.

15. Dickerman BA, Torfadottir JE, Valdimarsdottir UA, et al. Body fat distribution on computed tomography imaging and prostate cancer risk and mortality in the AGES-Reykjavik study. *Cancer.* 2019;125(16):2877–2885.

16. Shephard RJ. Physical activity and prostate cancer: an updated review. *Sports Med.* 2017;47:1055–1073.

17. Zuniga KB, Chan JM, Ryan CJ, Kenfield SA. Diet and lifestyle considerations for patients with prostate cancer. *Urol Oncol.* 2020;38(3):105–117.

18. Emilio S, Luigi V, Riccardo B, Carlo G. Lifestyle in urology: cancer. *Urologia.* 2019;86(3):105–114.

19. Gleason DF. Histologic grading of prostate cancer: a perspective. *Hum Pathol.* 1992;23:273–279.

20. Saitoh H, Hida M, Shimbo T, Nakamura K, Yamagata J, Satoh T. Metastatic patterns of prostatic cancer: correlation between sites and number of organs involved. *Cancer.* 1984;54(12):3078–3084.

21. Dow D, Whitaker RH. Prostatic contribution to normal serum acid phosphatase. *Brit Med J.* 1970;4(5733);470–472.

22. Gamble AR, Bell JA, Ronan JE, Pearson D, Ellis IO. Use of tumor marker immunereactivity to identify primary site of metastatic cancer. *BMJ.* 1993;306(6873):295–298.

23. Marques RB, Dits NF, Erkens-Schulze S, van Weerden WM, Jenster G. Bypass mechanisms of the androgen receptor pathway in therapy-resistant prostate cancer cell models. *PLoS One.* 2010;5(10):e13500.

24. Harris WP, Mostaghel EA, Nelson PS, Montgomery B. Androgen deprivation therapy: progress in understanding mechanisms of resistance and optimizing androgen depletion. *Nat Clin Pract Urol.* 2009;6(2):76–85.

25. Grozescu T, Popa F. Prostate cancer between prognosis and adequate/proper therapy. *J Med Life.* 2017;10(1):5–12.

26. Bross IDJ, Viadana E, Pickren J. Do generalized metastases occur directly from the primary? *J Chronic Dis.* 1975;28:149–159.

27. Bubendorf L, Schopfer A, Wagner U, et al. Metastatic patterns of prostate cancer: an autopsy study of 1589 patients. *Hum Pathol.* 2000;31(5):578–583.

28. Quinn FB Jr, McCabe BF. Laryngeal metastases from malignant tumors in distant organs. *Ann Otol Rhinol Laryngol.* 1957;66(1):139–143.

29. Batson OV. Function of the vertebral veins and their role in the spread of metastases. *Ann Surg.* 1940;112:138–149.

30. Fields JA. Renal carcinoma metastasis to the larynx. *Laryngoscope.* 1966;76:99–101.

31. Fisher B, Fisher ER. Significance of the interrelationships of lymph and blood vascular systems in tumor cell dissemination. *Prog Clinl Cancer.* 1970;4:84–96.

32. Butler JJ, Howe CD, Johnson DE. Enlargement of the supraclavicular lymph nodes as the initial sign of prostatic carcinoma. *Cancer.* 1971;27:1055–1063.

33. Welsh LW, Welsh JJ. Cervical lymphatics: pathologic conditions. *Ann Otol Rhinol Laryngol.* 1966;75:176–191.

34. Ehrlich A. Tumor involving the laryngeal cartilages. *AMA Arch Otolaryngol.* 1954;59(2):178–185.

35. Coakley JF, Ranson DL. Metastasis to the larynx from a prostatic carcinoma. A case report. *J Laryngol Otol.* 1984;98(8):839–842.

36. Batsakis JG, Luna MA, Byers RM. Metastases to the larynx. *Head Neck Surg.* 1985;7(6):458–460.

37. Hessan H, Strauss M, Sharkey FE. Urogenital tract carcinoma metastatic to the head and neck. *Laryngoscope.* 1986;96(12):1352–1356.

38. Ferlito A, Caruso G, Recher G. Secondary laryngeal tumors. Report of seven cases with review of the literature. *Arch Otolaryngol Head Neck Surg.* 1988;114(6):635–639.

39. McMenamin PG, Anderson JD, Baker JJ. Prostatic carcinoma presenting with neck metastasis. *J Otolaryngol.* 1989;18(3):119–124.

40. Grignon DJ, Ro JY, Ayala AG, Chong C. Carcinoma of prostate metastasizing to vocal cord. *Urology.* 1990;36(1):85–88.

41. Park YW, Park MH. Vocal cord paralysis from prostatic carcinoma metastasizing to the larynx. *Head Neck.* 1993;15(5):455–458.

42. Prescher A, Schick B, Stütz A, Brors D. Laryngeal prostatic cancer metastases: an underestimated route of metastases? *Laryngoscope.* 2002;112(8):1467–1473.

43. Escudero RM, Amo FH, Martinez MC, et al. Metastatic prostate cancer on the thyroid cartilage: unusual symptoms of prostatic adenocarcinoma. Case report. *Arch Esp Urol.* 2011;64(2):132–135.

44. Oliveira JA, Said Rde A, Cartaxo Rde S, Santos JA, Gondim RL. Laryngeal metastasis of a prostate carcinoma: one rare entity. *Braz J Otorhinolaryngol.* 2012;78(3):135.

45. Marchioni A, Lasagni A, Busca A, et al. Endobronchial metastasis: an epidemiologic and clinicopathologic study of 174 consecutive cases. *Lung Cancer.* 2014;84(3):222–228.

46. Lalli C, Gogia H, Raju L. Multiple endobronchial metastases from carcinoma of prostate. *Urology.* 1983;21(2):164–165.

47. Shen Q, Yao Y, Teng X, Zhou J. Endobronchial metastasis from prostate cancer mimicking primary lung cancer. *Intern Med.* 2010;49(15):1613–1615.

48. Asghar Nawaz M, Shackcloth M. Unusual endobronchial prostatic metastatic tumor occluding right main bronchus. *Asian Cardiovasc Thorac Ann.* 2019;27(3):228–230.

49. Cichoń S, Anielski R, Konturek A, Barczyński M, Cichoń W. Metastases to the thyroid gland: seventeen cases operated on in a single clinical center. *Langenbecks Arch Surg.* 2006;391(6):581–587.

50. Ro JY, Guerrieri C, el-Naggar AK, Ordonez NG, Sorge JG, Ayala AG. Carcinomas metastatic to follicular adenomas of the thyroid gland. Report of two cases. *Arch Pathol Lab Med.* 1994;118(5):551–556.

51. Michelow PM, Leiman G. Metastasis to the thyroid gland diagnosis by aspiration cytology. *Diagn Cytopathol.* 1995;13(3):209–213.

52. Momma T, Kimura S, Saito S, Onado N. Prostate cancer with high serum level of CEA and CA19-9: A case report. *Hinyokika Kiyo*. 1998;44(3):187–191.

53. Bayram F, Soyuer I, Atmaca H, et al. Prostatic adenocarcinoma metastasis in the thyroid gland. *Endocr J*. 2004;51(4):445–448.

54. Selimoglu H, Duran C, Saraydaroglu O, et al. Prostate cancer metastasis to thyroid gland. *Tumori*. 2007;93(3):292–295.

55. Albsoul NM, Obeidat FN, Hadidy AM, AlZoubi MN, Taib AA, Shahait AD. Isolated multiple bilateral thyroid metastases from prostatic adenocarcinoma: case report and literature review. *Endocr Pathol*. 2013;24(1):36–39.

56. Badawey MR, Punekar S, Zammit-Maempel I. Prospective study to assess vocal cord palsy investigations. *Otolaryngol Head Neck Surg*. 2008;138(6):788–790.

57. Riquet M, Berna P, Brian E, et al. Intrathoracic lymph node metastases from extrathoracic carcinoma: the place for surgery. *Ann Thorac Surg*. 2009;88(1):200–205.

58. Lindell MM, Doubleday LC, von Eschenbach AC, Libshitz HI. Mediastinal metastases from prostatic carcinoma. *J Urol*. 1982;128(2):331–334.

59. Yam LT, Winkler CF, Janckila AJ, Li CY, Lam KW. Prostatic cancer presenting as metastatic adenocarcinoma of undetermined origin. Immunodiagnosis by prostatic acid phosphatase. *Cancer*. 1983;51(2): 283–287.

60. Cho KR, Epstein JI. Metastatic prostatic carcinoma to supradiaphragmatic lymph nodes. A clinicopathologic and immunohistochemical study. *Am J Surg Pathol*. 1987; 11(6):457–463.

61. Old SE. Superior vena cava obstruction in prostate cancer. *Clin Oncol*. 1999;11(5): 352–354.

62. Oyan B, Engin H, Yalcin S. Generalized lymphadenopathy: a rare presentation of disseminated prostate cancer. *Med Oncol*. 2002;19(3):177–179.

63. Ikekubo K, Hino M, Ito H, Ohtsuka H, Saiki Y. A case report of distant lymph nodes metastases from prostate cancer imaged with 201Tl and 99mTc-MIBI. *Kaku Igaku*. 2003;40(4):439–443.

64. Roca Edreira A, Aguilera Tubet C, Villanueva Pena A, Ballestero Diego R, Zubillaga Guerrero S. Mediastinal lymph nodes during the course of a metastatic prostate cancer. *Actas Urol Esp*. 2007;31(6):693–695.

65. Perez NE, Maryala S, Seren S, Feng J, Pansare V, Dhar R. Metastatic prostate cancer presenting as mediastinal lymphadenopathy identified by EUS with FNA. *Gastrointest Endosc*. 2007;65(6):948–949.

66. Soydal C, Ozkan E, Yerlikaya H, Utkan G, Kucuk ON. Widespread metastatic prostate carcinoma shown by 68Ga-PSMA PET/CT. *Clin Nucl Med*. 2016;41(6):e294–e295.

67. Su HY, Chen ML, Hsieh PJ, Hsieh TS, Chao IM. Lung metastasis from prostate cancer revealed by 18F-FDG PET/CT without osseous metastasis on bone scan. *Clin Nucl Med*. 2016;41(5):392–393.

68. Hayashi S, Hamanaka Y, Sueda T, Yonehara S, Matsuura Y. Thymic metastasis from prostatic carcinoma: report of a case. *Surg Today*. 1993;23(7):632–634.

69. McGarry RC. Superior vena cava obstruction due to prostate carcinoma. *Urology*. 2000;55:436.

70. Montalban C, Moreno MA, Molina JP, Hernanz I, Bellas C. Metastatic carcinoma of the prostate presenting as a superior vena cava syndrome. *Chest*. 1993;104:1278–1280.

71. Moura FM, Garcia LT, Castro LP, Ferrari TC. Prostate adenocarcinoma manifesting as generalized lymphadenopathy. *Urol Oncol*. 2006;24:216–219.

72. Park Y, Oster MW, Olarte MR. Prostatic cancer with an unusual presentation: polymyositis and mediastinal adenopathy. *Cancer*. 1981;48:1262–1264.

73. Tohfe M, Baki SA, Saliba W, et al. Metastatic prostate adenocarcinoma presenting with pulmonary symptoms: a case report and review of the literature. *Cases J*. 2008;1(1):316.

74. Yun HD, Ershler WB. Superior vena cava syndrome as a presentation of metastatic prostate cancer. *BMJ Case Rep*. 2012 Sep 3: 2012. doi:10.1136/bcr-2012-006480

75. Jones H, Anthony PP. Metastatic prostatic carcinoma presenting as left-sided cervical lymphadenopathy: a series of 11 cases. *Histopathology.* 1992;21(2):149–154.

76. Wang HJ, Chiang PH, Peng JP, Yu TJ. Presentation of prostate carcinoma with cervical lymphadenopathy: report of three cases. *Chang Gung Med J.* 2004;27(11):840–844.

77. Tan-Shalaby J. Prostate carcinoma presenting with bulky mediastinal and cervical lymphadenopathy. *BMJ Case Rep.* 2013 Apr 22:2013. doi:10.1136/bcr-2013-008643

78. Hess KR, Varadhachary GR, Taylor SH, et al. Metastatic patterns in adenocarcinoma. *Cancer.* 2006;106(7):1624–1633.

79. Golub JS, Chen P, Otto K, Hapneer E, Johns MM 3rd. Prevalence of perceived dysphonia in a geriatric population. *J Am Geriatr Soc.* 2006;54(11):1736–1739.

80. Woo P, Casper J, Colton R, Brewer D. Dysphonia in the aging: physiology versus disease. *Laryngoscope.* 1992;102(2):139–144.

81. Turley R, Cohen S. Impact of voice and swallowing problems in the elderly. *Otolaryngol Head Neck Surg.* 2009;140(1):33–36.

82. Gregory ND, Chandran S, Lurie D, Sataloff RT. Voice disorders in the elderly. *J Voice.* 2012;26(2):254–258.

83. Kendall K. Presbyphonia: a review. *Curr Opin Otolaryngol Head Neck Surg.* 2007;15(3):137–140.

84. Honjo I, Isshiki N. Laryngoscopic and voice characteristics of aged persons. *Arch Otolaryngol.* 1980;106(3):149–150.

85. Kahane JC. Connective tissue changes in the larynx and their effects on voice. *J Voice.* 1987;1(1):27–30.

86. Segre R. Senescence of the voice. *Eye Ear Nose Throat Monthly.* 1971;50(6):223–227.

87. Kawai Y, Kishimoto Y, Sogami T, et al. Characterization of aged rat vocal fold fibroblasts. *Laryngoscope.* 2019;129(3):e94–e101.

88. Melcon MC, Hoit JD, Hixon TJ. Age and laryngeal airway resistance during vowel production. *J Speech Hear Disord.* 1989;54 (2):282–286.

89. Hodge FS, Colton RH, Kelley RT. Vocal intensity characteristics in normal and elderly speakers. *J Voice.* 2001;15(4):503–511.

90. Morris RJ, Brown WS Jr. Age-related differences in speech intensity among adult females. *Folia Phoniatr Logop.* 1994;46(2):64–69.

91. Baker KK, Ramig LO, Sapir S, Luschei ES, Smith ME. Control of vocal loudness in young and old adults. *J Speech Lang Hear Res.* 2001;44(2):297–305.

92. Couper JW, Bloch S, Love A, Duchesne G, Macvean M, Kissane DW. The psychosocial impact of prostate cancer on patients and their partners. *Med J Aust.* 2006;185(8):428–432.

93. Salvo N, Zeng L, Zhang L, et al. Frequency of reporting and predictive factors for anxiety and depression in patients with advanced cancer. *Clin Oncol.* 2012;24(2):139–148.

94. Watts S, Leydon G, Eyles C, et al. A quantitative analysis of the prevalence of clinical depression and anxiety in patients with prostate cancer undergoing active surveillance. *BMJ Open.* 2015;5(5):e006674.

95. Watts S, Leydon G, Birch B, et al. Depression and anxiety in prostate cancer: a systemic review and meta-analysis of prevalence rates. *BMJ Open.* 2014;4(3):e003901.

96. Pompe RS, Kruger A, Preisser F, et al. The impact of anxiety and depression on surgical and functional outcomes in patients who underwent radical prostatectomy. *Eur Urol Focus.* 2018 Dec 31. doi:10.1016/j.euf .2018.12.008

97. Burnet KL, Parker C, Deamaley D, Brewin CR, Watson M. Does active surveillance for men with localized prostate cancer carry psychological morbidity? *BJU Int.* 2007;100(3):540–543.

98. Chipperfield K, Fletcher J, Millar J, et al. Predictors of depression, anxiety and quality of life in patients with prostate cancer receiving androgen deprivation therapy. *Psychooncology.* 2013;22(10):2169–2176.

99. Rosen DC, Huer RJ, Sasso DA, Sataloff RT. Psychological aspects of voice disorders. In: Sataloff RT. *Professional Voice: The Science and Art of Clinical Care.* 4th ed. San Diego, CA: Plural Publishing; 2017:705–736.

100. Hamdan AL, Sataloff RT, Hawshaw MJ. In: Hamdan AL, Sataloff RT, Hawkshaw M, ed. *Laryngeal Manifestations of Systemic Diseases*. San Diego, CA: Plural Publishing; 2018:87–110.

101. Aronson AE. *Clinical Voice Disorders*. 3rd ed. New York, NY: Thieme; 1990:117–145, 314–315.

102. Ritch C, Cookson M. Recent trends in the management of advanced prostate cancer. *F1000Res*. 2018 Sep 21;7. doi:10.12688/f1000research.15382.1

103. Harris WP, Mostaghel EA, Nelson PS, Montgomery B. Androgen deprivation therapy: progress in understanding mechanisms of resistance and optimizing androgen depletion. *Nat Clin Urol*. 2009;6(2):76–85.

104. Rhoden EL, Averbeck MA, Teloken PE. Androgen replacement in men undergoing treatment for prostate cancer. *J Sex Med*. 2008;5(9):2202–2208.

105. Huggins C, Hodges CV. Studies on prostatic cancer: The effect of castration, of estrogen and androgen injection on serum phosphatases in metastatic carcinoma of the prostate. *Cancer Res*. 1941;1:293–297.

106. Sharifi N, Gulley JL, Dahut WL. Androgen deprivation therapy for prostate cancer. *JAMA*. 2005;294(2):238–244.

107. Seidenfeld J, Samson DJ, Hasselblad V, et al. Single-therapy androgen suppression in men with advanced prostate cancer: a systemic review and meta-analysis. *Ann Intern Med*. 2000;132(7):566–577.

108. Nowicki M, Bryc W, Kokot F. Hormonal regulation of appetite and body mass in patients with advanced prostate cancer treated with combined androgen blockade. *J Endocrinol Invest*. 2001;24(1):31–36.

109. Smith JC, Bennett S, Evans LM, et al. The effects of induced hypogonadism on arterial stiffness, body composition, and metabolic parameters in males with prostate cancer. *J Clin Endocrinol Metab*. 2001;86(9):4261–4267.

110. Smith MR, Finkelstein JS, McGovern FJ, et al. Changes in body composition during androgen deprivation therapy for prostate cancer. *J Clin Endocrinol Metab*. 2002;87(2):599–603.

111. Smith MR. Changes in fat and lean body mass during androgen-deprivation therapy for prostate cancer. *Urology*. 2004;63(4):742–745.

112. Nishiyama T, Ishizaki F, Anraku T, Shimura H, Takahashi K. The influence of androgen deprivation therapy on metabolism in patients with prostate cancer. *J Clin Endocrinol Metab*. 2005;90(2):657–660.

113. Hamilton EJ, Gianatti E, Strauss BJ, et al. Increase in visceral and subcutaneous abdominal fat in men with prostate cancer treated with androgen deprivation therapy. *Clin Endocrinol*. 2011;74(3):377–383.

114. Timilshina N, Breunis H, Alibhai SM. Impact of androgen deprivation therapy on weight gain differs by age in men with nonmetastatic prostate cancer. *J Urol*. 2012;188(6):2183–2188.

115. Seible DM, Gu X, Hyatt AS, et al. Weight gain on androgen deprivation therapy: which patients are at highest risk? *Urology*. 2014;83(6):1316–1321.

116. Mitsuzuka K, Kyan A, Sato T, et al. Influence of 1 year of androgen deprivation therapy on lipid and glucose metabolism and fat accumulation in Japanese patients with prostate cancer. *Prostate Cancer Prostatic Dis*. 2016;19(1):57–62.

117. Eri LM, Urdal P, Bechensteen AG. Effects of the luteinizing hormone-releasing hormone agonist leuprolide on lipoproteins, fibrinogen and plasminogen activator inhibitor in patients with benign prostatic hyperplasia. *J Urol*. 1995;154(1):100–104.

118. Smith MR, Lee H, Nathan DM. Insulin sensitivity during combined androgen blockade for prostate cancer. *J Clin Endocrinol Metab*. 2006;91(4):1305–1308.

119. Torimoto K, Samma S, Kagebayashi Y, et al. The effects of androgen deprivation therapy on lipid metabolism and body composition in Japanese patients with prostate cancer. *Jpn J Clin Oncol*. 2011;41(4):577–581.

120. Dockery F, Bulpitt CJ, Agarwal S, Donaldson M, Rajkumar C. Testosterone suppression in men with prostate cancer leads to an

increase in arterial stiffness and hyperinsulinaemia. *Clin Sci.* 2003;104(2):195–201.

121. Salvador C, Planas J, Agreda F, et al. Analysis of the lipid profile and atherogenic risk during androgen deprivation therapy in prostate cancer patients. *Urol Int.* 2013;90(1):41–44.

122. Maillefert JF, Sibilia J, Michel F, Saussine C, Javier RM, Tavernier C. Bone mineral density in men treated with synthetic gonadotropin-releasing hormone agonists for prostatic carcinoma. *J Urol.* 1999;161(4):1219–1222.

123. Berruti A, Dogliotti L, Terrone C, et al. Changes in bone mineral density, lean body mass and fat content as measured by dual energy x-ray absorptiometry in patients with prostate cancer without apparent bone metastases given androgen deprivation therapy. *J Urol.* 2002;167(6):2361–2367.

124. Daniell HW, Dunn SR, Ferguson DW, et al. Progressive osteoporosis during androgen deprivation therapy for prostate cancer. *J Urol.* 2000;163(1):181–186.

125. Newman SR, Butler J, Hammond EH, Gray SD. Preliminary report on hormone receptors in the human vocal fold. *J Voice.* 2000;14(1):72:81.

126. Voelter Ch, Kleinsasser N, Joa P, et al. Detection of hormone receptors in the human vocal fold. *Eur Arch Otorhinolaryngol.* 2008; 265(10):1239–1244.

127. Kahane JC. Growth of the human prepubertal and pubertal larynx. *J Speech Hear Res.* 1982;25:446–455.

128. Titze IR. *Principles of Vocal Production.* Englewood Cliffs, NJ: Prentice Hall; 1994.

129. Meuser W, Nieschlag E. Sex hormone and depth of voice in the male. *Dtsch Med Wochenschr.* 1977;102(08):261–264.

130. Pedersen MF, Moller S, Krabbe S, Bennett P. Fundamental voice frequency measured by electroglottography during continuous speech. A new exact secondary sex characteristic in boys in puberty. *Int J Pediatr Otorhinolaryngol.* 1986;11(1):21–27.

131. Dabbs JM, Mallinger A. High testosterone levels predict low voice pitch among men. *Pers Indiv Differ.* 1999;27:801–804.

132. Evans S, Neave N, Wakelin D, Hamilton C. The relationship between testosterone and vocal frequencies in human males. *Physiol Behav.* 2008;93(4–5):783–788.

133. Gugatschka M, Kiesler K, Obermayer-Pietsch B, et al. Sex hormones and the elderly male voice. *J Voice.* 2010;24(3):369–373.

134. Hamdan AL, Jabbour J, Saadeh R, Kazan I, Nassar J, Bulbul M. Vocal changes in patients with prostate cancer following androgen ablation. *J Voice.* 2012;26(6):812. e11-5.

135. Akcam T, Bolu E, Merati AL, Durmus C, Gerek M, Ozkaptan Y. Voice changes after androgen therapy for hypogonadotrophic hypogonadism. *Laryngoscope.* 2004;114(9): 1587–1591.

136. Sassoon D, Segil N, Kelley D. Androgen-induced myogenesis and chondrogenesis in the larynx of *Xenopus laevis. Dev Biol.* 1986;113(1):135–140.

137. American Cancer Society. Cancer facts and figures. Accessed September 2, 2019. http://www.cancer.org/research/cancer-facts-statistics/all-cancer-facts-figures/cancer-facts-figures-2019.html

138. NIH. Prostate Cancer Treatment (PDQ), Patient Version. National Cancer Institute. Accessed Sep 5, 2019. https://www.cancer.gov/types/prostate/hp/prostate-treatment-pdq

139. Jarzemski P, Brzoszczyk B, Popiolek A, et al. Cognitive function, depression and anxiety in patients undergoing radical prostatectomy with and without adjuvant treatment. *Neuropsychiatr Dis Treat.* 2019;15:819–829.

140. Albaugh JA, Sufrin N, Lapin BR, Petkewicz J, Tenfelde S. Life after prostate cancer treatment: a mixed methods study of the experiences of men with sexual dysfunction and their partners. *BMC Urol.* 2017;17(1):45.

141. Meissner VH, Herkommer K, Marten-Mittag B, Gschwend JE, Dinkel A. Prostate cancer-related anxiety in long-term survivors after radical prostatectomy. *J Cancer Surviv.* 2017;11(6):800–807.

142. Verdolini K, Min Y, Titze IR, et al. Biological mechanisms underlying voice changes due to dehydration. *J Speech Lang Hear Res.* 2002;45:268–281.

143. Solomon NP, DiMattia MS. Effects of a vocally fatiguing task and systemic hydration on phonation threshold pressure. *J Voice.* 2000;14(3):341–362.

144. Mattioni J, Opperman DA, Solimando DA Jr, Sataloff RT. Cancer chemotherapy: An overview and voice implications. In: Sataloff RT, *Professional Voice: The Science and Art of Clinical Care.* 4th ed. San Diego, CA: Plural Publishing; 2017:1137–1141.

8

Thyroid Cancer and Voice

Abdul-Latif Hamdan, Robert Thayer Sataloff, and Mary J. Hawkshaw

Epidemiology and Clinical Presentation

Thyroid cancer is the ninth most common cancer in the world.[1] There were an estimated 567 233 newly diagnosed cases in 2018, for 3.1% of all cancer incidence worldwide.[1] The highest incidence has been reported in the Republic of Korea, followed by North America, Australia, and Eastern Asia. In the United States, an estimated 52 070 new cases were diagnosed in 2019, with women being affected 3 times more commonly than men.[2] The risk peak for having thyroid cancer is between the ages of 40 and 59 years for women, and 60 and 79 years for men.[3] White Americans are more likely to develop thyroid cancer in comparison to black Americans.[4] The incidence is highest in non-Hispanic white and lowest in non-Hispanic black, while the death rate is the highest in Asian and Pacific Islanders and lowest in Native Americans, Indian people and Alaska natives.[3] The estimated number of thyroid-related deaths worldwide in 2018 was 41 071, accounting for 0.4% to 0.5% of all cancer-related deaths in men and women. In the United States, it is estimated that 2170 died of thyroid cancer in 2018, with equal death distribution among genders.[1]

The last 3 decades have witnessed a marked increase in the incidence of thyroid cancer among all age groups: children, adolescent, and adults.[2] This rise in incidence is ascribed primarily to overdiagnosis.[5–8] In a review by Vaccarella et al on the epidemic of thyroid cancer, the authors reported overdiagnosis in 50% to 90% of cases worldwide.[5] The overdiagnosis has been attributed to easy access to medical care and to the improvement in technology. In an epidemiologic study on the association between socioeconomic status and the rising incidence of thyroid cancer, Li et al reported a moderate increase in incidence of tumors less than 4 cm in high socioeconomic countries versus a steady increase in low socioeconomic countries.[9] The authors suggested that the increase in thyroid cancer incidence is related partly to the enhanced detection of small lesions using advanced radiologic imaging. In a study by Brito et al, 16% of thyroid cancer were diagnosed incidentally on computed tomography (CT) and/or magnetic resonance images.[10] Two-thirds of the detected thyroid nodules were less than 15 mm in size. The authors referred to the expanding gap between the increasing incidence of thyroid cancer and the constant death rate as evidence of overdiagnosis.[10] Similarly, Kent et al reported an increase in the incidence of differentiated thyroid cancer which they speculated was secondary to excessive usage of medical imaging. In their review of 7422 cases operated on over the course of 11 years, an increasing number of small nodules (less than 2 cm) had been diagnosed.[11] The authors concluded that overdiagnosis had led to an increase in the number of thyroid surgeries for small intrathyroid lesions. Udelsman and Zhang concurred. They reviewed cancer statistics in the United States and also found a significant correlation between the increased incidence of diagnosed thyroid cancer and the usage of cervical ultrasonography. The authors concluded that overdetection of occult thyroid disease has fostered unnecessary surgical intervention, with subsequent physical, emotional, and financial burdens on patients and health care providers.[12] Nevertheless, it is important to note that a rising diagnostic trend for large tumors greater than 2 cm also has been observed in both males and females in the United States.[8] A review by Enewold et al on the rising incidence of thyroid cancer highlighted the need to consider other contributing factors aside from heightened medical surveillance given that 50% of newly diagnosed thyroid cases had lesions greater than 1 cm in size.[13]

Other catalysts for the increase in prevalence of thyroid cancer include change in dietary habits, exposure to pollutants and environmental hazards, and genetic predisposition.[14-19] Among environmental factors, exposure to ionizing irradiation is the most significant, with consensus on its etiologic role in both follicular and papillary thyroid cancer. Other factors include xenobiotics also referred to as *endocrine-disrupting chemicals* (EDCs),[14] which are abundantly present in the environment. A plausible explanation for the association between these factors and thyroid cancer

is the autoimmune inflammatory response that is associated with a proliferative effect on the peripheral metabolism of thyroid hormones, thus leading to tissue hyperplasia and thyroid oncogenesis.[15] Gas and ash emission in volcanic areas also is considered carcinogenic by inducing genetic alterations and neoplastic transformation.[16] With regard to diet and thyroid cancer, the etiologic roles of several nutrients have been investigated in the literature. Marcello et al reported a strong association between high caloric intake, in particular protein and carbohydrate, and differentiated thyroid carcinoma.[17] The study, which evaluated 115 patients with differentiated thyroid cancer versus 103 healthy controls, advocated dietary control in the prevention of thyroid carcinoma. A strong link between excessive fruit juice intake and thyroid cancer also has been reported by Zamora-Ros et al. The authors reported a positive but borderline trend between the 2, with a hazard ratio of 1.23.[18] Another risk factor for thyroid cancer is obesity. In a study that included 1917 patients and 2127 cancer-free controls, Xu et al reported an association between risk of cancer, weight, fat percentage, and body mass index.[20]

Based on several histopathologic features, different types of thyroid cancer have been described, with papillary carcinoma and follicular carcinoma accounting for the majority of cases. Less frequent thyroid carcinomas are the oxyphilic cell carcinoma and anaplastic thyroid carcinoma.[21,22] The overall prognosis and survival rate of thyroid cancer depend on several factors among which are age and gender.[23-27] In a study by Nilubol et al which included 61 523 patients who were followed up for 4½ years, the authors showed that men are diagnosed with more advanced disease in comparison to women. Moreover, men displayed more aggressive pathology on histologic examination, which in turn has led to short disease-specific survival and an increased thyroid-cancer specific mortality.[24] Similarly, in a study by Tubiana et al which included 546 patients with differentiated thyroid cancer, elderly patients had lower total survival and relapse-free survival in comparison to younger patients.[25] Other important prognostic factors in patients with thyroid cancer are the size and histology of the tumor. In a review by Olson et al that included 343 386 patients with thyroid cancer, those with follicular carcinoma were less likely to be diagnosed at an advanced stage (stage IV) in comparison to patients with medullary/anaplastic carcinoma and patients with papillary carcinoma (16.9% versus 33.7% versus 49.4%, respectively). The review included all cases of thyroid cancer National Cancer Database between 2000 and 2013.[22] Moreover, patients with 2 or more comorbidities were more likely to be diagnosed with stage IV in comparison to those with no or 1 comorbidity. In another retrospective study on 499 patients with differentiated thyroid carcinoma, Jukkola et al reported that large tumors, extrathyroidal invasion, and nodal metastasis are poor prognostic factors associated with a higher recurrence rate. Similarly, the follicular type of carcinoma and the presence of local invasion were predictive of poor survival.[26] Sellers et al demonstrated that tumors larger than 3 cm, cervical lymph node metastasis, and distant metastasis are poor prognostic factors.[27]

Thyroid carcinoma is known to metastasize to cervical lymph nodes in 1 out of 2 patients. However, its metastasis to distant sites is rare and its prevalence varies across the literature.[28-31] In a study on the predictive factors of distant metastasis in 1023 patients with papillary thyroid cancer, Sugitami et al reported distant metastasis in 86 cases, half of whom had their

metastasis diagnosed at the time of their initial presentation.[31] In another review by Hoie et al of 731 cases with papillary thyroid carcinoma, 12.4% of whom had distant metastasis, the sites affected the most were the thoracic cavity, lungs, and mediastinum. Two patterns of chest metastasis were recognized: the granular type and the localized infiltrative type. Less frequently affected organs were skeletal structures such as ribs, long bones, and pelvis, as well as cerebrum and subcutaneous tissues.[29] Similarly, in a study on 444 patients with papillary and follicular carcinoma, Durante et al reported lung and bone metastasis in 223 and 115 patients, respectively.[30] Thyroid carcinoma also may spread to unusual sites such as the kidneys, adrenal glands, liver, and brain.[31-34] In patients with metastasis to the kidney, the diagnosis of renal metastasis may precede or follow that of the primary tumor. If diagnosed early, treatment usually is successful.[32] Similarly, in patients with a solitary cerebellar metastatic lesion, the need for early detection and neurosurgical intervention is paramount.[33] Skin is another rare site of distant metastasis that should not be overlooked in patients with thyroid carcinoma.[35,36] Lissak et al described 2 patients with thyroid microcarcinoma who developed cutaneous metastasis in the scalp. The diagnosis was confirmed using immunoperoxidase staining for thyroglobulin.[35] Similarly, Reusser et al described a 95-year-old man, diagnosed previously with thyroid and prostate cancer, who presented with a cervical cutaneous lesion measuring 1.3 × 0.9 cm and causing intermitted dysphagia. Immunohistochemical staining confirmed the diagnosis of metastatic papillary thyroid carcinoma.[36]

Laryngeal metastasis and/or invasion to the aerodigestive tract in patients with carcinoma of the thyroid gland warrants special attention. Affected patients who present with dysphonia need to be investigated thoroughly. This chapter summarizes the association between thyroid cancer and voice. Surgery-induced dysphonia with emphasis on neurogenic and nonneurogenic causes of dysphonia should be considered. This information is essential for laryngologists, speech-language pathologists, voice teachers, and internists involved in the care of patients with thyroid carcinoma.

Disease-Induced Dysphonia in Patients With Thyroid Carcinoma

Dysphonia is common in patients with thyroid disease. A diligent voice history and a thorough laryngeal examination reveal signs and symptoms of voice dysfunction in a high percentage of affected patients.[37] In a review by Pernambuco et al on patients with benign thyroid disease, the authors reported low voice-assessment scores and poor voice-related quality of life.[38] Patients with hypothyroidism often report deepening of their voice and loss of range secondary to excessive deposition of hyaluronic acid in the lamina propria, whereas patients with hyperthyroidism complain of a tremulous voice in addition to symptoms of excessive sweating, heart palpitations, and weight loss.[39,40] Thyroiditis may also affect phonation. Falhamar et al reported dysphonia and dysphagia as common symptoms in the clinical presentation of Reidel thyroiditis.[41] Similarly, Volpe and Johnston reported hoarseness in 8 of 56 patients with subacute thyroiditis.[42] These reports are in agreement with the study by Altman et al that proved the larynx as a hormone-end organ. The authors demonstrated the presence of thyroid hormones receptors, alpha and beta, in the lamina propria, glands, and laryngeal car-

tilages.[43] That strong link between thyroid hormones and voice is substantiated further by the reversibility of vocal symptoms in patients with hypothyroid treated with hormone replacement.[44]

Dysphonia in patients with thyroid disease also may result from compression on the aerodigestive tract. This is not surprising given the anatomical position of the thyroid gland in the lower anterior neck and its proximity to the laryngeal framework. In a review of 90 patients with goiter, Moumen et al reported a predominance of compressive symptoms in 82.5% of cases and dysphonia in 2 out of 3.[45] In another study on the prevalence of phonatory symptoms in 40 patients with goiter, Hamdan et al reported a significantly higher prevalence of voice strain in the study group in comparison to the control group. The most common voice symptom was voice fatigue, followed by globus sensation.[46] Alfonso et al reported tracheal and/or esophageal compression in one-third of patients with benign goiter. The prevalence of compressive symptoms was higher in patients with multinodular goiter and in patients with thyroiditis in comparison to those with colloid goiter. Moreover, the presence of tracheal deviation on radiologic imaging was predictive of dyspnea and dysphagia in two-thirds of patients.[47] The prevalence of dysphonia among other compressive symptoms varies with the histology of the disease and its local spread.[47-51] In a review by Banks et al which included 332 patients undergoing thyroidectomy, the prevalence of dysphonia was higher in patients with thyroid malignancies in comparison to patients with benign goiter. Dysphonia was reported in 100% of patients with medullary thyroid cancer and 71% of patients with anaplastic thyroid cancer.[48] Similarly, in a study by Caroline et al on 17 patients undergoing thyroidectomy, the authors emphasized the link between thyroid carcinoma and dysphonia before surgery.[51]

In conclusion, dysphonia is common in patients with benign and malignant thyroid disease. Its etiology is multifactorial. The change in voice quality can be secondary to vocal fold paresis and/or paralysis, to disease invasion of the aerodigestive tract with or without vocal fold fixation, or to thyroid cancer metastasizing to the larynx and related structures, to hormone changes, and to other factors.

Vocal Fold Paralysis or Paresis in Patients With Thyroid Carcinoma

Vocal fold paralysis or paresis in patients with thyroid carcinoma is not uncommon. In a study on the etiologic role of thyroid disease in laryngeal neuropathy, Heman-Ackah et al reported thyroid dysfunction in almost half the patients who presented with dysphonia and vocal fold paresis.[52] Affected patients usually present with hoarseness, inability to project the voice, voice fatigue, dysphagia, and aspiration.[53-57] In many instances, patients may be asymptomatic despite impairment in vocal fold mobility. In an investigation on 240 patients undergoing thyroidectomy, Farrag et al reported lack of phonatory symptoms in one-third of patients with preoperative vocal fold paralysis (32% of 22 patients). The positive and negative predictive values of voice symptoms in diagnosing impairment in vocal fold movement were 31% and 98%, respectively.[55] Similarly, in a study by Randolph et al on the clinical presentation of 365 patients undergoing thyroidectomy, two-thirds of patients diagnosed with vocal fold paralysis were asymptomatic.[56] The lack of phonatory symptoms in patients with thyroid carcinoma and vocal fold paralysis can be

attributed to the compensatory behavior of the opposite vocal fold, as compensatory muscle tension dysphonia often develops gradually as symptoms progress. Moreover, the slow enlargement of the thyroid gland allows progressive adaptation with minimal or no change in voice quality up to a point in certain patients. Another cause for the absence of phonatory symptoms in affected patients is a "favorable" medial position of the paralyzed vocal fold, allowing good glottic closure during phonation.

The inconsistent association between dysphonia and vocal fold paralysis highlights the importance of electromyographic evaluation to detect or exclude disease-induced recurrent laryngeal nerve (RLN) or superior laryngeal nerve (SLN) palsy,[58] although there is still controversy regarding laryngeal examination in the preoperative workup of patients undergoing thyroidectomy.[59,60] In an editorial report by Hodin et al, only patients with voice symptoms, history of prior surgery along the course of the RLN, and/or with a strong suspicion of thyroid cancer invasion to the contiguous structures were advised to undergo flexible or indirect laryngoscopy for the evaluation of vocal fold mobility prior to thyroidectomy.[61] Similarly, in a review by Chandrasekhar et al, preoperative laryngeal examination was advocated only in patients with voice impairment, history of prior neck surgery, and/or increased risk of RLN injury, or in patients with suspected extracapsular thyroid extension.[62] However, the American Academy of Otolaryngology-Head and Neck Surgery and the American Association of Endocrine Surgeons have endorsed the need for preoperative laryngeal examination of all patients undergoing thyroidectomy, even in the absence of phonatory symptoms, a consensus that has markedly increased the rate of preoperative diagnosis of vocal fold paralysis in clinical practice.[63]

The controversy about the need for preoperative laryngeal examination in patients with thyroid carcinoma undergoing surgery is consistent with the large range in the prevalence of disease-induced RLN and SLN palsy.[64-69] In a study by Chiang et al on 622 patients, among whom 156 had thyroid malignancies, the incidence of preoperative RLN palsy was reported as 3%. Of the 16 patients diagnosed with preoperative RLN palsy, 15 had malignant thyroid disease, the majority of whom had extracapsular disease invasion.[67] In a clinical study by McCaffrey et al that included 286 cases of thyroid tumors and 624 invasion sites, the RLN was the second most common site of invasion ($n = 131$). Tracheal and laryngeal invasion occurred in 109 and 30 cases, respectively.[68] Kay-Rivest et al reported the prevalence of preoperative vocal fold paralysis in 1.3% of 1923 consecutive patients who underwent thyroidectomy at McGill University teaching hospital. The majority of affected patients (76%) had malignant disease, the most common of which was papillary carcinoma.[63] In a study by Falk and McCaffrey, 123 of 262 patients with invasive papillary carcinoma had RLN invasion. Ten percent of those with preoperative vocal fold paralysis had perineural invasion in comparison to only 1.1% of those with no vocal fold paralysis.[69] In a study by Roh et al on 319 patients with papillary thyroid papillary carcinoma who had undergone thyroidectomy, 14 had unilateral vocal fold paralysis preoperatively. Intraoperatively, 8,8% had invasion of the RLN.[70] In a large review that included 365 consecutive patients undergoing thyroidectomy, RLN palsy was reported in two-thirds of patients with invasive thyroid malignancies ($n = 21$), in comparison to only 0.3% of those with noninvasive disease.[56] In the study by Farrag et al on 340 patients undergoing thyroid surgery, 6.4% had preoperative vocal fold paralysis (22 out of 340). Out of these, 13 had thyroid ma-

lignancy on histologic examination, 62% of whom had papillary carcinoma.[55]

Despite the previously mentioned research that suggests that vocal fold paralysis is an ominous sign of malignancy, it is important to emphasize that vocal fold paralysis is also common in patients with benign thyroid disease, with a high propensity for recovery.[71-75] Rowe et al examined the association between benign disease of the thyroid gland and vocal fold paralysis in 2408 patients admitted for thyroidectomy. A total of 29 patients with vocal fold paralysis were noted, 89% of whom had recovery in vocal fold function after surgical removal of the thyroid gland.[72] Fenton et al reported 3 patients with benign goiter who had vocal fold paralysis during the course of their disease. The authors highlighted the etiologic role of intraglandular hemorrhage in the development of RLN palsy in affected patients.[73] Moorthy et al described 5 patients with multinodular goiter with vocal fold paralysis, 2 of whom had full recovery of their vocal fold paralysis following thyroidectomy. The authors emphasized the need to spare the RLN during surgery despite the presence of preoperative vocal fold paralysis.[74] Interestingly, Collazo et al reported 4 patients with benign nodular thyroid disease and vocal fold paralysis, 2 of whom had the paralysis contralateral to the side of the thyroid nodules.[75] This emphasizes the fact that vocal fold paresis/paralysis diagnosed in conjunction with thyroid cancer is not always causally related to cancer (Figures 8–1 and 8–2).

The diagnosis of vocal fold paralysis in patients with thyroid cancer is extremely important, particularly in patients undergoing surgery. In addition to indirect laryngoscopy, flexible laryngoscopy, and stroboscopy, laryngeal electromyography (EMG) plays a key role in detecting subclinical vocal fold neurogenic disorders and in identifying other causes of dysphonia in affected patients.[58] In a large study

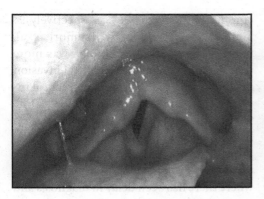

Figure 8–1. Fiberoptic laryngeal examination of a 73-year-old woman with retrosternal goiter who presented with history of dysphonia and aspiration. Right vocal fold paralysis in the paramedian position.

on 751 patients, Sataloff et al demonstrated 2 findings of high clinical relevance in the workup of patients with vocal fold paralysis; one is the limitation of laryngeal videostroboscopy in diagnosing impairment in vocal fold mobility. The second is the added value of laryngeal EMG in detecting neuromuscular dysfunction in the absence of impaired vocal fold mobility on laryngeal examination.[58] When vocal fold paralysis is diagnosed, the greatest care in the handling and dissection of the ipsilateral and contralateral RLN during thyroidectomy is advocated. Evidence-based documentation of the paralysis also is invaluable in regard to postoperative litigations in patients with neurogenic complications.[67]

In summary, vocal fold paresis/paralysis is not uncommon in patients with thyroid cancer. Based on the earlier reports, the mechanisms of injury include mass compression and/or neural infiltration by malignant cells. Important predictors are the size of the tumor and its histology. Preoperative diagnosis is crucial to optimal management of affected patients and for minimizing medicolegal liabilities.

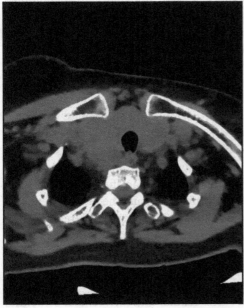

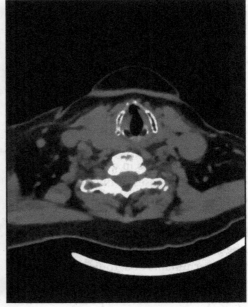

A   **B**

Figure 8–2. Computed tomography of the upper chest revealing an enlarged multinodular goiter with retrosternal extension causing mass effect on the right tracheaesophageal groove (**A**). A higher cut at the neck shows displacement of the larynx and trachea to the left (**B**).

Thyroid Carcinoma Invasion of the Upper Aerodigestive Tract and Dysphonia

Invasion of thyroid carcinoma to structures contiguous with the thyroid gland is not uncommon. Honings et al, in their review of 20 studies that included 10 251 patients with thyroid carcinoma, reported laryngotracheal invasion in 0.5% to 35% of cases.[76] The large range in the prevalence rate can be attributed primarily to the variable definition of the word "invasion." To some authors, invasion refers to the spread of thyroid tumor beyond the thyroid capsule, as in cases of adherence or attachment of the thyroid gland to adjacent structures. To other authors, invasion refers to tumor transgression or extension into the laryngeal or tracheal lumen. In a review of 859 patients with papillary carcinoma, McConahey et al reported external adherence to the thyroid gland in 9.9% of cases.[77] In a study by Djalilian et al on 2000 patients with thyroid disease, the authors reported endoluminal laryngeal and tracheal disease in only 0.9% of cases, all of whom had thyroid malignancies.[78] Another cause for the wide range in the prevalence of thyroid invasion is the disparity in the diagnostic method used.[79,80] In a radiologic review by Lawson et al that included 100 cases of thyroid carcinoma, the prevalence of airway involvement was 35%,[79] whereas in a pathologic review of 193 autopsy cases of thyroid carcinoma, direct extension beyond the capsule in combination with metastasis was reported in only 13% of cases.[80] The histology and stage of the thyroid carcinoma are important determinants of aerodigestive tract invasion.[77,80–85] In a clinical-pathologic study by Silliphant and Levitin, poorly differentiated thyroid carcinoma was more likely to invade local structures and to metastasize in comparison to well-differentiated carcinoma (96% versus 36%, respectively).[80] Similarly, in a review by Tsumori et al, poorly differentiated carcinoma was more prevalent in patients with tracheal invasion in comparison to those with no tracheal invasion.[83] In another review by Chala et al, 9 of 16 patients with laryngeal invasion had an aggressive type of papillary carcinoma. It is important to note that the risk of invasion also increases in neglected cases where there has been delay in diagnosis and treatment.[85]

Pathophysiology and Mechanisms of Invasion in Thyroid Carcinoma

Alterations in tumor-suppressing genes and genetic mutations responsible for tumor suppression and cell adhesion are some of the factors responsible for tumor growth beyond the capsule in patients with thyroid cancer.[86–88] An imbalance in metalloproteinases (MPPs) and other endopeptidases initiates a proteolytic degradation of the basement membrane and extracellular matrix, leading to tumor invasion to adjacent structures.[89–92] In addition, there are alterations in intercellular adhesion glycoprotein and intracytoplasmic molecules, with a decrease in the expression of adherent molecules E-cadherin and B-catenin.[93–95] In an immunohistochemical study by McCaffrey that included 42 paraffin-embedded samples of thyroid tissue, the authors reported a statistically significant difference in the concentration of E-cadherin in patients with invasive papillary thyroid tumor in comparison to those with no invasion and in comparison to controls.[68]

The cellular and intercellular structural alterations discussed earlier allow thyroid carcinoma to extend beyond the thyroid capsule to contiguous structures. Invasion into the larynx occurs through 3 main anatomical routes: One is the cricothyroid membrane and cricoid cartilage, the second is through the thyroid cartilage, and the third is through the paraglottic space posterolaterally.[68] On presentation, the symptoms and signs vary with the site of invasion and extent of the disease.[69,96-99] Both airway and phonatory symptoms may occur, although dysphonia is not always secondary to RLN or SLN palsy as discussed in the previous section. Other causes of dysphonia include alteration in vocal tract anatomy and resonance, hormonal and others, with or without fixation of vocal fold mobility. In a review of 16 patients with locally advanced thyroid tumor, Chala et al reported dysphonia in all patients, 5 of whom had no RLN palsy during their initial evaluation.[85] Additional symptoms included dysphagia, hemoptysis, dyspnea, and stridor. In a report of 3 patients with lymphoma of the thyroid gland, Graham et al emphasized that hoarseness may ensue secondary to lymphedema of the vocal folds even in the absence of vocal fold paralysis. The authors described 3 patients with thyroid lymphoma, all of whom had dysphonia and normal mobility of the vocal folds.[96] In a study by McCarty et al that included 40 patients with thyroid cancer and laryngotracheal invasion, only 20% had unilateral vocal fold paralysis. Hoarseness and hemoptysis were present in 22% and 11% of cases, respectively.[98] In a case report of a papillary thyroid carcinoma neglected for many years, Georgiades et al attributed dysphonia and obstructive symptoms to laryngeal edema and fixation of the right vocal fold. The patient underwent total laryngectomy, thyroidectomy, and neck dissection followed by radioactive iodine therapy.[97]

The diagnosis of laryngeal invasion is often a challenge, as the presenting symptoms can distract from recognizing the extent of invasion, particularly at the early stage of the disease. The most commonly used diagnostic modality is flexible laryngoscopy. In a study by Tomoda et al, the diagnostic yield of flexible laryngoscopy reached 85%, with only 6.5% of those examined having a false-positive reading.[100] In a review by Chala et al, flexible endoscopy confirmed laryngeal invasion in all patients with advanced thyroid cancer admitted for laryngectomy and thyroidectomy.[85] The most common findings on laryngeal examination were submucosal mass or bulge, mucosal ulceration, and narrowing of the airway with or without vocal fold fixation. The diagnosis of laryngotracheal invasion can be assessed further using CT.[101-103] In a radiologic study by Takashima et al on 19 patients with anaplastic thyroid carcinoma, CT correctly identified laryngeal invasion in 5 out of 6 cases, and tracheal invasion in 8 out of 10 cases. The authors alluded to the diagnostic role of CT and to its added value in the surgical planning of patients with thyroid carcinoma and metastasis.[101] In another study by Seo et al on 84 patients with thyroid carcinoma and extracapsular spread, CT was accurate in diagnosing tracheal invasion and RLN invasion in 83.2% and 85.5% of cases, respectively, with a specificity of 91.4% and 89.8%, respectively[102] (Figure 8–3).

The treatment of laryngotracheal invasion varies, with several surgical techniques being described in the literature. Partial resection of the aerodigestive tract is almost invariably advocated in order to preserve function. Ballantyne et al in their large series of 1098 patients, 46 of whom had partial resection of the upper aerodigestive tract, reported marked improvement in the 5-year survival rate.[104] More radical surgery is recommended often for better oncologic control in cases of extensive disease spread.

In summary, invasion of the aerodigestive tract is an ominous sign in patients

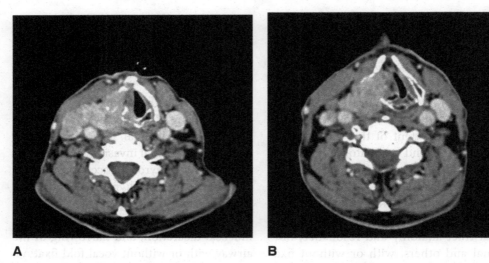

A   **B**

Figure 8–3. Axial cut of a computed tomography scan of an 80-year-old man presenting with papillary thyroid carcinoma showing evidence of laryngeal involvement with invasion of the thyroid cartilage (**A–B**).

with thyroid cancer. Dysphonia and/or airway symptoms are reported commonly. A change in voice quality is not always indicative of RLN palsy. Proper diagnosis of the extent of invasion is paramount for surgical planning as invasion of thyroid carcinoma to the laryngotracheal complex remains a significant predictor of survival rate and death.[68,105,106]

Laryngeal Metastasis in Patients With Thyroid Cancer

Thyroid cancer is known to metastasize to various structures in the body, in addition to its propensity to invade contiguous structures in the head and neck.[107] Lymphatic spread is the most frequent mode of metastasis with marked involvement of intrathyroid and cervical lymph nodes. Factors described commonly as determinants of metastasis include male gender, older age, and advanced stage of the disease.[108] In a study by Hoie et al, which included 90 patients with papillary carcinoma and distant

metastasis, men were more affected than women, and patients with advanced disease had more distant metastasis.[29] Another important determinant of distant metastasis in patients with thyroid cancer is extracapsular metastatic lymphadenopathy.[109] In a study by Yamashita et al comparing patients with thyroid papillary carcinoma with metastasis to those without metastasis, the authors reported higher prevalence of large lymph nodes and extranodal invasion in the former group. The odds ratio of extranodal invasion in patients with distant metastatic disease was reported as 9.[109]

Laryngeal metastasis in patients with thyroid carcinoma is rare. A review of the literature revealed only 2 cases of thyroid carcinoma with metastasis to the larynx. In 2003, Varghese et al described a 41-year-old man, diagnosed with papillary carcinoma of the thyroid gland, who presented with multinodular thyroid lesions and multiple cervical lymphadenopathies at levels II, III, and IV. On laryngeal examination, the patient had submucosal nodules on the posterior pharyngeal wall and right aryepiglottic fold, with normal mobility of the vocal folds. Histologic examination of punch biopsies from the suspected area confirmed the presence of metastatic papillary carcinoma. Metastatic workup failed to show any distant metastatic lesion. Given the local spread of the disease and its extensive nature, the patient underwent debulking surgery and concomitant radiotherapy.[110] In 2012, Hakeem et al reported a 50-year-old man who presented with a cervical mass and throat discomfort. The patient denied any symptoms related to swallowing or phonation. On examination, he had a 4 × 3 cm thyroid nodule and 2 lymph nodes on the right side. Indirect laryngoscopy using a 70° rigid scope showed a nodular lesion in the right pyriform sinus and aryepiglottic fold. Fine-needle aspiration using ultrasound guidance revealed papillary thyroid carcinoma, and histopathologic examination of the laryngeal lesion was consistent with metastatic disease from the primary papillary neoplastic lesion. Radiologic imaging using CT failed to show direct extension between the thyroid tumor and that observed in the larynx. The patient underwent total thyroidectomy, neck dissection, and microlaryngeal excision of the laryngeal mass using carbon dioxide laser.[111]

In both reported cases, the course of the disease was indolent, and patients did not complain of dysphonia, dysphagia, or airway obstructive symptoms that are reported commonly in patients with thyroid carcinoma and/or invasion into the aerodigestive tract.[112] Similar to other cases of laryngeal metastasis, the laryngeal findings were non-specific with no differentiating criteria. The supraglottis is affected most commonly, and the lesion is almost invariably submucosal with an intact overlying mucosa. The treatment consists primarily of surgery with or without radiotherapy. Although prognosis is usually poor, the 5-year survival in patients with thyroid laryngeal metastasis is

uncertain. In the review by Sugitami et al, factors associated with worse prognosis in patients with thyroid cancer metastasis included metastatic lesions above 2 cm in size, metastatic sites aside from lungs, the presence of metastatic lymphadenopathy greater than 3 cm, and older age.[31] In another study by Dinneen et al looking at predictive factors of survival in 100 papillary carcinoma patients, 6% of whom had metastasis, the 5- and 10-year survival rates were better in patients with low-grade disease and who had undergone complete surgical resection of their tumor.[113]

Surgery-Induced Dysphonia in Patients With Thyroid Carcinoma

As noted in the American Thyroid Association guidelines, management of patients with thyroid carcinoma consists primarily of surgical resection, radioiodine therapy, and thyroid hormonal suppression. Various types of surgeries have been described, the most common of which are lobectomy, subtotal thyroidectomy, and total thyroidectomy with or without lymph node dissection.[114] The type of surgery is chosen based on the histology of the disease, the site and size of the tumor, the presence or absence of extracapsular spread, and/or invasion of structures contiguous with the thyroid gland. When the aerodigestive tract is invaded, tailoring the surgical resection is essential for oncologic disease control and safe preservation of function. In cases of extraluminal invasion, shaving techniques that spare the function of the larynx and pharynx have been advocated highly. In patients with tumor invasion into the lumen of the laryngotracheal complex, more radical surgery including partial or complete laryngectomy and sleeve or step tracheal resection, with or without muscle flap reconstruction, are recommended.[99,115,116]

In all surgeries of thyroid carcinoma, the phonatory system is in jeopardy. A study by Solomon et al on 70 patients who underwent thyroidectomy showed both perceptual and acoustic vocal changes postoperatively. Spectral peak performance was the strongest variable among other acoustic parameters in following-up on vocal changes after thyroidectomy.[117] In another study looking at the morbidity of thyroidectomy from the patient's perspective, 40% of the study group reported subjective worsening of their voice following surgery. Moreover, there was an increase in the voice handicap index (VHI) score, with poor to fair voice-related quality of life in 38% and 14,3% of cases, respectively.[118] These results are not surprising given the intimate proximity of the thyroid gland to the phonatory apparatus. A thorough review of the literature indicates that surgical resection of thyroid malignancies can lead to dysphonia in many ways. These include injury to the RLN, injury to the external branch of the SLN, dysfunction in the strap muscles with or without scarring of the laryngeal framework, transient or permanent hypoparathyroidism, scarring of the skin to the larynx with restriction of vertical laryngeal motion, and endotracheal tube–related injuries. A summary of the mechanisms by which thyroid surgery can induce a change in voice helps highlight issues of which clinicians should be aware.

Surgery-Induced Injury to the Recurrent Laryngeal Nerve in Patients With Thyroid Cancer

Notwithstanding the major evolution in surgical technique with direct visualization of the RLN during thyroidectomy, injury to the RLN is still a challenging complication encountered commonly in laryngology practice. In a study by Chiang et al that included 521 patients who underwent thyroidectomy, 2.0% and 0.7% had temporary and permanent vocal fold paralysis, though the RLN was directly visualized intraoperatively.[119] Similarly, in another study by Bergenfelz et al, RLN injury had been recognized intraoperatively in only 1 of 6 patients who developed bilateral vocal fold paralysis.[120] The insult is usually more frequent on the left side given the longer course of the RLN on the left in comparison to the right. In a study by Kay-Rivest et al, the rate of left-sided RLN injury was almost twice (72%) that reported on the right side,[63] similar to what has been reported by other authors.[121,122]

The overall prevalence of RLN palsy following thyroidectomy varies across the literature, depending whether the paralysis is reported as transient or permanent. The prevalence of temporary RLN palsy ranges between 1.4% and 38.4%, whereas that of permanent RLN palsy ranges between 0 and 18.6%.[59,123–131] In a large study by Hayward et al that included 2422 thyroid surgeries, 53 patients developed RLN palsy, of whom only 6 had permanent vocal fold paralysis.[126] In another review of 1020 thyroidectomy patients by Goncalves-Filho et al, the prevalence of permanent vocal fold paralysis was only 0.4% in comparison to transient vocal fold paralysis in 1.4% of cases.[127] This leads us to conclude that the recovery rate of RLN injury following thyroidectomy is very high, more so when the RLN is left intact during surgery. Another important determinant of the prevalence of RLN palsy is the mode of laryngeal assessment. In a systematic review by Jeannon et al that included 25 000 patients who underwent thyroidectomy, the authors reported a heterogeneous rate in the prevalence of permanent and temporary RLN palsy using different diagnostic methods. For indirect laryngoscopy, the prevalence of permanent RLN palsy ranged between 0.4% and 18.6%, whereas for flexible laryngoscopy, the range was between 0 and 3.5%. When using the stroboscope with indirect laryngoscopy or flexible laryngoscopy, the prevalence increased to 0.9%.[130] In a large study by Erbil et al on 3250 patients who had thyroid surgeries, 520 of whom had thyroid malignancies, the overall rate of RLN palsy using indirect laryngoscopic examination was 2.3%.[128] In another study by Kocak et al, laryngeal videostroboscopy had higher sensitivity in detecting vocal fold paralysis than clinical evaluation and flexible laryngeal examination (100% versus 81% versus 67%, respectively).[131] These results are in partial agreement with the 2016 consensus statement of the American Head and Neck Society, which recommends the usage of flexible laryngeal examination as the optimal mode of laryngeal assessment for patients undergoing thyroidectomy.[132]

What are the risk factors for RLN injury? Intraoperative injury to the RLN may occur secondary to compression, traction, clamping, ligation, and/or thermal injury. In a study that included 380 patients who underwent thyroidectomies, Snyder et al reported traction to the anterior branch of the RLN as the most common cause of RLN palsy present in 28% of cases. The second and third causes were paratracheal lymph node dissection and ligature, occurring in 24% and 16% of cases, respectively.[133] Several risk factors for RLN palsy following thyroidectomy have been described in the literature. From the physician's perspective, the impact of the surgeon's experience on the prevalence of RLN palsy is controversial. In a large review of 3250 thyroidectomy patients, the rate of RLN palsy in the group of patients who had their surgery performed by an experienced surgeon was comparable to the rate in the group operated upon by

residents (1.8% versus 1.9%, respectively), with no statistical significance between the 2. It is noteworthy that residents did more subtotal thyroidectomies and lobectomies than the experienced surgeon.[128] However, in a large study by Dralle et al that included 16 448 thyroid operations, a low-volume surgeon was considered a risk factor for RLN palsy, with an odds ratio of 1.2.[134] Similarly, in a review on the importance of the surgeon's experience in patients undergoing thyroidectomy, Sosa et al reported the lowest complication rate in high-volume, experienced surgeons (more than 100 cases over the course of 6 years), in comparison to surgeons with lower volumes.[135] From the patient's perspective, the most important risk factors for RLN palsy following thyroidectomy are the histology of the disease, size and location of the tumor, extent of surgery performed, revision or primary surgery, identification of the RLN during surgery, and anatomical variations of the RLN. More detailed discussion of each of these factors follows.

Histology of the Disease

Based on numerous reports, the histology of thyroid disease is a major determinant of RLN palsy. Patients with thyroid malignancies are at a higher risk of developing RLN palsy following thyroid surgery than patients with benign thyroid disease. In a study by Dralle et al in which 29 998 nerves were at risk, thyroid malignancy doubled the risk of RLN injury in patients who underwent thyroidectomy.[134] In another study by Chiang et al, the rate of permanent RLN injury was higher in patients with thyroid cancer in comparison to patients with benign disease (0.7% versus 0.2%, respectively). The review included 521 patients who underwent thyroidectomy during which the recurrent laryngeal was routinely

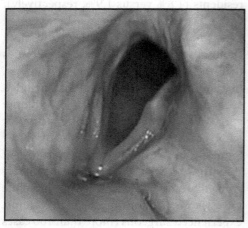
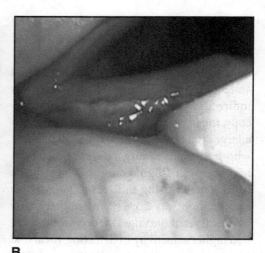

A   **B**

Figure 8–4. A 72-year-old man presented with dysphonia and aspiration following thyroidectomy for medullary carcinoma. On laryngeal examination, he had a left vocal fold paralysis in the paramedian position (**A**). Patient underwent injection laryngoplasty under local anesthesia using the transnasal fiberoptic approach. Hyaluronic acid, 0.7 cc, was injected in the paralyzed vocal fold (**B**).

identified.[119] In a review by Karamanakos et al on the complications of thyroidectomy, the odds ratio of vocal fold paralysis in patients with thyroid malignancy was 1.7.[136] Similarly, in another review of vocal fold paralysis following thyroidectomy, Lo et al reported malignant neoplasms as a risk factor for permanent RLN palsy. The study group consisted of 500 patients, all of whom had evaluation of vocal fold mobility before and after surgery[137] (Figure 8–4).

Size and Position of the Thyroid Gland

The association between the size/position of the thyroid gland and RLN palsy has been discussed thoroughly in the literature. In a study by Zambudio et al that included 301 patients with multinodular goiter, the authors reported size of the gland, in particular the intrathoracic component, as an independent risk factor (relative risk [RR]

1.5) for postoperative RLN palsy among other complications. One of the 3 patients with definitive complications had an intrathoracic goiter with symptoms of compression to the aerodigestive tract.[138] In another study by Lo et al on the rate of RLN palsy following thyroidectomy, the authors demonstrated an association between RLN paresis/paralysis and recurrent retrosternal goiter. Vocal fold mobility was assessed periodically for 1 year following surgery in a group of 213 patients.[137] In a report by Erbil et al, the incidence of transient RLN palsy was the highest in patients with retrosternal goiter (2.4%) in comparison to other subgroups of patients, except for those with recurrent goiter.[128] Similarly, in an investigation by Testini et al on substernal goiter as a risk factor for RLN palsy in patients undergoing thyroidectomy, the authors showed that mediastinal extension of goiter and its surgical access were significantly associated with higher prevalence of RLN palsy in comparison to conventional thyroidectomy. The study was multi-institutional and included 14 993 patients.[139]

Extent of Thyroid Surgery Performed

The association between the extent of thyroid surgery performed and the prevalence of RLN injury is controversial. In a large study on the complications of thyroid surgery that included 2043 consecutive patients, Karamanakos et al reported extended resection as an independent risk factor for transient RLN paralysis with an odds ratio of 1.6.[136] Similarly, Thomusch et al, in their review of 7266 thyroidectomy patients, demonstrated that extended surgical resection is a significant risk factor for RLN palsy with a RR of 1.5 to 2.1.[140] In another review on the predictive factors of RLN palsy, Erbil et al reported a 12-fold increase in the odds of RLN palsy in cases of extended thyroidectomy.[128] The study included 3250 patients who underwent thyroid surgery for different thyroid pathologies (Figure 8–5). However,

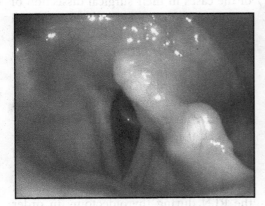

Figure 8–5. A fiberoptic laryngeal examination showing evidence of left vocal fold paralysis in a 59-year–old woman following a left neck dissection. Patient had history of thyroidectomy with cervical lymph node metastasis 1 year ago.

in a study by Roh et al that included 319 patients who underwent thyroidectomy or lobectomy, with or without neck dissection, the extent of surgical resection and neck dissection did not affect the rate of injury to the RLN. The prevalence of temporary and permanent RLN palsy in patients who underwent lobectomy versus total thyroidectomy were 2.4% and 0, respectively, versus 2.2% and 0.4%, respectively ($p = .999$). Thirteen patients had shaving of the tumor from the RLN, only 2 of whom ended up with permanent paralysis.[70] Similarly, in a study by Hermann et al, the rate of RLN injury was higher in the group who had localized dissection in comparison to those who had partial or complete dissection, alluding to an inverse relation between the extent of surgery and prevalence of RLN injury.[141]

Primary or Revision Surgery

Patients with recurrent thyroid cancer are considered at high risk of RLN palsy following thyroidectomy. Revision thyroidectomy is a challenging surgery associated with a higher rate of complications, among which is RLN palsy.[142,143] In a large study that included 2043 patients with various thyroid diseases undergoing thyroidectomy, Karamanakos et al showed that recurrent goiter is an independent risk factor for postoperative transient and permanent RLN palsy with odds ratios of 2.3 and 1.7, respectively.[136] Similarly, in a large multicenter study by Thomusch investigating postoperative complications in benign goiter surgery, recurrent goiter was a significant risk factor for RLN palsy with a RR of 1.8 to 3.4.[140] In a study on 500 thyroidectomy patients, Lo et al demonstrated an association between recurrent substernal goiter and an increased risk of permanent RLN palsy.[137] Patients were evaluated preoperatively and postoperatively during a period that ranged from 1 to 9 months, Similarly, in a study by Erbil et al on 6250 thyroidectomy patients, among whom 125 had recurrent disease, revision surgery was associated with a higher rate of RLN palsy in comparison to primary thyroid surgery (17.8% versus 5.9%).[128] In a study by Seiler et al on 1318 patients who underwent thyroidectomy, revision surgery trended toward being a significant risk factor for permanent RLN palsy. Higher rates were reported in secondary operations versus primary operations (3.5%–5.6% versus 0.7%–1.7%, respectively).[142]

Intraoperative Identification of the Recurrent Laryngeal Nerve

Dissection/identification of the RLN during thyroid surgery is a revolutionary step that has markedly reduced the prevalence of vocal fold paralysis following thyroidectomy. This technique has been endorsed by many surgeons with improvement in the preservation of the RLN. In a review of 803 thyroid surgeries in which the RLN was at risk in 797 cases, Jatzko et al reported a significant difference in the rate of RLN palsy in the group of patients who had the nerve identified during surgery in comparison to those who did not have identification of the nerve.[129] The rate of permanent RLN palsy was 0.5%, and the recovery rate was 86%. The added value of RLN identification during surgery for benign and malignant thyroid disease has also been emphasized by Dralle et al. The authors reported no nerve identification, among other factors, as a risk factor for RLN paralysis with an odds ratio of 1.4.[134] Similarly, Hermann et al, in their large review of 26 413 nerves at risk during thyroidectomies, reported a marked decrease in the rate of RLN injury from 0.9% to 0.1% when the RLN had been visualized and dissected along its course during surgery. The authors emphasized the need to

identify the RLN in order to reduce the rate of RLN injury.[141]

Anatomical Variations of the Recurrent Laryngeal Nerve

The RLN is at risk during thyroid surgery along its course in the neck, particularly above the inferior thyroid artery and under the ligament of Berry.[144,145] Anatomical variations in its course put it at even higher risk, particularly in the presence of bifurcation or trifurcation before its entry into the larynx. In a study by Serpell et al on the prevalence of RLN anatomical variants, the authors reported bifurcations on the right in 25.7%, bifurcation on the left in 22.9% of cases, and bilateral bifurcation in 8.9% of cases.[146] Rustad, in the dissection of 200 nerves in 100 cadavers, reported branching of the RLN before its entry in the larynx in 43% of cases.[147] Ardito et al in their intraoperative study on 1543 thyroidectomies where 2626 RLNs were observed, reported bifurcation in 70.6% of the cases and trifurcation in 23 cases.[148] Beneragama and Serpell described bifurcation or trifurcation in 36% of the cases in their surgical dissection of 213 nerves in 137 patients. The majority had unilateral bifurcation, mostly on the right side, and only 8 patients identified with trifurcation.[149] In a study on 1177 RLNs by Katz and Nemiroff, 63% had either bifurcation or trifurcation around 0.5 cm caudal to the cricoid cartilage. The nerve bifurcation was bilateral in 170 cases.[150] In another study by the same authors, the high rate of bifurcation was ascertained with emphasis on the need to preserve all branches of the RLN during thyroidectomy in order to reduce the rates of dysphonia and dysphagia.[151] The anatomical variation in the course of the RLN, particularly within 2 cm before its entry into the larynx, carries important surgical implications in patients undergoing thyroidectomy. Identification of only one branch of the RLN during surgical dissection puts the other branch at jeopardy if the surgeon is not aware of this common anatomical variation. The posterior branch innervating the posterior cricoarytenoid muscle can be mistaken for the whole nerve, thus leaving the anterior branch unrecognized and prone to injury.

Role of Intraoperative Nerve Monitoring

Despite the advancement in surgical technique with direct visualization of the RLN during thyroidectomy, permanent RLN palsy remains a major concern. A low prevalence rate of injury is still alarming given the consensus that surgical preservation of the RLN is highly advocated even in patients with preoperative vocal fold paralysis.[119] To that end, alternatives to further reduce the risk of nerve injury have emerged. Intraoperative nerve monitoring (IONM) is one of them. IONM allows assessment of the function of the RLN intraoperatively via direct or indirect nerve stimulation. It is a viable technique that provides direct feedback to the surgeon as to when injury has occurred during the surgical dissection, thus allowing better understanding of the mechanism by which RLN palsy could have occurred.[152–154] Its main added value has been emphasized mostly in revision surgery where scarring and fibrosis may mask the anatomical course of the RLN.[152] A similar situation may be encountered in patients with thyroiditis and chronic inflammation of the thyroid gland, which again may lead to perineural fibrosis and put the nerve at risk. The added value of IONM is apparent also in cases of thyroid cancer invasion to structures contiguous with the thyroid gland.

The role of IONM as an adjuvant tool in dissecting the RLN during thyroidectomy has been supported by many authors, but with some debate on its validity in significantly reducing the rate of RLN palsy. In a study by Snyder et al, IONM was helpful in identifying the RLN before visual identification in 19.4% of cases. In 7.5% of cases where the nerve was at risk of injury, the usage of IONM has also assisted the surgeon in its identification.[133] Thomusch et al examined the rate of transient and permanent RLN palsy in thyroidectomy patients who underwent intraoperative neuromonitoring versus those who did not. The authors reported lower rates in the former group, 1.4% versus 2.1% for permanent RLN palsy and 0.4% versus 0.8% for transient RLN palsy. In conclusion, the authors advocated the usage of IONM given the significant difference in the rate of injury between the 2 groups.[155] In another study by Barczynski et al that included 1000 nerves at risk, the authors also reported a significant decrease in the incidence of transient RLN palsy using IONM. The negative predictive value of IONM for postoperative RLN palsy was 98.9%.[156] However, in a large review by Dralle et al, no significant difference was found in the frequency of RLN palsy between those who had nerve monitoring versus those who had only visual identification of the nerve. The lack of significant difference between the 2 groups was attributed to the low frequency of RLN paralysis.[134]

What are the prognostic factors for recovery in patients with RLN palsy? Which patient with vocal fold paralysis is more likely to recover is a challenging question that surgeons often face in counseling patients with vocal fold paralysis following thyroidectomy. Several clinical, acoustic, aerodynamic, and electrophysiologic parameters can assist the caring physician in predicting the recovery rate in affected patients. In a study that included 63 patients with unilateral vocal fold paralysis following thyroidectomy, 58% of whom have had full recovery, Choi et al demonstrated that small tumors, lower jitter, and higher maximum phonation time correlated significantly with recovery. Additional factors that correlated with recovery included lack of compensatory supraglottic behavior, incomplete paralysis, and absence of arytenoid tilting seen on laryngeal videostroboscopy. Only lack of compensatory laryngeal behavior was a significant predictor of recovery ($p = .022$).[157] Laryngeal EMG also plays an important role in predicting recovery. In a study by Wang et al on the prognostic indicators of unilateral vocal fold paralysis, the positive predictive and negative predictive values of laryngeal EMG were 78.9% and 71.4%, respectively, and the specificity and sensitivity were 38.5% and 77.8%, respectively. The study was conducted on 45 patients, and laryngeal EMG was performed until 6 months from the date of onset of symptoms. The authors concluded that laryngeal EMG provides additional information regarding prognosis of vocal fold paralysis, more so if performed during the early first 8 weeks following surgery.[158] In another large study on the usefulness of laryngeal EMG in predicting long-term prognosis, the same authors concurred with their previous conclusion and reported a positive predictive value of 97.9%. Prognosis was considered poor when there was absence of fibrillation and reduction in recruitment of less than 20%.[159] Similarly, in an investigation by Sittel et al on the prognostic value of laryngeal EMG in vocal fold paralysis, the prediction of defective recovery (i.e., absence of vocal fold mobility) was 94.4%, whereas the prediction of complete recovery was 12.8%. The study group consisted of 98 patients with 111 vocal fold paralyses, 53 of whom had previous thyroid surgery.[54] Caroline et al also reported an important predictor of postoperative laryngeal nerve function. All

of their patients had undergone preoperative laryngeal EMG. Although recovery of preoperative paresis occurred in some patients with benign disease, no patient with cancer and preoperative paresis improved after surgery.[51]

Management of vocal fold paresis or paralysis varies depending on whether the injury is transient or permanent, and whether it is unilateral or bilateral. In patients with unilateral RLN palsy and with symptoms of dysphonia and aspiration, early surgical intervention (often a temporary medialization) is advocated, notwithstanding the invaluable role of voice and swallowing therapy in the course of recovery. The reform in laryngology practice has allowed laryngologists to perform unsedated office-based medialization procedures, namely, injection laryngoplasty using different augmentation materials.[160,161] When the RLN has been sacrificed, more permanent early medialization procedures are recommended such as thyroplasty type I with or without arytenoid adduction or adjuvant reinnervation.[162] In cases of bilateral vocal fold paralysis with compromise of the airway, a lateralization procedure is often needed to secure the airway,[163,164] or another surgical procedure is required, such as arytenoidectomy.

Surgery-Induced Injury to the External Branch of the Superior Laryngeal Nerve

Injury to the external branch of the SLN is an often-overlooked complication of thyroidectomy. Given its intimate anatomical position in relation to the superior thyroid artery, the external branch of the SLN is commonly injured while dissecting the superior pole of the thyroid gland and/or ligating its superior vascular bundle. In a study by McIvor et al, 10% of patients who underwent thyroidectomy for various thyroid pathologies had injury to the external laryngeal nerve.[37] In another review by Stojadinovic et al that included 54 patients, 14% of whom had persistent dysphonia at 3-months' follow-up, 2% had been diagnosed with injury to the SLN.[165] Similarly, a study by Kark et al that included 325 patients who underwent thyroidectomy demonstrated that injury to the external branch of the SLN is the most common cause of permanent vocal dysfunction, the rate of which was higher in those who underwent subtotal thyroidectomy in comparison to those who underwent lobectomy.[166] Affected patients may be asymptomatic in one-third of the cases,[167] or may complain of deepening of their voice, breathiness, and loss of intonation. The effect on voice is more noticeable in professional voice users who often describe an inability to reach the high notes, a loss of range, volume disturbance, trouble projecting the voice during speech, and loss of control of soft mid-range notes during singing. Based on a study by Dursen et al on 126 patients with laryngeal EMG–confirmed SLN paresis or paralysis, the most common symptom was voice fatigue in 82.5%, followed by hoarseness in 75.4% in 124 out of 126 patients in whom SLN paresis had been confirmed. Volume disturbance and loss of range were reported in 75.4% and 69% of cases, respectively.[168] These symptoms are not surprising given that the cricothyroid muscle is a tensor muscle, the contraction of which results in tensing and elongating the vocal folds with subsequent decrease in mass per unit length. Inadvertent injury to the external branch of the SLN can cause dysfunction of that tensor muscle.

The prevalence of SLN injury varies in the literature depending on the diagnostic method used to evaluate suspected patients.[167–174] The signs said to be seen on laryngeal endoscopy are vocal fold bowing and twisting of the larynx toward the injured site. However, these are less common than sluggishness in adduction during rapidly repeated phonatory gestures, commonly mistaken for RLN paresis. Additional diagnostic tests such as laryngeal videostroboscopy often are recommended, particularly in patients in whom laryngeal signs are subtle or unnoticeable. The usefulness of laryngeal videostroboscopy including flexible laryngoscopy in diagnosing SLN palsy has been proven by many authors. In the study by Dursen et al that included 124 out of 126 patients with confirmed SLN injury, the most common findings were asymmetry in amplitude and phase in 84.9% and 73% of cases, respectively. Incomplete closure of the vocal folds during phonation was observed in 55.5%, and decrease in mucosal waves occurred in two-thirds of cases.[168] In another study by Aluffi et al, the most common laryngeal stroboscopic findings were decrease in mucosal waves and incomplete closure in 9% and 7% of cases, respectively. A less commonly reported finding was vocal fold bowing.[173] Laryngeal EMG is invaluable in detecting SLN injury. In studies in which laryngeal EMG was performed in addition to stroboscopic evaluation, the prevalence rate of injury to the external branch of the SLN reached up to 68% of cases,[167,171,173,174] except for the study by Dursen et al in which it reached 98.4%.[168] Decrease in recruitment and polyphasic potentials are indicative of partial denervation and reinnervation, whereas absence of recruitment and presence of fibrillation are signs of complete paralysis.[166] In a study by Aluffi et al in which EMG of the cricothyroid muscle was performed on 21 patients with changed voice quality out of 45 patients who had thyroidectomy, the authors reported injury to the external branch of the RLN in 14% of cases. The most commonly reported symptoms were voice fatigue and contracted pitch range.[173] The role of laryngeal EMG and laryngeal videostroboscopy in the diagnosis of SLN injury also has been emphasized by Teitelbaum and Wenig. Their study on the incidence of SLN injury included 20 thyroidectomy patients who were evaluated during the 3 months following surgery.[174]

The management of patients with injury to the external branch of the SLN relies primarily on voice therapy. Medialization procedures using injection laryngoplasty or laryngeal framework surgery are advocated mostly for symptomatic patients who do not achieve satisfactory results after expert conservative treatment. Notwithstanding the beneficial role of voice therapy, prevention remains paramount. This is achieved best by identifying and skeletonizing the superior thyroid vessels prior to ligation, keeping in mind the anatomical locations of the external branch of the SLN.[175-177] In a study by Lekacos et al, the prevalence of SLN injury was markedly higher in the subgroup of patients who had high ligation of the superior bundle in comparison to those who had separate ligation of the superior thyroid artery (6% versus 0%, respectively).[171] Proper understanding of the variations in the anatomical distribution of the external branch of the SLN is crucial in preventing injury. In the anatomical study by Chuang et al on 43 cadavers, the authors highlighted the importance of the inferior cornu of the thyroid cartilage as a surgical landmark.[177] Intraoperative nerve monitoring is often helpful in avoiding injury given the various courses of the nerve.[172,178-180] In a study on 76 patients who underwent superior thyroid pole dissection, Cernea et al reported 12% to 28% sustained injury to the external branch of the superior laryngeal nerve (EBSLN) when dissection was carried without visualization of the nerve versus no injury when the nerve was identified using a nerve stimulator.[178] Similarly, Glover et al investigated the added value of a nerve integrity monitor (NIM) in identifying the external branch of the SLN in 228 thyroidectomy/or hemithyroidectomy cases. The authors concluded that NIM assists the surgeon in better identifying the nerve intraoperatively.[179] The contribution of NIM in identifying and preserving the external branch of the SLN was further supported in a study by Gurleyik et al.[180]

Nonneurogenic Causes of Dysphonia Following Thyroidectomy

A change in voice quality following thyroid surgery is not always neurogenic in origin.[181-185] Despite preserving the laryngeal neural structures, surgeons still encounter patients who complain of dysphonia following thyroidectomy. In a study by Hong and Kim on 54 patients who had both subjective and objective voice evaluation before and after thyroidectomy, the authors reported a drop in the mean speaking fundamental frequency (SFo) although no injury to the external branch of the SLN or to the RLN was noted. The mean value of the SFo decreased from 205.4 to 177.6 Hz 3 months after surgery. Moreover, there was a decrease in the highest notes of the vocal range in 86% of cases. The authors emphasized the role of strap muscles and the vertical movement of the laryngeal framework in pitch control.[181] Periera et al investigated the prevalence of nonspecific symptoms of the upper aerodigestive system in patients who underwent uncomplicated thyroidectomy ($n = 38$) or subtotal thyroidectomy ($n = 22$), in comparison to a control group. Dysphonia and dysphagia occurred in 28% and 15% of cases, respectively, and were associated with a feeling of neck strangling.

The authors attributed these symptoms to injury to the perithyroidal neural plexus during surgery,[182] although there is no evidence to support that speculation. In another study by Mclvor et al that included 50 patients who underwent thyroidectomy, the authors reported subjective deterioration in voice quality in 20% of cases postoperatively. Although 10 patients had subjective deterioration of their voice, only 2 patients had temporary vocal fold paralysis, and 4 patients had paresis of the external laryngeal nerve postoperatively.[37] Similarly, in a review by Stojadinovic et al on 54 patients who underwent thyroidectomy, 50 of whom were evaluated at 1 week and 46 at 3 months after surgery, the authors reported early and late subjective changes in voice quality in 30% and 14% of cases, respectively. About 1 in 10 (12%) had objective changes in 3 vocal parameters, which correlated with postoperative voice symptoms. The 2 voice parameters with predictive value on persistent vocal changes were alterations in maximum phonation frequency range and jitter. More than a 100% increase in jitter had a sensitivity and specificity for long-term voice symptoms of 71% and 91%, respectively.[165] The lack of RLN injury in the study group implied nonneurogenic causes for dysphonia in patients following thyroidectomy, among which is laryngotracheal fixation, as first reported by Sataloff et al in 1992.[185] Similarly, in a study on 100 thyroidectomy patients, Pedro-Netto et al reported subjective voice changes in 29.7% of the cases despite having normal vocal fold mobility. Moreover, there was a significant increase in the VHI score and voice turbulence index in the study group in comparison to the control group.[183] In the study by Aluffi et al on 45 patients who underwent thyroidectomy, 42 of whom had no injury to the external branch of the RLN, a significant difference in the degree of subharmonics after surgery

was reported. The authors suggested other causes for dysphonia aside from neural injury, namely, fixation of the laryngotracheal complex due to scarring, and/or division of the strap muscles.[173] In a study on the long-lasting phonatory symptoms in the absence of RLN palsy following thyroidectomy, Kim et al demonstrated that professional voice users are less likely to recover than nonprofessional voice users. The study included 68 patients stratified as those who recovered versus those who did not, based on a periodic voice assessment over the course of 1 year.[184] Sataloff et al reported a 63-year-old man who presented 2 years following thyroidectomy with a drastic change in his vocal pitch. Both laryngeal videostroboscopic examination and laryngeal electromyography were normal. CT showed narrowing of the cricothyroid space suggestive of cricothyroid scarring and approximation. The patient underwent surgical exploration with release of the cricothyroid scar and restoration of the visor angle. Postoperatively there was a substantial drop in his speaking fundamental frequency from 214 Hz preoperatively to 104 Hz.[185]

In addition to dysfunction in the strap muscles which can cause laryngeal tilting and motion asymmetries that lead to dysphonia, another important cause of dysphonia in thyroidectomy patients with normal vocal fold mobility and intact SLNs is endotracheal tube–related injury. Endotracheal injuries are well-known causes of dysphonia in patients undergoing general anesthesia, particularly in patients with an enlarged thyroid gland. In a review of 200 consecutive thyroidectomies, Randolph et al reported bilateral cervical goiter as a significant risk factor for endotracheal intubation injury.[186] The change in voice quality following endotracheal intubation usually is due either to laryngeal/vocal fold mucosal injuries or to dislocation of the arytenoid cartilage or to vocal process avulsion. In a study by Echternach et al on laryngeal complications following thyroidectomy in 761 patients, intubation-induced vocal fold injury was more frequent than RLN injury (31.3% versus 6.6%, respectively). The authors emphasized the importance of patient counselling, particularly for professional voice users.[187] In a large study on the changing etiology of vocal fold paralysis, Benninger et al reported intubation injuries as the etiology of unilateral and bilateral vocal fold immobility/paralysis in 7.5% and 15.4% of cases, respectively. Intubation-induced injuries exceeded thyroidectomy-induced injuries, which accounted for only 8.2% of the cases.[121] In a review on the mortality rate following thyroidectomy that included 30 495 cases, 65% of whom had thyroid malignancies, Gomez-Ramirez et al demonstrated that tracheal injuries accounted for 15% of the deaths.[188]

Surgery-Induced Hypothyroidism and Dysphonia

Hypothyroidism is a forgotten complication of thyroid surgery. Despite advocating hemithyroidectomy for patients with microcancer in an attempt to preserve thyroid tissue and hence function, postoperative hypothyroidism remains an impediment that is often unanticipated.[189] The delay in its occurrence following surgery more often than not masks its true prevalence. In most studies, hypothyroidism developed within the course of 1 year, though many cases were diagnosed even up to 3 years postoperatively.[190–192] In a review by Kevin et al on biochemical hypothyroidism in 263 patients who underwent thyroid surgery, 24% of those who developed hypothyroidism were diagnosed later than a year following their surgery.[191] Moreover, hypothyroidism is often self-limited. In a review by Piper et al that included 66 patients,

18% of whom had postoperative hypothyroidism, one-third reverted back to normal without medical intervention.[193] Similarly, in a study by Su et al, 12.5% of patients who were diagnosed with hypothyroidism following hemithyroidectomy recovered without the need for thyroid hormone replacement. The authors attributed the recovery rate to the compensatory hypertrophy of the residual thyroid tissue.[192]

Despite the self-recovery in many instances, hypothyroidism following thyroid surgery remains common. Based on several reviews, the prevalence of hypothyroidism varies with the duration of follow-up and the frequency of testing for thyrotropin (TSH) level. The estimated range is between 9% and 43%.[193–198] In a retrospective review that included 233 euthyroid patients who had undergone hemithyroidectomy, the majority of whom were diagnosed with papillary carcinoma (100 out of 233), Tomoda et al reported hypothyroidism in 1 out of 4 patients. Patients' TSH levels were assessed every 3 to 6 months for a period of 3 years following surgery.[190] In a study by Elmas et al on the incidence and symptoms of hypothyroidism in 127 patients who underwent hemithyroidectomy, 43% developed hypothyroidism, and the majority were diagnosed within the first 8 weeks following surgery. What is important to note is that 60% of those who developed hypothyroidism, based on a TSH level greater than 4 mU/L, were asymptomatic.[199] However, it also is important to note that these patients were not screened for subtle voice dysfunction. In professional voice users, the incidence of symptoms might be higher. In a study by McHenry and Slusarczyk on the incidence of hypothyroidism following hemithyroidectomy, the authors reported hypothyroidism in 35% of the patients, two-thirds of whom were also subclinical.[197]

The delay in the occurrence of hypothyroidism and its subclinical presentation have put into question the time and need to start treatment after thyroidectomy. This reluctance has spurred the urge to detect predictors of hypothyroidism in order to identify patients at high risk and in true need of hormonal replacement. Several clinical and pathologic variables have been linked to the prevalence of hypothyroidism, most common of which are lymphocytic infiltration on histologic examination, and/or high titers of autoimmune antibodies. In a study by Volokh et al on 1231 patients who underwent thyroid surgery for various thyroid pathologies, the authors highlighted that lymphocytic infiltration on histologic examination and prior autoimmune disease are risk factors for the development of hypothyroidism, which occurred in 6.17% of their cases postoperatively.[200] In another study by Buchanan and Lee, carried out on 158 patients who had thyroid surgery, the authors reported high levels of thyroid autoantibodies (TAAs) preoperatively in 75.6% of patients who developed hypothyroidism postoperatively (38 out of 158 patients). The authors concluded that there is an association between preoperative TAA and the risk of developing hypothyroidism.[198] In a review of 294 patients who underwent hemithyroidectomy, Su et al in 2009 reported hypothyroidism in 10.9% of cases. Patients with elevated thyroid antibodies levels preoperatively were more likely to develop hypothyroidism. Moreover, the presence of thyroiditis on histologic examination was more common in patients with postoperative hypothyroidism in comparison to those with no hypothyroidism (46.8% versus 11.8%, respectively).[192] These findings were further concurred by McHenry and Slusarczyck, who also proved a higher prevalence of lymphocytic infiltration in patients with hypothyroidism in comparison to patients who were euthyroid (40% versus 22%, respectively).[197] Other important predictors of hypothyroidism are age, preoperative TSH

level, and the weight of resected thyroid tissue. In a study by Tomoda et al in 2011 on 260 patients, 233 of whom were euthyroid preoperatively, both age and preoperative TSH levels were associated with a high prevalence of hypothyroidism. The prevalence of hypothyroidism was higher in patients with TSH level greater than 2.5 microIU/mL in comparison to those with a TSH level less than 1 microIU/mL (58.9% versus 6%, respectively). Similarly, patients above the age of 55 years had higher prevalence of hypothyroidism in comparison to patients below the age of 55 years (42.3% versus 18.2%, respectively).[190] In another study by Kevin et al on 263 patients who underwent thyroid surgery, the authors demonstrated that the light weight of the tissue resected in addition to thyroiditis are independent risk factors for hypothyroidism. Other important clinical-pathologic factors that were associated with hypothyroidism included older age, elevated preoperative TSH level, and positive antimicrosomal antibodies.[191]

The diagnosis of hypothyroidism as a postoperative complication following thyroid surgery is important. Given that 90% of hypothyroidism is diagnosed within the first year, frequent TSH monitoring during that period should allow timely diagnosis of patients lacking hormonal replacement and should also prevent unnecessary treatment of patients who are euthyroid postoperatively. Initiation of thyroid hormone replacement not only alleviates clinical symptoms of hypothyroidism but also reduces the rate of reoperation in patients who had undergone primary thyroid surgeries, particularly in patients with goiter. In a study by Miccoli et al who compared 84 thyroidectomy patients who were treated with suppressive dosage of levothyroxine, versus 92 patients who were not, the authors showed that suppressive therapy reduced the time interval between primary thyroidectomy and revision surgery.[201] Early identification and treatment of patients at risk of hypothyroidism following surgery are also imperative in professional voice users who are more vulnerable to alterations in thyroid hormonal level. The well-known laryngeal manifestations of hypothyroidism may adversely affect their performance.[202] Affected patients may suffer from loss of the high notes, contracted range, excessive vocal fatigue. and most typically muffling or a sensation of a "veil" over the voice. Diligent laryngeal examination of professional voice users undergoing thyroidectomy is highly recommended to avoid the phonatory adverse events of hypothyroidism.

In conclusion, hypothyroidism is common after thyroid surgery for benign and malignant thyroid disease. In reference to Manfredi et al, hypothyroidism is "a predictable consequence" rather than a complication.[203] Leaving sufficient thyroid tissue behind and addressing autoimmune disorders and abnormal preoperative TSH levels are some of the measures advocated to reduce the prevalence of hypothyroidism following surgery.[200] Patients at high risk are those with high preoperative TSH levels, history of thyroiditis, elevated antibody titers, and/or evidence of lymphocytic infiltrates on histologic examination. Selective monitoring of high-risk patients using serial testing of TSH level is highly advocated.[192] Symptomatic patients should be placed on hormonal replacement keeping in mind that the self-recovery rate is 12.5%.[192]

Surgery-Induced Hypoparathyroidism and Its Impact on Voice

Hypoparathyroidism is a biochemical condition characterized by a low level of intact parathyroid hormone (PTH) with or without symptoms of hypocalcemia.[204] Affected patients often complain of perioral numbness, paraesthesia and tingling sensation in the extremities, muscle cramps, and seizures. The prevalence of hypoparathyroidism following thyroidectomy is high.[204-206] The etiology is mostly ischemia and devascularization to the parathyroid gland during surgical dissection. Other causes include hemorrhage within the parathyroid gland or its inadvertent removal during surgical resection of the thyroid gland. Based on the American Thyroid Association, it can be either transient lasting less than 6 months after surgery, or permanent.[204] In a large review by Bergenfelz et al that included 4828 patients who underwent thyroidectomy, the rate of permanent hypoparathyroidism associated with long-term morbidity was 5%.[207] In a multicenter study of 1792 thyroidectomy patients, Diez et al reported hypoparathyroidism at time of discharge in 48.3% of cases. This prevalence gradually decreased along the course of 1 year to 16.7%, and to 14.5% at the last patient's visit. In conclusion, the authors emphasized the relatively high prevalence of permanent hypoparathyroidism and the need for diligent follow-up of affected patients.[208] Similarly, in another study by Goncalves-Filho et al that included 1020 thyroidectomy cases, transient and permanent hypocalcemia were reported in 13.1% and 2.5% of cases, respectively.[127]

Several risk factors for hypoparathyroidism have been described in the literature, among which are the size of the thyroid gland, presence of thyroid malignancy, extent of resection, revision surgery, thyrotoxicosis, Graves' disease, prior radioiodine therapy, history of diabetes mellitus, and female gender.[209-213] In a study by Wu et al on 118 consecutive patients who underwent thyroidectomy for thyroid malignancies, extrathyroidal disease extension and central neck dissection predicted hypoparathyroidism, with odds ratios of 4.9 and 4.3, respectively.[214] In the study by Serpell and Phan, the risk of temporary hypocalcemia was higher in patients with Graves' disease in comparison to other thyroid pathologies, with permanent hypocalcemia reported in 1.8% of cases.[215] In a review by Paduraru et al, preoperative low calcium level, hypovitaminosis D, and low level of PTH correlated with symptoms of hypocalcemia and were considered as additional risk factors for post-thyroidectomy hypoparathyroidisms.[216]

Laryngeal and phonatory manifestations of hypoparathyroidism and hypocalcemia are rare. In a study on the impact of thyroidectomy on voice, Borel et al reported an association between postoperative hypocalcemia and an increased risk of self-perceived impairment in voice. The study included 800 patients who had completed the voice handicap index questionnaire 2 and 6 months following thyroidectomy.[217]

Van Veelen et al reported a 51-year-old man who presented with change in voice quality described as pinched voice, in addition to laryngeal spasm and QT interval change on electrocardiography (ECG). The patient was diagnosed with hypoparathyroidism for which he received adequate treatment.[205] Similarly, Abrantes et al reported a 58-year-old man who also presented with laryngeal spasm in addition to generalized muscle spasms and dyspnea. The patient was diagnosed with DiGeorge/velocardiofacial/22q11/2 and refractory hypocalcemia.[206] Srivastava and Ravindran reported an 85-year-old man who presented with stridor secondary to laryngeal spasm. Laryngeal examination failed to show any signs of edema or vocal fold paralysis. The patient was diagnosed with hypocalcemia based on the clinical picture and laboratory testing. His calcium deficiency was rectified, and the patient was decannulated successfully.[218]

The management of hypoparathyroidism following thyroidectomy remains empirical with lack of consensus or evidence-based guidelines for treatment.[213] In view of the high prevalence of temporary hypocalcemia postoperatively, patient supplements of calcium and vitamin D are prescribed after surgery in order to reduce symptoms of hypocalcemia and to reduce hospital stay.[204] The presence of low magnesium level below 1.6 mg/mL has mandated the use of additional magnesium supplements.[219] With respect to the need for hospital admission and duration of stay, several predictive factors have been described in the literature. Saad et al, in their study on 429 patients who underwent thyroidectomy, showed that a drop in calcium level of 1 mg/mL over the course of 12 hours has a sensitivity and specificity of 71% and 73%, respectively, of predicting symptoms of hypocalcemia following thyroidectomy.[220] Sala et al, in their investigation of 134 patients, demonstrated that intact PTH level of less than 11.2 pg/mL and serum calcium levels of less than 8.05 mg/dL were associated with a 10.77 and 99 higher risk of developing symptoms of hypocalcemia, respectively. Moreover, these were significant predictors for the timing of safe discharge from the hospital after surgery.[221]

Radioiodine-Induced Dysphonia in Patients With Thyroid Carcinoma

Radioiodine therapy is commonly used in the management of patients with thyroid diseases and carcinoma. The main indications include disease refractory to treatment with antithyroid drugs for 1 year, high-risk patients for surgical intervention, and drug incompatibility.[222] The success rate is very high, with hypothyroidism achieved in the majority of patients even several years after treatment. In a study by Harrison et al conducted on 232 patients treated with I-131, hypothyroidism was reported in 20% to 35% of cases during the 6 to 8 years following treatment. The results were based on a computer-generated questionnaire that proved high sensitivity and specificity to voice changes.[223] Radioactive iodine acts by penetrating and destroying follicular and adjacent cells within the thyroid gland. The acute inflammatory process characterized initially by edema and lymphocytic infiltration is followed by necrosis of the follicular cells and subsequent tissue destruction.[222,223] Despite the safety of radioactive iodine therapy, there are many side effects to it, some of which are related to the larynx and upper airway.

In 1978, Synder described a 61-year-old woman who presented with an enlarged goiter and symptoms of hyperthyroidism with an elevated TSH level. The patient was started on 7.3 mCI of I-131 following which she developed hoarseness. Laryngeal examination showed evidence of right vocal fold paralysis. Radiologic imaging of the neck and chest failed to show any other cause for the RLN palsy.[224] In 1981, Robson reported a 65-year-old man who presented with symptoms of thyrotoxicosis and an elevated total serum thyroxine (196 nmol/mL). The patient was started on carbimazole and later given iodine therapy (222 MBq [6 mCi]). Two days after initiation of radioiodine therapy, the patient developed hoarseness. Laryngeal examination showed right vocal fold paralysis. The symptoms disappeared, and the vocal fold mobility recovered to normal 4 months after cessation of treatment.[225] In 1999, Coover reported a 75-year-old woman, diagnosed with hyperthyroidism, who developed hoarseness 1 week following treatment with 29.3 mCi

I-131. On laryngeal examination, she had right vocal fold paralysis that persisted for 6 months after cessation of therapy.[226] In 2007, Kinuya et al reported 2 patients with Graves' disease who developed airway symptoms following treatment with radioiodine. The first case was a 59-year-old woman who was diagnosed with Graves' disease 18 years after having undergone hemilobectomy for papillary thyroid carcinoma. The patient was refractory to antithyroid medications and hence was referred for iodine therapy. Six hours following treatment with 1.11 GBq (30 mCi) of I131, the patient developed neck discomfort and hoarseness. The second patient was a 19-year-old who had Graves' disease and also had diffuse goiter and was started on the same dose of radioiodine mentioned earlier. The patient complained of difficulty breathing 33 hours after initiation of therapy. Both patients were treated with chlorpheniramine maleate and hydrocortisone.[227] In 2008, Isolan-Cury et al investigated the effect of radioiodine therapy on voice in 13 patients diagnosed with Graves' disease. The authors reported no statistically significant difference in acoustic parameters or in the laryngeal findings before and after treatment. The phonatory measures were limited to vowel /ɑ/ and s/z ratio, and the laryngeal examination looked for the presence of vocal fold edema, supraglottic edema, and incomplete closure of the vocal folds.[228] In 2019, Hong et al investigated voice characteristics before and after radioiodine therapy in patients who underwent thyroidectomy. These were stratified into 2 groups, those who received recombinant human TSH and those who did not. The study showed that the mean, high, and low fundamental frequencies decreased before and after radioiodine therapy in comparison to postsurgery, but the difference between the before and after surgery radioiodine therapy was not significant (mFo 174.26 Hz pre-radioiodine therapy (Pre-RIT) versus 178.08 Hz post-radioiodine therapy (Post-RIT). Similarly, there was a nonsignificant decrease in shimmer (6.03 pre-RIT versus 3.84 post-RIT) and in jitter (1.60 pre-RIT versus 1.1 post-RIT).[229]

In summary, the effect of radioiodine therapy on the larynx should be well recognized by physicians for better patient counselling. Dysphonia can be due to vocal fold paralysis, to compression secondary to the transient increase in the size of the thyroid gland, or to exacerbation of thyrotoxicosis.

Conclusion

The thyroid gland is associated intimately with voice anatomically and hormonally. Thyroid cancers occur commonly in association with other thyroid pathology/dysfunction and must be managed globally. Thyroid cancer can affect the voice structurally by invasion, metastasis, and paralysis. However, response to treatment and to total loss of endogenous thyroid hormone can be equally devastating. Laryngologists need to be familiar not only with the structural aspects of thyroid cancer but also with its many other complexities.

References

1. Bray F, Ferlay J, Soerjomataram I, Siegel R, Torre LA, Jemal A. Global cancer statistics 2018: GLOBOCAN estimates of incidence and mortality worldwide for 36 countries in 185 countries. *CA Cancer J Clin.* 2018;68(6):394–424.

2. Thyroid Cancer: Statistics. Cancer.net. Updated January 2019. Accessed November 8, 2019. https://www.cancer.net/cancer-types/thyroid-cancer/statistics

3. Thyroid Cancer Risk Factors. American Cancer Society. Updated March 14, 2019. Accessed November 8, 2019. https://www.cancer.org/cancer/thyroid-cancer/causes-risks-prevention/risk-factors.html#references

4. Tang J, Kong D, Cui Q, et al. Racial disparities of differentiated thyroid carcinoma: clinical behavior, treatments, and long-term outcomes. *World J Surg Oncol.* 2018;16(1):45.

5. Vaccarella S, Franceschi S, Bray F, Wild CP, Plummer M, Dal Maso L. Worldwide thyroid-cancer epidemic? The increasing impact of overdiagnosis. *N Engl J Med.* 2016; 375(7):614–617.

6. Davies L, Welch HG. Increasing incidence of thyroid cancer in the United States, 1973–2002. *JAMA.* 2006;295(18):2164–2167.

7. Morris LG, Myssiorek D. Improved detection does not fully explain the rising incidence of well-differentiated thyroid cancer: a population-based analysis. *Am J Surg.* 2010;200(4):454–461.

8. Vergamini LB, Frazier AL, Abrantes FL, Ribeiro KB, Rodriguez-Galindo C. Increase in the incidence of differentiated thyroid carcinoma in children, adolescents, and young adults: a population-based study. *J Pediatr.* 2014;164(6):1481–1485.

9. Li N, Du XL, Reitzel LR, Xu L, Sturgis EM. Impact of enhanced detection on the increase in thyroid cancer incidence in the United States: review of incidence trends by socioeconomic status within the surveillance, epidemiology, and end results registry, 1980–2008. *Thyroid.* 2013;23(1):103–110.

10. Brito JP, Morris JC, Montori VM. Thyroid cancer: zealous imaging has increased detection and treatment of low risk tumours. *BMJ.* 2013;347:f4706.

11. Kent WD, Hall SF, Isotalo PA, Houlden RL, George RL, Groome PA. Increased incidence of differentiated thyroid carcinoma and detection of subclinical disease. *CMAJ.* 2007;177(11):1357–1361.

12. Udelsman R, Zhang Y. The epidemic of thyroid cancer in the United States: the role of

endocrinologists and ultrasounds. *Thyroid.* 2014;24(3):472–479.

13. Enewold L, Zhu K, Ron E, et al. Rising thyroid cancer incidence in the United States by demographic and tumor characteristics, 1980–2005. *Cancer Epidemiology Biomarkers Prev.* 2009;18(3):784–791.

14. van der Veen I, de Boer J. Phosphorous flame retardants: properties, production, environmental occurrence, toxicity and analysis. *Chemosphere.* 2012;88(10):1119–1153.

15. Capen CC. Mechanistic data and risk assessment of selected toxic end points of the thyroid gland. *Toxicol Pathol.* 1997;25(1): 39–48.

16. Vigneri R, Malandrino P, Giani F, Russo M, Vigneri P. Heavy metals in the volcanic environment and thyroid cancer. *Mol Cell Endocrinol.* 2017;457:73–80.

17. Marcello MA, Sampaio AC, Geloneze B, Vasques AC, Assumpcao LV, Ward LS. Obesity and excess protein and carbohydrate consumption are risk factors for thyroid cancer. *Nutr Cancer.* 2012;64(8): 1190–1195.

18. Zamora-Ros R, Beraud V, Franceschi S, et al. Consumption of fruits, vegetables and fruit juices and differentiated thyroid carcinoma risk in the European Prospective Investigation into Cancer and Nutrition (EPIC) study. *Int J Cancer.* 2018;142(3): 449–459.

19. Nettore IC, Colao A, Macchia PE. Nutritional and environmental factors in thyroid carcinogenesis. *Int J Environ Res Public Health.* 2018;15(8):1735.

20. Xu L, Port M, Landi S, et al. Obesity and the risk of papillary thyroid cancer: a pooled analysis of three case-control studies. *Thyroid.* 2014;24(6):966–974.

21. Haugen BR, Alexander EK, Bible KC, et al. 2015 American Thyroid Association Management Guidelines for Adult Patients with Thyroid Nodules and Differentiated Thyroid Cancer: the American Thyroid Association Guidelines Task Force on Thyroid Nodules and Differentiated Thyroid Cancer. *Thyroid.* 2016;26(1):1–133.

22. Olson E, Wintheiser G, Wolfe KM, Droessler J, Silberstein PT. Epidemiology of thyroid cancer: a review of the National Cancer Database, 2000–2013. *Cureus.* 2019;11(2): e4127.

23. Pathak KA, Leslie WD, Klonisch TC, Nason RW. The changing face of thyroid cancer in a population-based cohort. *Cancer Med.* 2013;2(4):537–544.

24. Nilubol N, Zhang L, Kebebew E. Multivariate analysis of the relationship between male sex, disease-specific survival, and features of tumor aggressiveness in thyroid cancer of follicular cell origin. *Thyroid.* 2013;23(6):695–702.

25. Tubiana M, Schlumberger M, Rougier P, et al. Long-term results and prognostic factors in patients with differentiated thyroid carcinoma. *Cancer.* 1985;55(4):794–804.

26. Jukkola A, Bloigu R, Ebeling T, Salmela P, Blanco G. Prognostic factors in differentiated thyroid carcinomas and their implications for current staging classifications. *Endocr Relat Cancer.* 2004;11(3):571–579.

27. Sellers M, Beenken S, Blankenship A, et al. Prognostic significance of cervical lymph node metastases in differentiated thyroid cancer. *Am J Surg.* 1992;164(6):578–581.

28. Somoza AD, Bui H, Samaan S, Dhanda-Patil R, Muasim DF. Cutaneous metastasis as the presenting sign of papillary thyroid carcinoma. *J Cutan Pathol.* 2013;40(2): 274–278.

29. Høie J, Stenwig AE, Kullmann G, Lindegaard M. Distant metastases in papillary thyroid cancer. A review of 91 patients. *Cancer.* 1988;61(1):1–6.

30. Durante C, Haddy N, Baudin E, et al. Long-term outcome of 444 patients with distant metastases from papillary and follicular thyroid carcinoma: benefits and limits of radioiodine therapy. *J Clin Endocrinol Metab.* 2006;91(8):2892–2899.

31. Sugitami I, Fujimoto Y, Yomamoto N. Papillary thyroid carcinoma with distant metastases: survival predictors and the importance of local control. *Surgery.* 2008;143(1): 35–42.

32. Graham LD, Roe SM. Metastatic papillary thyroid carcinoma presenting as a primary renal neoplasm. *Am Surg*. 1995;61(8): 732–734.

33. Pacak K, Sweeney DC, Wartofsky L, et al. Solitary cerebellar metastasis from papillary thyroid carcinoma: a case report. *Thyroid*. 1998;8(4):327–335.

34. McCaffrey TV, Bergstralh EJ, Hay ID. Locally invasive papillary thyroid carcinoma:1940–1990. *Head Neck*. 1994;16: 165–172.

35. Lissak B, Vannetzel JM, Gallouedec N, Berrod JL, Rieu M. Solitary skin metastasis as the presenting feature of differentiated thyroid microcarcinoma: report of two cases. *J Endocrinol Invest*. 1995;18(10):813–816.

36. Reusser NM, Holcomb M, Krishnan B, Rosen T, Orengo IF. Cutaneous metastasis of papillary thyroid carcinoma to the neck: a case report and review of the literature. *Dermatol Online J*. 2014;21(2).

37. McIvor NP, Flint DJ, Gillibrand J, Morton RP. Thyroid surgery and voice-related outcomes. *Aust N Z J Surg*. 2000;70(3):179–183.

38. Pernambuco Lde A, de Almeida MN, Matias KG, Costa EB. Voice assessment and voice-related quality of life in patients with benign thyroid disease. *Otolaryngol Head Neck Surg*. 2015;152(1):116–121.

39. Ficarra BJ. Myxedematous hoarseness. *Arch Otolaryngol*. 1960;72:75–76.

40. Kadakia A, Carlson A, Sataloff RT. The effect of hormones on the voice. *JOS*. 2013; 69(5):571–574.

41. Falhammar H, Juhlin CC, Barner C, Catrina SB, Karefylakis C, Calissendorff J. Riedel's thyroiditis: clinical presentation, treatment and outcomes. *Endocrine*. 2018;60(1):185–192.

42. Volpe R, Johnston MW. Subacute thyroiditis: a disease commonly mistaken for pharyngitis. *Can Med Assoc J*. 1957;77(4): 297–307.

43. Altman KW, Haines GK 3rd, Vakkalanka SK, Keni SP, Kopp PA, Radosevich JA. Identification of thyroid hormone recep-

tors in the human larynx. *Laryngoscope*. 2003;113(11):1931–1934.

44. Birkent H, Karacalioglu O, Merati AL, Akcam T, Gerek M. Prospective study of the impact of thyroid hormone replacement on objective voice parameters. *Ann Otol Rhinol Laryngol*. 2008;117(7):523–527.

45. Moumen M, Mehhane M, Kadiri B, Mawfik H, el Fares F. Compressive goiters. Apropos of 80 cases. *J Chir* (Paris). 1989; 126(10):521–526.

46. Hamdan AL, Dowli A, Jabbour J, Sabri A, Azar ST. Phonatory symptoms and impact on quality of life in female patients with goiter. *Ear Nose Throat J*. 2016;95(7):E5–E10.

47. Alfonso A, Christoudias G, Amaruddin Q, Herbsman H, Gardner B. Tracheal or esophageal compression due to benign thyroid disease. *Am J Surg*. 1981;142(3): 350–354.

48. Banks CA, Ayers CM, Hornig JD, et al. Thyroid disease and compressive symptoms. *Laryngoscope*. 2012;122(1):13–16.

49. Lacoste L, Gineste D, Karayan J, et al. Airway complications in thyroid surgery. *Ann Otol Rhinol Laryngol*. 1993;102(6):441–446.

50. McHenry CR, Piotrowski JJ. Thyroidectomy in patients with marked thyroid enlargement: airway management, morbidity, and outcome. *Am Surg*. 1994;60(8): 586–591.

51. Caroline M, Joglekar S, Mandel S, Sataloff R, Herman-Ackah YD. The predictors of postoperative laryngeal nerve paresis in patients undergoing thyroid surgery: a pilot study. *J Voice*. 2012;26(2):262–266.

52. Heman-Ackah YD, Joglekar SS, Caroline M, et al. The prevalence of undiagnosed thyroid disease in patients with symptomatic vocal fold paresis. *J Voice*. 2011;25(4):496–500.

53. Rubin AD, Sataloff RT. Vocal fold paresis and paralysis. In: Sataloff RT. *Professional Voice: The Science and Art of Clinical Care*. San Diego, CA: Plural Publishing; 2017: 1059–1076.

54. Sittel C, Stennert E, Thumfart WF, Dapunt U, Eckel HE. Prognostic value of laryngeal

electromyography in vocal fold paralysis. *Arch Otolaryngol Head Neck Surg.* 2001;127: 155–160.

55. Farrag TY, Samlan RA, Lin FR, Tufano RP. The utility of evaluating true vocal fold motion before thyroid surgery. *Laryngoscope.* 2006;116(2):235–238.

56. Randolph GW, Kamani D. The importance of preoperative laryngoscopy in patients undergoing thyroidectomy: voice, vocal cord function, and the preoperative detection of invasive thyroid malignancy. *Surgery.* 2006;139(3):357–362.

57. Agu KA, Nwosu JN, Akpeh JO. Evaluation of vocal cord function before thyroidectomy: experience from a developing country. *Indian J Surg.* 2018;80(3):211–215.

58. Sataloff RT, Praneetvatakul P, Heuer RJ, et al. Laryngeal electromyography: clinical application. *J Voice.* 2010;24(2):228–234.

59. Yeung P, Erskine C, Mathews P, Crowe PJ. Voice changes and thyroid surgery: is preoperative indirect laryngoscopy necessary? *Aust N Z J Surg.* 1999;69(9):632–634.

60. Steurer M, Passler C, Denk DM, Schneider B, Niederle B, Bigenzahn W. Advantages of recurrent laryngeal nerve identification in thyroidectomy and parathyroidectomy and the importance of preoperative and postoperative laryngoscopic examination in more than 1000 nerves at risk. *Laryngoscope.* 2002;112(1):124–133.

61. Hodin R, Clark O, Doherty G, Grant C, Heller K, Weigel R. Voice issues and laryngoscopy in thyroid surgery patients. *Surgery.* 2013;154(1):46–47.

62. Chandrasekhar SS, Randolph GW, Seidman MD, et al. Clinical practice guideline: improving voice outcomes after thyroid surgery. *Otolaryngol Head Neck Surg.* 2013;148(6 suppl):S1–S37.

63. Kay-Rivest E, Mitmaker E, Payne RJ, et al. Preoperative vocal cord paralysis and its association with malignant thyroid disease and other pathological features. *J Otolaryngol Head Neck Surg.* 2015;44(1):35.

64. Miyauchi A, Inoue H, Tomoda C, et al. Improvement in phonation after recon-struction of the recurrent laryngeal nerve in patients with thyroid cancer invading the nerve. *Surgery.* 2009;146(6):1056–1062.

65. McCall AR, Ott R, Jarosz H, Lawrence AM, Paloyan E. Improvement of vocal cord paresis after thyroidectomy. *Am Surg.* 1987;53(7):377–379.

66. Mitchell AL, Gandhi A, Scott-Coombes D, Perros P. Management of thyroid cancer: United Kingdom national multi-disciplinary guidelines. *J Laryngol Otol.* 2016;130(S2):S150–S160.

67. Chiang FY, Lin JC, Lee KW, et al. Thyroid tumors with preoperative recurrent laryngeal nerve palsy: clinicopathologic features and treatment outcome. *Surgery.* 2006;140(3):413–417.

68. McCaffrey JC. Aerodigestive tract invasion by well-differentiated thyroid carcinoma: diagnosis, management, prognosis, and biology. *Laryngoscope.* 2006;116(1):1–11.

69. Falk SA, McCaffrey TV. Management of the recurrent laryngeal nerve in suspected and proven thyroid cancer. *Otolaryngol Head Neck Surg.* 1995;113(1):42–48.

70. Roh JL, Yoon YH, Park CI. Recurrent laryngeal nerve paralysis in patients with papillary thyroid carcinomas: evaluation and management of resulting vocal dysfunction. *Am J Surg.* 2009;197(4):459–465.

71. Holl-Allen RT. Laryngeal nerve paralysis and benign thyroid disease. *Arch Otolaryngol.* 1967;85(3):335–337.

72. Rowe-Jones JM, Rosswick RP, Leighton SE. Benign thyroid disease and vocal cord palsy. *Ann R Coll Surg Engl.* 1993;75(4):241–244.

73. Fenton JE, Timon CI, McShane DP. Recurrent laryngeal nerve palsy secondary to benign thyroid disease. *J Laryngol Otol.* 1994;108(10):878–880.

74. Moorthy R, Balfour A, Jeannon JP, Simo R. Recurrent laryngeal nerve palsy in benign thyroid disease: can surgery make a difference? *Eur Arch Otorhinolaryngol.* 2012;269(3):983–987.

75. Collazo-Clavell ML, Gharib H, Maragos NE. Relationship between vocal cord paral-

ysis and benign thyroid disease. *Head Neck.* 1995;17(1):24–30.

76. Honings J, Stephen AE, Marres HA, Gaissert HA. The management of thyroid carcinoma invading the larynx or trachea. *Laryngoscope.* 2010;120(4):682–689.

77. McConahey WM, Hay ID, Woolner LB, van Heerden JA, Taylor WF. Papillary thyroid cancer treated at the Mayo Clinic, 1946 through 1970: initial manifestations, pathologic findings, therapy, and outcome. *Mayo Clin Proc.* 1986;61(12):978–996.

78. Djalilian M, Beahrs OH, Devine KD, Weiland LH, DeSanto LW. Intraluminal involvement of the larynx and trachea by thyroid cancer. *Am J Surg.* 1974;128(4):500–504.

79. Lawson VG. The management of airway involvement in thyroid tumors. *Arch Otolaryngol.* 1983;109(2):86–90.

80. Silliphant WM, Klinck GH, Levitin MS. Thyroid carcinoma and death: a clinicopathological study of 193 autopsies. *Cancer.* 1964;17:513–525.

81. Batsakis JG. Laryngeal involvement by thyroid disease. *Ann Otol Rhinol Laryngol.* 1987;96(6):718–719.

82. Clark RL, Ibanez ML, White EC. What constitutes an adequate operation for carcinoma of the thyroid? *Arch Surg.* 1966;92(1):23–26.

83. Tsumori T, Nakao K, Miyata M, et al. Clinicopathologic study of thyroid carcinoma infiltrating the trachea. *Nihon Geka Gakkai Zasshi.* 1985;86(4):404–410.

84. Brauckhoff M. Classification of aerodigestive tract invasion from thyroid cancer. *Langenbecks Arch Surg.* 2014;399(2):209–216.

85. Chala AI, Vélez S, Sanabria A. The role of laryngectomy in locally advanced thyroid carcinoma. Review of 16 cases. *Acta Otorhinolaryngol Ital.* 2018;38(2):109–114.

86. Pecina-Slaus N. Tumor suppressor gene E-cadherin and its role in normal and malignant cells. *Cancer Cell Int.* 2003;3(1):17.

87. Campbell RJ, Pignatelli M. Molecular histology in the study of solid tumours. *Mol Pathol.* 2002;55(2):80–82.

88. Ito Y, Yoshida H, Tomoda C, et al. Maspin expression is directly associated with biological aggressiveness of thyroid carcinoma. *Thyroid.* 2004;14(1):13–18.

89. Ueno H, Nakamura H, Inoue M, et al. Expression and tissue localization of membrane-types 1, 2, and 3 matrix metalloproteinases in human invasive breast carcinomas. *Cancer Res.* 1997;57(10):2055–2060.

90. Nomura H, Fujimoto N, Seiki M, Mai M, Okada Y. Enhanced production of matrix metalloproteinases and activation of matrix metalloproteinase 2 (gelatinase A) in human gastric carcinomas. *Int J Cancer.* 1996;69(1):9–16.

91. Demeure MJ, Damsky CH, Elfman F, Goretzki PE, Wong MG, Clark OH. Invasion by cultured human follicular thyroid cancer correlates with increased beta 1 integrins and production of proteases. *World J Surg.* 1992;16(4):770–776.

92. Kusunoki T, Nishida S, Kimoto-Kinoshita S, Murata K, Satou T, Tomura T. Type IV collagen, type IV collagenase activity and ability of cell proliferation in human thyroid tumours. *Asian J Surg.* 2002;25(4):304–308.

93. Rocha AS, Soares P, Seruca R, et al. Abnormalities of the E-cadherin/catenin adhesion complex in classical papillary thyroid carcinoma and in its diffuse sclerosing variant. *J Pathol.* 2001;194(3):358–366.

94. Serini G, Trusolino L, Saggiorato E, et al. Changes in integrin and E-cadherin expression in neoplastic versus normal thyroid tissue. *J Natl Cancer Inst.* 1996;88(7):442–449.

95. Nagafuchi A, Takeichi M. Transmembrane control of cadherin-mediated cell adhesion: a 94 kDa protein functionally associated with a specific region of the cytoplasmic domain of E-cadherin. *Cell Regul.* 1989;1(1):37–44.

96. Graham JC. Hoarseness associated with lymphoma of the thyroid gland. *South Med J.* 1982;75(12):1566–1567.

97. Georgiades F, Vasiliou G, Kyrodimos E, Thrasyvoulou G. Extensive laryngeal infiltration from a neglected papillary thyroid

carcinoma: A case report. *World J Clin Cases*. 2016;4(7):187–190.

98. McCarty TM, Kuhn JA, Williams WL Jr, et al. Surgical management of thyroid cancer invading the airway. *Ann Surg Oncol*. 1997;4(5):403–408.

99. Gaissert HA, Honings J, Grillo HC, et al. Segmental laryngotracheal and tracheal resection for invasive thyroid carcinoma. *Ann Thorac Surg*. 2007;83(6):1952–1959.

100. Tomoda C, Uruno T, Takamura Y, et al. Ultrasonography as a method of screening for tracheal invasion by papillary thyroid cancer. *Surg Today*. 2005;35(1):819–822.

101. Takashima S, Morimoto S, Ikezoe J, et al. CT evaluation of anaplastic thyroid carcinoma. *AJR Am J Roentgenol*. 1990;154(5):1079–1085.

102. Seo YL, Yoon DY, Lim KJ, et al. Locally advanced thyroid cancer: can CT help in prediction of extrathyroidal invasion to adjacent structures? *AJR Am J Roentgenol*. 2010;195(3):W240–W244.

103. Takashima S, Takayama F, Wang J, Kobayashi S, Kadoya M. Using MR imaging to predict invasion of the recurrent laryngeal nerve by thyroid carcinoma. *AJR Am J Roentgenol*. 2003;180(3):837–842.

104. Ballantyne AJ. Resections of the upper aerodigestive tract for locally invasive thyroid cancer. *Am J Surg*. 1994;168(6):636–639.

105. Shin DH, Mark EJ, Suen HC, Grillo HC. Pathologic staging of papillary carcinoma of the thyroid with airway invasion based on the anatomic manner of extension to the trachea: a clinicopathologic study based on 22 patients who underwent thyroidectomy and airway resection. *Hum Pathol*. 1993;24(8):866–870.

106. Czaja JM, McCaffrey TV. The surgical management of laryngotracheal invasion by well-differentiated papillary thyroid carcinoma. *Arch Otolaryngol Head Neck Surg*. 1997;123(5):484–490.

107. Morton RP, Ahmad Z. Thyroid cancer invasion of neck structures: epidemiology, evaluation, staging and management. *Curr Opin Otolaryngol Head Neck Surg*. 2007;15:89–94.

108. Rosai J, Zampi G, Carcangui ML. Papillary carcinoma of the thyroid: A discussion of its several morphological expressions, with particular emphasis on the follicular variant. *Am J Surg Pathol*. 1983;7(8):809–817.

109. Yamashita H, Noguchi S, Murakami N, Kawamoto H, Watanabe S. Extracapsular invasion of lymph node metastasis is an indicator of distant metastasis and poor prognosis in patients with thyroid papillary carcinoma. *Cancer*. 1997;80(12):2268–2272.

110. Varghese BT, Mathews A, Pandey M, Pradeep VM. Unusual metastasis of papillary thyroid carcinoma to larynx and hypopharynx a case report. *World J Surg Oncol*. 2003;1(1):7.

111. Hakeem AH, Pradhan SA, Bhele S, Tubachi J. Metastasis of papillary thyroid cancer to the larynx and pharynx: unusual case report. *Eur Arch Otorhinolaryngol*. 2012; 269(12):2585–2587.

112. Moosa M, Mazzaferri EL. Disorders of the Thyroid Gland. In: Cummings CW, Fredrickson JM, Harker LA, Krause CJ, Richardson MA, Schuller DE. *Otolaryngology Head and Neck Surgery*. 3rd ed. St. Louis, MO, Mosby; 1998.:2450–2479.

113. Dinneen SF, Valimaki MJ, Bergstralh EJ, Goellner JR, Gorman CA, Hay ID. Distant metastases in papillary thyroid carcinoma: 100 cases observed at one institution during 5 decades. *J Clin Endocrinol Metab*. 1995;80(7):2041–2045.

114. American Thyroid Association Guidelines Taskforce, Cooper DS, Doherty GM, et al. Revised American Thyroid Association management guidelines for patients with thyroid nodules and differentiated thyroid cancer. *Thyroid*. 2009;19(11):1167–1214.

115. Musholt TJ, Musholt PB, Behrend M, Raab R, Scheumann GF, Klempnauer J. Invasive differentiated thyroid carcinoma: tracheal resection and reconstruction procedures in the hands of the endocrine surgeon. *Surgery*. 1999;126(6):1078–1087.

116. Nishida T, Nakao K, Hamaji M. Differentiated thyroid carcinoma with airway invasion: indication for tracheal resection based

on the extent of cancer invasion. *J Thorac Cardiovasc Surg*. 1997;114(1):84–92.

117. Solomon NP, Awan SN, Helou LB, Stojadinovic A. Acoustic analyses of thyroidectomy-related changes in vowel phonation. *J Voice*. 2012;26(6):711–720.

118. Grover G, Sadler GP, Mihai R. Morbidity after thyroid surgery: patient perspective. *Laryngoscope*. 2013;123(9):2319–2323.

119. Chiang FY, Wang LF, Huang YF, Lee KW, Kuo WR. Recurrent laryngeal nerve palsy after thyroidectomy with routine identification of the recurrent laryngeal nerve. *Surgery*. 2005;137(3):342–347.

120. Bergenfelz A, Jansson S, Kristoffersson A, et al. Complications to thyroid surgery: results as reported in a database from a multicenter audit comprising 3,660 patients. *Langenbecks Arch Surg*. 2008;393(5):667–673.

121. Benninger MS, Gillen JB, Altman JS. Changing etiology of vocal fold immobility. *Laryngoscope*. 1998;108(9):1346–1350.

122. Spataro EA, Grindler DJ, Paniello RC. Etiology and time to presentation of unilateral vocal fold paralysis. *Otolaryngol Head Neck Surg*. 2014;151(2):286–293.

123. Röher HD, Goretzki PE, Hellmann P, Witte J. Complications in thyroid surgery. Incidence and therapy. *Chirurg*. 1999;70(9):999–1010.

124. Kube R, Horschig P, Marusch F, Horntrich J, Gastinger I. Postoperative recurrent nerve paralysis after initial interventions for benign goiter. *Zentralbl Chir*. 1998;123(1):11–16.

125. Miller W, Butters M, Leibl B, Bittner R. Quality assurance in goiter surgery by rate of recurrent nerve paralysis. *Chirurg*. 1995;66(12):1210–1214.

126. Hayward NJ, Grodski S, Yeung M, Johnson WR, Serpell J. Recurrent laryngeal nerve injury in thyroid surgery: a review. *ANZ J Surg*. 2013;83(1–2):15–21.

127. Goncalves-Filho J, Kowalski LP. Surgical complications after thyroid surgery performed in a cancer hospital. *Otolaryngol Head Neck Surg*. 2005;132(3):490–494.

128. Erbil Y, Barbaros U, Işsever H, et al. Predictive factors for recurrent laryngeal nerve palsy and hypoparathyroidism after thyroid surgery. *Clin Otolaryngol*. 2007;32(1):32–37.

129. Jatzko GR, Lisborg PH, Müller MG, Wette VM. Recurrent nerve palsy after thyroid operations—principal nerve identification and a literature review. *Surgery*. 1994;115(2):139–144.

130. Jeannon JP, Orabi AA, Bruch GA, Abdalsalam HA, Simo R. Diagnosis of recurrent laryngeal nerve palsy after thyroidectomy: a systematic review. *Int J Clin Pract*. 2009;63(4):624–629.

131. Koçak S, Aydıntug S, Özbaş S, Koçak İ, Küçük B, Baskan S. Evaluation of vocal cord function after thyroid surgery. *Eur J Surg*. 1999;165(3):183–186.

132. Sinclair CF, Bumpous JM, Haugen BR, et al. Laryngeal examination in thyroid and parathyroid surgery: An American Head and Neck Society consensus statement. *Head Neck*. 2016;38(6):811–819.

133. Snyder SK, Lairmore TC, Hendricks JC, Roberts JW. Elucidating mechanisms of recurrent laryngeal nerve injury during thyroidectomy and parathyroidectomy. *J Am Coll Surg*. 2008;206(1):123–130.

134. Dralle H, Sekulla C, Haerting J, et al. Risk factors of paralysis and functional outcome after recurrent laryngeal nerve monitoring in thyroid surgery. *Surgery*. 2004;136(6):1310–1322.

135. Sosa JA, Bowman HM, Tielsch JM, Powe NR, Gordon TA, Udelsman R. The importance of surgeon experience for clinical and economic outcomes from thyroidectomy. *Ann Surg*. 1998;228(3):320–330.

136. Karamanakos SN, Markou KB, Panagopoulos K, et al. Complications and risk factors related to the extent of surgery in thyroidectomy. Results from 2,043 procedures. *Hormones (Athens)*. 2010;9(4):318–325.

137. Lo CY, Kwok KF, Yuen PW. A prospective evaluation of recurrent laryngeal nerve paralysis during thyroidectomy. *Arch Surg*. 2000;135(2):204–207.

138. Zambudio AR, Rodríguez J, Riquelme J, Soria T, Canteras M, Parrilla P. Prospective study of postoperative complications after

total thyroidectomy for multinodular goiters by surgeons with experience in endocrine surgery. *Ann Surg.* 2004;240(1):18–25.

139. Testini M, Gurrado A, Bellantone R, et al. Recurrent laryngeal nerve palsy and substernal goiter. An Italian multicenter study. *J Visc Surg.* 2014;151(3):183–189.

140. Thomusch O, Machens A, Sekulla C, et al. Multivariate analysis of risk factors for postoperative complications in benign goiter surgery: prospective multicenter study in Germany. *World J Surg.* 2000;24(11): 1335–1341.

141. Hermann M, Alk G, Roka R, Glaser K, Freissmuth M. Laryngeal recurrent nerve injury in surgery for benign thyroid diseases: effect of nerve dissection and impact of individual surgeon in more than 27 000 nerves at risk. *Ann Surg.* 2002;235(2):261–268.

142. Seiler C, Glaser C, Wagner HE. Thyroid gland surgery in an endemic region. *World J Surg.* 1996;20(5):593–597.

143. Calò PG, Pisano G, Medas F, Tatti A, Tuveri M, Nicolosi A. Risk factors in reoperative thyroid surgery for recurrent goiter: our experience. *G Chir.* 2012;33(10):335–338.

144. Sataloff RT. Clinical anatomy and physiology of the voice. In: Sataloff RT. *Professional Voice: The Science and Art of Clinical Care.* 4th ed. San Diego, CA: Plural Publishing; 2017:157–196.

145. Randolph GW. Surgical anatomy of the recurrent laryngeal nerve. In: Randolph GW, ed. *Surgery of the Thyroid and Parathyroid Glands.* Philadelphia, PA: Saunders; 2003:300–342.

146. Serpell JW, Yeung MJ, Grodski S. The motor fibers of the recurrent laryngeal nerve are located in the anterior extralaryngeal branch. *Ann Surg.* 2009;249(4):648–652.

147. Rustad WH. Revised anatomy of the recurrent laryngeal nerves: surgical importance, based on the dissection of 100 cadavers. *J Clin Endocrinol Metab.* 1954;14(1):87–96.

148. Ardito G, Revelli L, D'Alatri L, Lerro V, Guidi ML, Ardito F. Revisited anatomy of the recurrent laryngeal nerves. *Am J Surg.* 2004;187(2):249–253.

149. Beneragama T, Serpell JW. Extralaryngeal bifurcation of the recurrent laryngeal nerve: a common variation. *ANZ J Surg.* 2006;76(10):928–931.

150. Katz AD, Nemiroff P. Anastamosis and bifurcations of the recurrent laryngeal nerve—report of 1177 nerves visualized. *Am Surg.* 1993;59(3):188–190.

151. Katz AD. Extralaryngeal division of the recurrent laryngeal nerve. Report on 400 patients and the 721 nerves measured. *Am J Surg.* 1986; 152(4):407–410.

152. Wong KP, Mak KL, Wong CK, Lang BH. Systematic review and meta-analysis on intraoperative neuromonitoring in high-risk thyroidectomy. *Int J Surg.* 2017;38:21–30.

153. Chan W, Lang BH, Lo CY. The role of intraoperative neuromonitoring of the recurrent laryngeal nerve during thyroidectomy: a comparative study on 1000 nerves at risk. *Surgery.* 2006;140(6):866–873.

154. Thomusch O, Sekulla C, Machens A, Neumann HJ, Timmermann W, Dralle H. Validity of intraoperative neuromonitoring signals in thyroid surgery. *Langenbecks Arch Surg.* 2004;389(6):499–503.

155. Thomusch O, Sekulla C, Walls G, Machens A, Dralle H. Intraoperative neuromonitoring of surgery for benign goiter. *Am J Surg.* 2002;183(6):673–678.

156. Barczyński M, Konturek A, Cichoń S. Randomized clinical trial of visualization versus neuromonitoring of recurrent laryngeal nerves during thyroidectomy. *Br J Surg.* 2009;96(3):240–246.

157. Choi YS, Joo YH, Park YH, Kim SY, Sun DI. Factors predicting the recovery of unilateral vocal fold paralysis after thyroidectomy. *World J Surg.* 2018;42(7):2117–2122.

158. Wang CC, Chang MH, Wang CP, Liu SA. Prognostic indicators of unilateral vocal fold paralysis. *Arch Otolaryngol Head Neck Surg.* 2008;134(4):380–388.

159. Wang CC, Chang MH, De Virgilio A, et al. Laryngeal electromyography and prognosis of unilateral vocal fold paralysis—a long-term prospective study. *Laryngoscope.* 2015;125(4):898–903.

160. Reiter R, Brosch S. Laryngoplasty with hyaluronic acid in patients with unilateral vocal fold paralysis. *J Voice*. 2012;26(6):785–791.

161. King JM, Simpson CB. Modern injection augmentation for glottic insufficiency. *Curr Opin Otolaryngol Head Neck Surg*. 2007; 15(3):153–158.

162. Zimmermann TM, Orbelo DM, Pittelko RL, Youssef SJ, Lohse CM, Ekbom DC. Voice outcomes following medialization laryngoplasty with and without arytenoid adduction. *Laryngoscope*. 2019;129(8): 1876–1881.

163. Remacle M, Lawson G, Mayne A, Jamart J. Subtotal carbon dioxide laser arytenoidectomy by endoscopic approach for treatment of bilateral cord immobility in adduction. *Ann Otol Rhinol Laryngol*. 1996;105(6):438–445.

164. Ossoff RH, Sisson GA, Duncavage JA, Moselle HI, Andrews PE, McMillan WG. Endoscopic laser arytenoidectomy for the treatment of bilateral vocal cord paralysis. *Laryngoscope*. 1984;94(10):1293–1297.

165. Stojadinovic A, Shaha AR, Orlikoff RF, et al. Prospective functional voice assessment in patients undergoing thyroid surgery. *Ann Surg*. 2002;236(6):823–832.

166. Kark AE, Kissin MW, Auerbach R, Meikle M. Voice changes after thyroidectomy: role of the external laryngeal nerve. *Br Med J (Clin Res Ed)*. 1984;289(6456):1412–1415.

167. Jansson S, Tisell LE, Hagne I, Sanner E, Stenborg R, Svensson P. Partial superior laryngeal nerve (SLN) lesions before and after thyroid surgery. *World J Surg*. 1988;12(4): 522–527.

168. Dursun G, Sataloff RT, Spiegel JR, Mandel S, Heuer RJ, Rosen DC. Superior laryngeal nerve paresis and paralysis. *J Voice*. 1996;10(2):206–211.

169. Lore JM, Kim DJ, Elias S. Preservation of the laryngeal nerves during total thyroid lobectomy. *Ann Otol Rhinol Laryngol*. 1977;86(6 pt1):777–788.

170 Lennquist S, Cahlin C, Smeds S. The superior laryngeal nerve in thyroid surgery. *Surgery*. 1987;102(6):999–1008.

171. Lekacos NL, Miligos ND, Tzardis PJ, Majiatis S, Patoulis J. The superior laryngeal nerve in thyroidectomy. *Am Surg*. 1987; 53(10):610–612.

172. Keseroglu K, Bayir O, Umay EK, et al. Laryngeal electromyographic changes in postthyroidectomy patients with normal vocal cord mobility. *Eur Arch Otorhinolaryngol*. 2017;274(4):1925–1931.

173. Aluffi P, Policarpo M, Cherovac C, Olina M, Dosdegani R, Pia F. Post-thyroidectomy superior laryngeal nerve injury. *Eur Arch Otorhinolaryngol*. 2001;258(9):451–454.

174. Teitelbaum BJ, Wenig BL. Superior laryngeal nerve injury from thyroid surgery. *Head Neck*. 1995;17(1):36–40.

175. Aina EN, Hisham AN. External laryngeal nerve in thyroid surgery: recognition and surgical implications. *ANZ J Surg*. 2001; 71(4):212–214.

176. Cernea CR, Ferraz AR, Nisho S, Dutra A, Hojaij FC, dos Santos LR. Surgical anatomy of the external branch of the superior laryngeal nerve. *Head Neck*. 1992;14(5):380–383.

177. Chuang FJ, Chen JY, Shyu JF, et al. Surgical anatomy of the external branch of the superior laryngeal nerve in Chinese adults and its clinical applications. *Head Neck*. 2010; 32(1):53–57.

178. Cernea CR, Ferraz AR, Fulani J, et al. Identification of the external branch of the superior laryngeal nerve during thyroidectomy. *Am J Surg*. 1992;164(6):634–639.

179. Glover AR, Norlén O, Gundara JS, Morris M, Sidhu SB. Use of the nerve integrity monitor during thyroid surgery aids identification of the external branch of the superior laryngeal nerve. *Ann Surg Oncol*. 2015;22(6):1768–1773.

180. Gurleyik E, Dogan S, Cetin F, Gurleyik G. Visual and electrophysiological identification of the external branch of superior laryngeal nerve in redo thyroid surgery compared with primary thyroid surgery. *Ann Surg Treat Res*. 2019;96(6):269–274.

181. Hong KH, Kim YK. Phonatory characteristics of patients undergoing thyroidectomy

without laryngeal nerve injury. *Otolaryngol Head Neck Surg.* 1997;117(4):399–404.

182. Pereira JA, Girvent M, Sancho JJ, Parada C, Sitges-Serra A. Prevalence of long-term upper aerodigestive symptoms after uncomplicated bilateral thyroidectomy. *Surgery.* 2003;133(3):318–322.

183. de Pedro Netto I, Fae A, Vartanian JG, et al. Voice and vocal self-assessment after thyroidectomy. *Head Neck.* 2006;28(12):1106–1114.

184. Kim CS, Park JO, Bae JS, et al. Long-lasting voice-related symptoms in patients without vocal cord palsy after thyroidectomy. *World J Surg.* 2018;42(7):2109–2116.

185. Sataloff RT, Spiegel JR, Carroll LM, Heuer RJ. Male soprano voice: a rare complication of thyroidectomy. *Laryngoscope.* 1992;102(1):90–93.

186. Randolph GW, Shin JJ, Grillo HC, et al. The surgical management of goiter: part II. Surgical treatment and results. *Laryngoscope.* 2011;121(1):68–76.

187. Echternach M, Maurer C, Mencke T, Schilling M, Verse T, Richter B. Laryngeal complications after thyroidectomy: is it always the surgeon? *Arch Surg.* 2009;144(2):149–153.

188. Gómez-Ramírez J, Sitges-Serra A, Moreno-Llorente P, et al. Mortality after thyroid surgery, insignificant or still an issue? *Langenbecks Arch Surg.* 2015;400(4):517–522.

189. Ito Y, Miyauchi A, Inoue H, et al. An observational trial for papillary thyroid microcarcinoma in Japanese patients. *World J Surg.* 2010;34(1):28–35.

190. Tomoda C, Ito Y, Kobayashi K, Miya A, Miyauchi A. Subclinical hypothyroidism following hemithyroidectomy: a simple risk-scoring system using age and pre-operative thyrotropin level. *ORL.* 2011;73(2):68–71.

191. Chu KK, Lang BH. Clinicopathologic predictors for early and late biochemical hypothyroidism after hemithyroidectomy. *Am J Surg.* 2012;203(4):461–466.

192. Su SY, Grodski S, Serpell JW. Hypothyroidism following hemithyroidectomy:

a retrospective review. *Ann Surgery.* 2009;250(6):991–994.

193. Piper HG, Bugis SP, Wilkins GE, Walker BA, Wiseman S, Baliski CR. Detecting and defining hypothyroidism after hemithyroidectomy. *Am J Surg.* 2005;189(5):587–591.

194. De Carlucci D Jr, Tavares MR, Obara MT, Martins LA, Hojaij FC, Cernea CR. Thyroid function after unilateral total lobectomy: risk factors for postoperative hypothyroidism. *Arch Otolaryngol Head Neck Surg.* 2008;134(10):1076–1079.

195. Moon HG, Jung EJ, Park ST, et al. Thyrotropin level and thyroid volume for prediction of hypothyroidism following hemithyroidectomy in an Asian patient cohort. *World J Surg.* 2008;32(11):2503–2508.

196. Koh YW, Lee SW, Choi EC, et al. Prediction of hypothyroidism after hemithyroidectomy: a biochemical and pathological analysis. *Eur Arch Otorhinolaryngol.* 2008;265(4):453–457.

197. McHenry CR, Slusarczyk SJ. Hypothyroidism following hemithyroidectomy: incidence, risk factors, and management. *Surgery.* 2000;128(6):994–998.

198. Buchanan MA, Lee D. Thyroid auto-antibodies, lymphocytic infiltration and the development of post-operative hypothyroidism following hemithyroidectomy for nontoxic nodular goitre. *J R Coll Surg Edinb.* 2001;46(2):86–90.

199. Elmas F, Lauber F, Linder T, Mueller W. Hypothyreosis after hemithyroidectomy—surprisingly frequent complication in aftercare. *Laryngorhinootologie.* 2018;97(1):24–29.

200. Volokh I, Pak VP, Osipov DP. Causes, prevention and treatment of postoperative hypothyroidism. *Vestn Khir Im I I Grek.* 1988;141(8):134–136.

201. Miccoli P, Frustaci G, Fosso A, Miccoli M, Materazzi G. Surgery for recurrent goiter: complication rate and role of the thyroid-stimulating hormone-suppressive therapy after the first operation. *Langenbecks Arch Surg.* 2015;400 (2):253–258.

202. Pfaff JA, Caruso-Sales H, Jaworek A, Sataloff RT. The vocal effects of thyroid disorders and their treatment. In: Sataloff RT. *Professional Voice: The Science and Art of Clinical Care*. San Diego, CA: Plural Publishing; 2017:671–681.

203. Manfredi A, Soliani P, Lombardi M, Goffrini PA. Pathophysiology and predictivity of postoperative hypothyroidism. *Ital J Surg Sci*. 1988;18(2):143–149.

204. Orlof LA, Wiseman SM, Bernet VJ, et al. American Thyroid Association statement on postoperative hypoparathyroidism: diagnosis, prevention, and management in adults. *Thyroid*. 2018;28(7):830–841.

205. van Veelen MJ, Visser MF, Baggen MG, Dees A. Hypocalcaemic laryngospasm in the emergency department. *BMJ Case Rep*. 2011 Feb 17;2011. doi:10.1136/bcr.11.2010.3555

206. Abrantes C, Brigas D, Casimiro HJ, Madeira M. Hypocalcaemia in an adult: the importance of not overlooking the cause. *BMJ Case Rep*. 2018 Apr 5;2018. doi:10.1136/bcr-2017-224108

207. Bergenfelz A, Nordenström E, Almquist M. Morbidity in patients with permanent hypoparathyroidism after total thyroidectomy. *Surgery*. 2020;167(1):124–128.

208. Díez JJ, Anda E, Sastre J, et al. Prevalence and risk factors for hypoparathyroidism following total thyroidectomy in Spain: a multicentric and nation-wide retrospective analysis. *Endocrine*. 2019;66(2):405–415.

209. Harris AS, Prades E, Tkachuk O, Zeitoun H. Better consenting for thyroidectomy: who has an increased risk of postoperative hypocalcaemia? *Eur Arch Otorhinolaryngol*. 2016;273(12):4437–4443.

210. Pelizzo MR, Bernante P, Toniato A, Piotto A, Grigoletto R. Hypoparathyroidism after thyroidectomy. Analysis of a consecutive, recent series. *Minerva Chir*. 1998;53(4):239–244.

211. Al-Dhahri SF, Mubasher M, Mufarji K, Allam OS, Terkawi AS. Factors predicting post-thyroidectomy hypoparathyroidism recovery. *World J Surg*. 2014;38(9):2304–2310.

212. Prazenica P, O'Driscoll K, Holy R. Incidental parathyroidectomy during thyroid surgery using capsular dissection technique. *Otolaryngol Head Neck Surg*. 2014;150(5):754–761.

213. Edafe O, Mech CE, Balasubramanian SP. Calcium, vitamin D or recombinant parathyroid hormone for managing post-thyroidectomy hypoparathyroidism. *Cochrane Database Syst Rev*. 2019;(5):CD012845.

214. Wu SY, Chiang YJ, Fisher SB, et al. Risks of hypoparathyroidism after total thyroidectomy in children: A 21-year experience in a high-volume cancer center. *World J Surg*. 2020;44(2):442–451.

215. Serpell JW, Phan D. Safety of total thyroidectomy. *ANZ J Surg*. 2007;77(1–2):15–19.

216. Păduraru DN, Ion D, Carsote M, Andronic O, Bolocan A. Post-thyroidectomy hypocalcemia—risk factors and management. *Chirurgia (Bucur)*. 2019;114(5):564–570.

217. Borel F, Tresallet C, Hamy A, et al. Self-assessment of voice outcomes after total thyroidectomy using the Voice Handicap Index questionnaire: results of a prospective multicenter study. *Surgery*. 2020;167(1):129–136.

218. Srivastava A, Ravindran V. Stridor secondary to hypocalcemia in the elderly: an unusual presentation. *Eur J Int Med*. 2008;19(3):219–220.

219. Minuto MN, Reina S, Monti E, Ansaldo GL, Varaldo E. Morbidity following thyroid surgery: acceptable rates and how to manage complicated patients. *J Endocrinol Invest*. 2019;42(11):1291–1297.

220. Saad RK, Boueiz NG, Akiki VC, Fuleihan GH. Rate of drop in serum calcium as a predictor of hypocalcemic symptoms post total thyroidectomy. *Osteoporos Int*. 2019;30(12):2495–2504.

221. Sala DT, Muresan M, Voidazan S, et al. First day serum calcium and parathyroid hormone levels as predictive factors for safe discharge after thyroidectomy. *Acta Endocrinol (Buchar)*. 2019;15(2):225–230.

222. Reiners C. Radioiodine therapy of Graves' disease—quality assurance and radiation

protection. *Z Arztl Fortbild Qualitatssich.* 1999;93(suppl 1):61–66.

223. Harrison LC, Buckley JD, Martin FI. Use of a computer-based postal questionnaire for the detection of hypothyrodism following radioiodine therapy for thyrotoxicosis. *Aust N Z J Med.* 1977;7(1):27–32.

224. Snyder S. Vocal cord paralysis after radioiodine therapy. *J Nucl Med.* 1978;19(8): 975–976.

225. Robson AM. Vocal-cord paralysis after treatment of thyrotoxicosis with radioiodine. *Br J Radiol.* 1981;54(643):632.

226. Coover LR. Vocal cord paralysis after 131 I therapy for solitary toxic nodule. *J Nucl Med.* 1999;40(3):505.

227. Kinuya S, Yoneyama T, Michigishi T. Airway complication occurring during radioiodine treatment for Graves' disease. *Ann Nucl Med.* 2007;21(6):367–369.

228. Isolan-Cury RW, Monte O, Cury AN, et al. Acute effects of radioiodine therapy on the voice and larynx of Basedow-Graves' patients. *Braz J Otorhinolaryngol.* 2008;74(2): 224–229.

229. Hong YT, Lim ST, Hong KH. Voice outcome of total thyroidectomy in comparison with administration of recombinant human TSH. *J Voice.* 2019. doi:10.1016/j .jvoice.2019.08.021

9

Non-Hodgkin Lymphoma and Voice

Abdul-Latif Hamdan, Robert Thayer Sataloff, and Mary J. Hawkshaw

Epidemiology and Clinical Presentation

Non-Hodgkin lymphoma (NHL) accounts for 4.2% of all cancer cases diagnosed in the United States. The estimated number in 2019 is 74 200, averaging 19.6 per 100 000 men and women per year.[1] Its incidence is on the rise partially due to the worldwide epidemic of human immunodeficiency virus, the increasing number of organs transplant surgeries, and obesity, although obesity remains controversial. Infectious agents significantly associated with NHL include Epstein-Barr virus, human T-cell leukemia virus, herpes virus 8, and hepatitis C.[2-5] Other precipitating factors include autoimmune diseases such as rheumatoid arthritis, and exogenous factors such as smoking and exposure to irradiation.[6] The number of deaths from non-Hodgkin lymphoma is 5.6 per 100 000 men and women per year, with an estimated 19 970 deaths in 2019.[1] Based on a review by Hong et al in 2018, female gender and low Ann Arbor staging are favorable prognostic indicators for survival.[7]

Non-Hodgkin lymphoma accounts for 90% of all lymphomas.[8] It is more common in patients over the age of 65 years and affects men more frequently than women (41 090 versus 33 110 estimated new cases in 2019).[9] Based on the World Health Organization classification that relies on molecular and immunologic cell characteristics, NHL can be subdivided into numerous types, the most common of which is the diffuse large B-cell lymphoma (DLBCL). Less common subtypes include lymphocytic follicular lymphoma and small lymphocytic lymphoma. These indolent lymphomas often present with cervical and systemic lymphadenopathy that fluctuates with spontaneous regression, making the diagnosis more challenging. Rare and more aggressive lymphomas include lymphoblastic and Burkitt lymphoma, both of which may follow a very aggressive course leading to life-threatening conditions.[6]

The head and neck manifestations of non-Hodgkin lymphoma can be either nodal or extranodal. Unlike Hodgkin lymphoma that affects predominantly the lymph nodes, NHL has extranodal manifestations in 30% of cases.[10] The extranodal sites affected most commonly are the Waldeyer ring, nasopharynx, oral cavity, salivary glands, thyroid, and paranasal sinuses.[11,12] In a study of 156 cases of NHL of the head and neck, the tonsils and

179

nasopharynx were affected in 18% and 16% of the cases, respectively. Other affected organs were the salivary glands and paranasal sinuses in 13% of the cases.[13] In another investigation on the clinical presentations of 53 patients with NHL of the sinonasal tract, Hatta et al reported involvement of the nasal cavity in 67.8% of the cases, followed by the maxillary sinus in 20.8% of the cases.[14] All patients had a diffuse growth pattern, and 41.5% had symptoms of weight loss, fever, and night sweats. Usually, more than one site is affected, and patients have worse 5-year survival in comparison to other sites of primary NHL lymphomas.[12] Yoon et al reported a case of DLBCL that involved both the ethmoid sinus and epiglottis, and alluded to the need for a thorough examination of the head and neck in patients with lymphomas.[15] Other rare extranodal sites of NHL include the periorbital and temporal bones. Elisei et al described a 51-year-old patient with diffuse, well-differentiated lymphocytic lymphoma who presented with proptosis and submandibular swelling, in addition to other systemic complaints.[16] Similarly, Ogasawara et al described 3 cases of diffuse B-cell lymphomas, 2 of whom had involvement of the temporal fossa.[17] Radiologic evaluation is commonly requested in the workup of affected patients. Magnetic resonance imaging (MRI) is needed for assessment of fascial planes and intracranial extension, whereas computed tomography (CT) is recommended for the evaluation of bone destruction.[18] The diagnosis of NHL is usually made by tissue examination and immunohistochemistry, and only 1 out of 4 has a favorable histology.[12]

In view of systemic manifestations of NHL, this chapter explores the impact of this disease on the phonatory apparatus. A thorough review of the most common laryngeal lymphomas is presented. Treatment-induced dysphonia is reviewed as well. This information is of paramount importance in the evaluation of patients with NHL complaining of dysphonia.

Disease-Induced Dysphonia in Patients With Non-Hodgkin Lymphoma

Primary Laryngeal Non-Hodgkin Lymphoma

The larynx is rarely the target of NHL.[19] Men are predominantly affected with a male-to-female (M:F) ratio reaching up to 3.4:1.[7,20] The mean age at diagnosis varies across different geographic areas. In the United States, it is reported as 64.2 years,[7] whereas in China it is reported as 46.10 years for men and 42.38 years for women.[20] The scarcity of laryngeal NHL is commensurate with the scarcity of hematopoietic laryngeal neoplasms, which account for less than 1% of laryngeal malignancies.[21] Laryngeal NHL often is masked by systemic diseases, most common of which are the autoimmune diseases. In a case report by Korst in 2007, primary B-cell lymphoma of the airway coexisted with Sjögren syndrome and led to severe circumferential subglottic stenosis.[22] In another report by Patiar et al in 2005, advanced rheumatoid arthritis was considered a risk factor for the development of non-Hodgkin laryngeal lymphoma (NHLL).[23] NHLL may occur in isolation or with involvement of other organs in the head and neck, most commonly the tonsils, thyroid, and salivary glands.[24,25]

The clinical presentation of laryngeal NHLL is nonspecific and lacks any differentiating criteria. Patients may complain of dysphonia, dysphagia, dyspnea, globus sensation, or simply feeling a neck mass.[26-28] In rare cases, patients may present with airway obstruction secondary to subglottic or tracheal involvement. Other rare clinical symptoms include cough and wheezing simulating asthma.[29,30] On laryngeal examination, the findings can be very misleading and ill defined. In a report by Word et al in 2006, the only laryngeal finding that led to the diagnosis of B-cell laryngeal lymphoma was asymmetry of the false vocal folds.[31] When a laryngeal lesion is present, it is usually submucosal and smooth. In rare cases it can be polypoid or ulcerative.[21] The left side of the larynx is affected more often than the right side with a predilection to the supraglottis and aryepiglottic folds. The diagnosis of laryngeal NHLL is frequently missed, which mandates a high level of suspicion. Diagnosis requires multiple deep biopsies because a substantial quantity of tissue is needed for staining.[19,31-33] The 5-year survival in affected patients varies with the type of lymphoma, the grade of the disease, and its systemic presentation. T-cell lymphoma has a worse prognosis than B-cell lymphoma, and patients with extranodal disease have lower 5-year survival compared to those with nodal disease only. Therapy usually consists of radiation in isolation or in conjunction with chemotherapy and/or immunotherapy.[34]

Several types of NHL can affect the larynx, the most common of which is DLBCL. Other rate entities include mucosa-associated lymphoid tissue (MALT) lymphoma, natural killer T-cell (NK/T) lymphoma, and T-cell lymphoma. In this section, the authors summarize cases of isolated and nonisolated laryngeal NHL with emphasis on the clinical presentation of these tumors and the importance of immunostaining for proper diagnosis.

Diffuse Large B-Cell Lymphoma of the Larynx

DLBCL has nodal and extranodal manifestations in the head and neck. Extranodal involvement is present in 1 out of 5 patients

with the sites most commonly affected being the Waldeyer ring, upper and lower jaw, and paranasal sinuses.[6] In rare cases, DLBCL may affect the larynx and usually arises from lymphoid tissues present in the supraglottic region. Similar to other types of laryngeal lymphoma, the diagnosis of laryngeal DLBCL requires immunostaining using specific monoclonal antibodies against B-cell surface antigens. The prognosis is usually favorable in comparison to other types of NHLL.[6] In a review of 110 patients with DLBCL, Lee et al reported longer survival in patients with extranodal involvement in the head and neck in comparison to those with only nodal involvement, more so in patients with negative staining for CD10, B16, and MUM1.[35] The improved prognosis was associated with tumor markers such as CD10 and Bc16. Laryngeal DLBCL is usually sensitive to radiation therapy. Patients are started on radiotherapy with or without chemotherapy depending on the stage of the disease and the extent of tumor dissemination.[36-38]

Laryngeal DLBCL has been thoroughly described in the literature. Since the early report by Mackenty and Faulkner in 1934[39] and that of Mills et al in 1947,[40] numerous cases have been published. In 1989, Morgan et al reported 4 cases of diffuse, high-grade B-cell laryngeal lymphoma. Different laryngeal sites were involved, including the true vocal fold, false vocal fold, epiglottis, and aryepiglottic fold. In all cases, the lesions were smooth, nonulcerative, and confined to the larynx.[41] In 1996, Kawaida et al reported an 86-year-old man who presented with dysphagia and foreign-body sensation. On laryngeal examination, he had a large supraglottic pedunculated mass arising from the aryepiglottic fold and obscuring the glottis. Histopathologic examination of the lesion was consistent with NHL, and immunostaining was positive for CD25 and negative for CD45R. The patient was diagnosed with laryngeal DLCBL and was treated with chemotherapy using the CHOP regimen (cyclophosphamide, doxorubicin, vincristine, and prednisone).[27] In 2001, Cavalot et al reported a 79-year-old man who presented with foreign-body sensation, dysphagia, and change in voice quality. Laryngeal endoscopy and imaging showed a lesion in the posterior commissure that extended to the right vocal fold and obliterated the perilaryngeal space. Histopathologic examination of the lesion was consistent with DLBCL. The patient was treated with 6 courses of chemotherapy that resulted in complete remission.[26] That same year, Ohta et al reported a 76-year-old man who presented with throat discomfort secondary to laryngeal DLBCL. The authors emphasized the added value of gene rearrangement in the diagnosis of these lesions.[42] In 2003, Nayak et al highlighted the use of a new diagnostic approach, namely, "chromosomal aberrations using banded karyotyping"[43(p1)] in differentiating DLBCL from MALT lymphoma. The authors reported a 64-year-old man who presented with dysphagia, dysphonia, and left referred otalgia. Laryngeal examination and CT of the larynx showed a 3 × 3 cm mass that involved the epiglottis and left aryepiglottic fold. The lesion was smooth, polypoid, and nonulcerative. Histologic evaluation of a biopsy taken showed dense lymphoid infiltrates, and immunohistochemical staining of neoplastic cells was positive for CD20 B-cell marker. Moreover, 40% of CD19+ cells co-expressed CD10 which is a marker of germinal center B cells.[43] In 2005, Agada et al described a 52-year-old man who presented with history of choking and globus sensation in the throat. On laryngeal examination, he had a large cystic mass originating from the posterior aspect of the supraglottis and extending to the right pyriform sinus. Biopsy from that mass revealed atypical lymphoid cell

infiltrates, which on immunohistochemistry staining were consistent with DLBCL. The patient was staged as 3a and was treated with the CHOP regimen.[44] In 2005, Roca et al described an 80-year-old woman with large B-cell non-Hodgkin lymphoma who presented with dysphagia and throat discomfort. The patient was treated successfully with radiotherapy with complete regression of the laryngeal tumor. The authors alluded to the "benign" behavior of large B-cell NHL of the larynx in comparison to other sites.[45] In 2012, Cui et al reported a rare case of a patient with primary composite laryngeal lymphoma who presented with dysphagia and subglottic tracheoesophageal fistula. On CT examination, the patient had soft tissue thickening in the vocal tract and esophagus, with signs of subglottic tracheal fistulae. Initial biopsies showed only signs of chronic inflammation; however, examination of the laryngeal specimen following a total laryngectomy revealed DLBCL and peripheral T-cell lymphoma.[46] In 2013, Revanappa et al reported a 73-year-old female who had laryngeal DLBCL lymphoma in addition to extranodal involvement of the salivary glands, buccal mucosa, and Waldeyer ring. The authors elaborated on the added value of imaging in diagnosing, staging, and treating affected patients.[47] In 2013, Yoon et al reported a case of large B-cell lymphoma that affected both the larynx and paranasal sinuses. The authors described a 26-year-old man who presented with visual disturbance and protrusion of the right eye. On examination, he had a polypoid, smooth epiglottic mass in addition to a right middle meatal lesion. Biopsies from both sites confirmed the diagnosis of DLBCL. The patient was staged as IIEA and was managed with 6 cycles of rituximab with CHOP (R-CHOP). The authors emphasized the rarity of multicentric lesions in patients with extranodal NHL and the need for diligent staging of the disease prior to treatment.[15] In 2014, Akhtar et al, in their review of the literature on polypoidal, pedunculated lymphomas of the upper aerodigestive tract, reported a 16-year-old female who presented with dysphonia, foreign-body sensation, and dyspnea. On laryngeal examination, she had a pedunculated mass arising from the left tonsillar fossa with isodense texture on CT. Immunohistologic staining of the biopsy tested positive for CD20, CD10, and MUM. The final diagnosis was DLBCL.[48] In 2017, Rahman et al described a patient with DLCBL who presented with wheezing and upper airway obstruction. The symptoms were attributed to primary laryngeal lymphoma. The patient was treated with chemoradiation in addition to immunotherapy.[30] In 2018, Sharma et al reported a 43-year-old patient who presented with a neck mass in addition to change in voice quality. Laryngeal examination revealed a submucosal mass arising from the aryepiglottic fold and pyriform sinus with an immobile left vocal fold. Biopsy of the lesion was consistent with DLBCL, and the patient was treated with chemotherapy.[49]

In summary, patients with laryngeal DLBCL can present with dysphonia, dysphagia, and airway obstructive symptoms. Any site of the larynx may be affected, and the lesion is usually submucosal. Diagnosis is confirmed by biopsy and tissue staining for specific B-cell markers. Laryngeal DLBCL should be considered as an extranodal site of involvement when suspected.

Mucosa-Associated Lymphoid Tissue Laryngeal Lymphoma

MALT lymphoma is a rare subtype of NHL of B-cell lineage. It is characterized histopathologically by the presence of centrocyte-like cells with infiltration of reactive lymphoid follicles.[50] The immunophenotype is positive for CD19, CD20, CD22, sIgM+ and immunoglobulin D.[50,51] MALT lymphoma most commonly affects the gastrointestinal system, with the first case being described by Isaacson et al in 1983.[52] Other organs affected include the lungs and urinary tract. In the head and neck, the thyroid, salivary glands, and orbit are often the target.[53] The larynx is affected rarely, and composite lymphoma may be present.[54] MALT laryngeal lymphoma can be triggered by a chronic inflammatory process. Based on a review by Kania et al, chronic laryngitis secondary to gastroesophageal reflux disease or other stimuli can prompt the formation of submucosal laryngeal lymphoid tissue.[32] Wotherspoon et al reported the strong association between *Helicobacter pylori* gastritis and gastric MALT lymphoma, and highlighted the importance of treating or curing the underlying inflammatory disorder before the formation of MALT lymphoma.[55] Early diagnosis is very important given the high success rate of radiotherapy in the early stages of the disease.[56]

Many reports of MALT laryngeal lymphoma have appeared in the literature. In 1990, Diebold et al reported a 46-year-old man who presented with hoarseness of 1-year duration. On laryngeal examination, he had a submucosal, left, paralaryngeal mass that extended to the glottis and supraglottis. The mass was removed through a left pharyngolaryngectomy approach, and histologic examination of that mass revealed a low-grade centrocytic and lymphoplasmacytic MALT-type lymphoma.[57] In 1992, Kobayashi et al reported a 44-year-old woman who presented with dysphonia and shortness of breath that necessitated a tracheotomy. Tracheo-laryngo-fiberoscopy revealed the presence of submucosal polypoid lesions abutting the right vocal fold. Pathologic examination of the lesion showed centrocyte-like cells similar to those observed in malignant lymphoma of MALT.[58] In 1994, Hisashi et al reported a 66-year-old man who presented with history of dysphonia of 4 weeks' duration that was attributed to papillary lesions of the vocal folds and ventricles. CT examination showed involvement of the thyroid cartilage with extralaryngeal spread. The patient was diagnosed with MALT-type lymphoma and was treated with radiation therapy. Following partial response to treatment, the patient developed another left vocal fold tumor that extended to the left false vocal fold. Biopsy of the tumor revealed squamous cell carcinoma. The patient received chemotherapy to no avail and subsequently underwent total laryngectomy.[59] In 1996, Horny et al described the histologic features of low-grade MALT lymphoma and the similarities of the features with those seen in marginal zone B cells, also called pseudolymphoma. The authors emphasized the need to consider the intersection in the cytologic characteristics of these lesions in the description of lymphomas of the upper aerodigestive system.[50] In 1997, Kato et al described 3 cases of NHL of the larynx, 2 of whom had low-grade B-cell-lymphoma of the small cell type. The first case was 54-year-old woman who presented with a 1-year history of dysphonia in the absence of systemic symptoms. On examination, she had a supraglottic polypoid mass arising from the epiglottis. Immunohistologic examination of that mass confirmed the diagnosis of non-Hodgkin lymphoma with B-cell–associated antigens. The patient was treated with 2 courses of chemotherapy (CHOP) followed by radiotherapy, which led to complete regression of the tumor. The second case was a 77-year-old woman who presented with dysphonia that was attributed to vocal fold submucosal swelling. Initial biopsies failed to demonstrate the presence of neoplasia. However, following her

diagnosis with ovarian cystadenocarcinoma, repeated laryngeal biopsy showed non-Hodgkin lymphoma, small lymphocytic with plasmacytoid differentiation, that is considered as a low-grade B-cell lymphoma of the small cell type.[60] In 1998, de Bree et al reported a 36-year-old woman with a history of hoarseness secondary to right ventricular fold submucosal swelling. Biopsy of the lesion revealed low-grade, B-cell non-Hodgkin lymphoma of MALT. The patient was treated successfully by local radiation to the larynx.[61] In 1999, Cheng et al described a 58-year-old woman with history of globus and dysphonia of 2 months' duration. On laryngeal examination, she had a 1.5 cm right aryepiglottic fold mass. Biopsy and immunohistochemistry of that mass showed malignant lymphoma, B-cell lineage, arising from the MALT. The patient received radiotherapy of 3000 cGy and had complete regression of the tumor.[33] In the same year, Zinzani et al reviewed 75 cases of nongastrointestinal MALT lymphoma, among which a case of laryngeal lymphoma. All patients were treated with radiation and local interferon-α and/or chemotherapy and had partial or complete regression of the tumor. The authors highlighted the good prognosis of this type of lymphoma and the positive response to the conventionally used therapies.[53] In 2000, Usui et al described a 25-year-old female who presented with hoarseness and cervical pain of 1-year duration. On laryngeal examination, she had a left false vocal fold mass, the histologic examination of which confirmed the diagnosis of MALT-type lymphoma. The tumor cells were CD5[-], CD20[+], and CD79a[+].[62] In 2002, Fung et al described a 78-year-old man who presented with a history of dysphonia, dysphagia, and intermittent dyspnea. On examination, he had a supraglottic mass that was causing a "Ball-valve" effect. Histologic examination showed marginal zone B-cell lymphoma of MALT with Hodgkin-like transformation.[54] Another case of subglottic MALT-type lymphoma in a 79-year-old woman was reported by Puig Garces et al. The authors concurred with the rare laryngeal manifestations of hematopoietic neoplasms and the need to incorporate lymphomas in the differential diagnosis of subglottic tumors.[63] In 2003, Caletti et al reported a patient with gastric and laryngeal MALT lymphoma who responded to *H pylori* treatment with regression of the lesion and no recurrence on follow-up. The authors recommended routine gastroscopy in patients presenting with extragastric MALT and the need to initiate early treatment of the precursor *H pylori*.[64] In 2003, Kuhnt et al reported a 56-year-old woman who presented with laryngeal MALT lymphoma many years after being diagnosed with and treated for low-grade B-cell lymphoma of the eyelid. The patient was staged as IE A and managed with locoregional radiation following laser resection.[65] In 2003, Dabaja et al, in their review on the role and diagnostic yield of esophagogastroduodenoscopy in patients with nongastric MALT lymphoma, described 1 case of laryngeal lymphoma out of 36 cases. Although 12 of the 36 cases had gastric involvement, the patient with laryngeal lymphoma had normal esophagogastroduodenoscopy.[66] In 2004, Aiyer et al reported a 70-year-old woman who presented with dysphagia, dysphonia, and dyspnea. On laryngeal examination, she had a polypoid mass arising from the epiglottis and aryepiglottic fold. The mass was excised, and histochemical examination confirmed the diagnosis of marginal B-cell lymphoma of the MALT type.[67] In 2005, Andratschke et al reported a 58-year-old man who developed dyspnea secondary to subglottic stenosis. A biopsy taken from the stenotic area showed signs of MALT-type lymphoma. The patient was treated with

radiation after his airway was secured.[68] In 2005, Kania et al reported a 46-year-old man with a history of dysphonia of a few months' duration. On laryngeal examination, he had a left false vocal fold submucosal mass with normal mobility of the vocal folds. CT of the neck showed a 10×15 mm mass filling the left paraglottic space. The patient underwent suspension microlaryngoscopy and excision of the mass using the CO_2 laser. Histopathologic examination revealed centrocyte-like lymphocytes with a mixture of monocytoid B cells, and lymphoplasmacytoid cells. Immunohistochemical staining proved that the centrocytes-like lymphocytes were B cells; hence, the diagnosis of MALT-type lymphoma was confirmed.[32] In 2007, Steffen et al reported a 62-year-old man who presented with dyspnea, cough, and stridor. On bronchoscopy, he had evidence of a subglottic lesion, the biopsy of which revealed lymphoid cells consistent with extranodal, marginal zone B-cell lymphoma. The patient was treated successfully with several courses of R-CHOP chemotherapy.[69] In 2007, Arndt et al described a case of laryngeal MALT lymphoma with gastric involvement and *H pylori* infection. The patient had only subjective improvement on conservative management. The authors emphasized the need for a comprehensive evaluation for possible laryngeal MALT lymphoma in the search for multifocal extranodal involvement.[70] In 2009, Markou et al reported a 76-year-old man who presented with stridor and dysphonia. On laryngeal examination, he had a supraglottic lesion that involved both vocal folds. Immunohistochemical staining of the biopsy specimen confirmed the diagnosis of marginal zone lymphoma of MALT type. The patient received 6 courses of chemotherapy with improvement in symptoms and complete regression of the lesion.[21] In 2011, Kuo et al reported a

50-year-old woman who presented with hoarseness and difficulty in breathing secondary to multiple subglottic nodular lesions. Examination of the biopsy specimen taken from the subglottic region demonstrated MALT lymphoma. The authors highlighted the need to include laryngeal lymphoma in the diagnostic workup of patients presenting with subglottic stenosis.[71] In 2012, Zhao et al reported a 35-year-old woman who presented with a history of progressive dysphonia. The patient was diagnosed with MALT lymphoma and was treated with CHOP therapy and radiation. The authors emphasized the usefulness of positron emission tomography (PET)/CT in the diagnosis and follow-up of affected patients.[72] In 2012, Yilmaz et al reported a 41-year-old woman who presented with dysphonia and dysphagia in the absence of systemic complaints. On examination, she had a submucosal left aryepiglottic mass that extended to the pyriform sinus. Biopsy and immunohistochemical examination of that mass confirmed the diagnosis of marginal zone lymphoma of MALT type. The patient was treated successfully with chemotherapy.[73] In 2014, Bielinski et al reported an 88-year-old woman who presented with stridor attributed to subglottic narrowing. Direct laryngoscopy showed spongy submucosal thickening. A biopsy taken was positive for CD20 and for monoclonal B-cell population, all indicative of marginal zone lymphoma of MALT type. The patient was treated with Rituxan, which led to widening of the subglottic stenosis and improvement in breathing.[74] In 2014, Gonzalez-Murillo et al reported a 41-year-old woman who presented with dyspnea and dysphonia of 1-year duration. On laryngeal examination, she had a subglottic mass 2.5 × 1.5 cm occluding 70% of the airway with signs of supraglottic mucosal inflammation. Biopsy of the lesion was consistent with MALT lymphoma. The patient was treated with 6 cycles of R-CHOP followed by local radiation and surgical resection.[75] In 2014, Hua et al described a 63-year-old woman with dysphonia secondary to a supraglottic mass that involved the left false vocal fold. Biopsy and histochemical examination of the mass confirmed the diagnosis of MALT lymphoma. Afterward the patient developed cutaneous lesions that necessitated 6 courses of chemotherapy.[76] In 2014, Zapparoli et al reported a 73-year-old woman who presented with chronic cough, dysphonia, and nocturnal dyspnea, which were treated with systemic steroids to no avail. Bronchoscopy was performed and showed a subglottic concentric submucosal mass. Biopsy of the lesion revealed small B-cell lymphocytic infiltration with positive staining for CD20, BCL-2, and IgD. The diagnosis of MALT lymphoma was confirmed, and the patient was started on radiotherapy that resulted in marked regression of the disease.[29] In 2015, Liu et al reported a 58-year-old woman who had persistent hoarseness of a few months' duration. On laryngeal examination, she had enlargement of the left false vocal fold, the histologic examination of which following laser resection was consistent with MALT lymphoma. The authors advocated radiotherapy as the first line of treatment for early stage laryngeal MALT lymphoma.[77]

In summary, MALT laryngeal lymphoma has histologic features often misdiagnosed as low-grade malignant lymphoma. They originate from the lymphoid tissue of the vocal fold edge and are confined usually to the site of origin. The presenting symptoms can be either phonatory or airway related. In cases of obstructive symptoms, subglottic involvement should be ruled out. These tumors are radiosensitive and carry a better prognosis than other types of laryngeal lymphoma.

Laryngeal NK/T-Cell Lymphoma

NK/T-cell lymphoma is a separate clinical-pathologic entity characterized by a broad morphological spectrum with predominant histochemical markers, namely, CD2 and CD56. It is associated with Epstein-Barr viral infection.[78,79] In a review of the clinical and pathologic features of 32 cases of NK-cell phenotype, Nakamura et al reported Epstein-Barr virus (EBV)–encoded RNA in 27 out of the 32 cases.[80] In the head and neck, many sites may be affected. Based on a review of 49 cases of nonnasal NK/T-cell lymphomas by Chan et al, the skin, the palate, nasopharynx, salivary glands, and tonsils were the sites most commonly affected in the head and neck. There was only one patient with laryngeal involvement that recurred in the terminal ilium, and one patient with skin tumor, misdiagnosed as vasculitis, who later developed laryngeal disease.[78] In 2001, Moke et al reported 2 cases of laryngeal NK/T-cell lymphoma. The first patient was a 35-year-old woman who presented with dysphonia and dysphagia in addition to generalized symptoms of weight loss and fever. On laryngeal examination, she had supraglottic necrotic tissues. The biopsies taken from these tissues were positive for NK/T-cell markers, including CD2, CD3, CD45RO, and CD56. The second patient was a 44-year-old woman who presented with dysphonia and sore throat secondary to swelling of the supraglottic region. Biopsy confirmed the diagnosis of NK/T-cell lymphoma, and the patient was referred for chemotherapy.[81] In 2008, Tardio et al described a rare case of laryngeal NK/T-cell lymphoma, nasal type, who presented with sore throat and globus sensation. On laryngeal examination, he had ulceration of the epiglottis and aryepiglottic fold. Initial biopsies taken in the office under local anesthesia showed only inflammatory debris. Later, the patient

developed multiple cervical lymphadenopathies that necessitated limited excision. Repeated biopsy of the laryngeal lesion and immunohistochemical staining confirmed the diagnosis of NK/T-cell lymphoma, nasal type. The lesion progressed aggressively despite the administration of polychemotherapy.[82] In 2008, Monobe et al reported a 73-year-old man with a history of dysphonia that was attributed to granulomatous lesions of the false vocal folds. The initial biopsies taken from these lesions were nonrevealing. One year after his initial presentation, the patient developed progression of the lesion together with fever. A repeat biopsy under general anesthesia revealed atypical cells that stained positive for CD56 and CD3, granzyme B. The patient was diagnosed with extranodal NK/T-cell lymphoma, nasal type. Treatment with chemotherapy resulted in partial regression of the laryngeal lesion, but the patient died of his systemic disease.[83] In 2011, Friedmann et al reported a 22-year-old man who presented with dysphonia, odynophagia, night sweats, fever, and weight loss. On laryngeal examination, he had thickened and polypoid supraglottic mucosa, biopsy of which showed NK/T-cell lymphoma, nasal type.[84] In 2011, de la Rosa Astacio et al described a 22-year-old woman who presented with dysphonia and hemoptysis secondary to erosion of the laryngotracheal complex as shown on CT evaluation. Biopsy of the lesion and immunohistochemical staining revealed NK/T-cell lymphoma with positive staining for CD2, CD56, and cytoplasmic CD3. The patient died prior to initiation of therapy.[85] In 2011, Hirai et al described a 33-year-old man who complained of sore throat of 1 month's duration that was attributed to epiglottic swelling and plaque formation. Repeated laryngeal biopsies confirmed the diagnosis of malignant epiglottic NK/T-cell lymphoma.[86] In 2012, Cikojevic et al reported a 77-year-old man with a history of dysphagia, foreign-body sensation, and cough. On examination, he had a mass over the left aryepiglottic fold, biopsy of which showed lymphatic cells of various sizes that stained positive for CD3, CD2, and CD56. The patient was diagnosed with NK/T-cell lymphoma and was started on chemotherapy followed by radiation therapy. The patient improved markedly on treatment with complete regression of the laryngeal pathology.[87] In 2012, Uri et al described a 45-year-old man with a history of dysphonia, sore throat, otalgia, and intermittent shortness of breath. Flexible nasolaryngoscopy showed a lesion on the right true vocal fold with involvement of the arytenoid. Biopsy of that lesion stained positive for CD3, CD56, CD43, CD30, and granzyme B. The patient was diagnosed with NK/T-cell lymphoma and was treated with 2 courses of chemotherapy (CHOP).[88] In 2014, Zhou et al reported a 59-year-old man who presented initially with a nasal mass resulting in obstruction and bleeding. Biopsy of the mass revealed extranodal NK/T-cell lymphoma for which he received radiotherapy. On follow-up, the patient developed hoarseness and sore throat in addition to his nasal obstruction. Laryngeal examination showed an anterior subglottic lesion with high uptake on PET/CT. Immunohistochemical staining of a biopsy taken in the operating room confirmed the diagnosis of laryngeal NK/T-cell lymphoma. The authors highlighted the superior role of PET/CT in the evaluation of laryngeal involvement and in staging these tumors.[89] In that same year, Koybasi et al reported a 45-year-old woman who presented with hoarseness and dysphagia. The patient was found to have hypertrophy of the lymphoid tissues in the nasopharynx and hypopharynx together with a supraglottic lesion that extended from the epiglottis to the ventricular folds. The lesion appeared granulomatous and eroded the mucosal lin-

ing. Histologic and immunohistochemical staining of a punch biopsy confirmed the diagnosis of extranodal NK/T-cell lymphoma.[90] In 2016, Zhu et al reported 2 cases of NK/T-cell lymphoma of the larynx and highlighted the difficulty in differentiating the symptoms of laryngeal involvement. Moreover, the authors alluded to the added value of combined chemoradiation to chemotherapy alone in the treatment of these tumors.[91] In 2016, Gungor et al reported a 14-year-old male diagnosed with extranodal NK/T-cell lymphoma (nasal) who, despite the improvement in nasal symptoms following treatment with chemoradiation, presented with dysphonia, difficulty in swallowing, and stridor. The upper aerodigestive symptoms were secondary to a subglottic and postcricoid exophytic lesion, the biopsy of which confirmed recurrence in the larynx.[92] In 2018, Meleca et al described a 27-year-old female who developed a supraglottic exophytic lesion that resulted in marked narrowing of the airway. Pathologic examination of that lesion confirmed NK/T-cell lymphoma. The patient received several courses of chemotherapy followed by radiation therapy and serial tracheal dilatation in order to secure the airway.[93] In 2019, Xiang et al reviewed their clinical experience with 31 cases of laryngeal extranodal NK/T-cell lymphoma over the course of 9 years. The authors reported hoarseness in 16 of 31 cases, laryngalgia in 10 of 31 cases, dyspnea in 5 of 31 cases, and dysphagia in 2 of 31 cases. Only one-third had B symptoms, namely, fever, weight loss, and night sweats. The laryngeal site most commonly affected was the supraglottis in 58.1%, and pseudoepitheliomatosis was found in 30.8% of the cases. The overall 5-year survival rate in this study group was 29.6%.[94]

In summary, NK/T-cell laryngeal lymphomas are aggressive tumors. The symptoms can be very subtle, ill defined, and of long duration before the patient seeks medical attention. The diagnosis is challenging because of the angio-destructive nature of these lesions that often leads to coagulative necrosis. Another challenge is the large spectrum of cell size which makes it hard to differentiate reactive inflammatory cells from neoplastic ones.[81] The disease is very aggressive, and conventional treatment consists of chemoradiation.

T-cell Laryngeal Lymphoma

T-cell lymphoma is an aggressive subtype of NHL characterized by malignant proliferation of T cells. It affects mainly the gastrointestinal system, lungs, and central nervous system.[95] Patients usually present with systemic complaints such as fever, weight loss, and night sweats. T-cell lymphoma in the head and neck region is rare and varies in incidence between 1% and 17% based on different geographic areas.[96–98] In a review of 62 patients with non-Hodgkin lymphoma of the head and neck, only 7 were diagnosed with T-cell lymphoma in comparison to 52 with B-cell lymphoma.[98] Extranodal T-cell lymphoma presenting in the head and neck is even rarer and carries no differentiating clinical signs. In a review of 11 cases by Broadwater et al, the sites most commonly affected were the sinonasal area in 45% of the cases, followed by the tonsils and tongue in 27% and 18% of the cases, respectively. Patients usually present with a mass at the site of involvement, and only a few complain of B symptoms. The disease has an aggressive course with a 3-year median overall survival. Following a thorough immune-phenotype evaluation for proper diagnosis, patients are started often on chemotherapy with or without adjuvant radiation.[99]

Laryngeal T-cell lymphoma has scarcely been described in the literature. In 1996,

Smith et al reported a 36-year-old man who presented with dysphonia of 4 weeks' duration that was attributed initially to fungal laryngitis. Despite antifungal treatment, the dysphonia persisted, and the patient developed an ulcerative lesion on the right aryepiglottic fold that prolapsed into the airway and led to right vocal fold paralysis. Histopathologic examination of that mass following excision confirmed the diagnosis of T-cell NHL. The patient was treated by irradiation that resulted in disease regression but persistence of the vocal fold paralysis.[100] In 1997, Kato et al reported a 36-year-old man who presented with sore throat secondary to an epiglottic mass noted on direct laryngoscopy. Biopsy and immunohistologic examination of that mass revealed atypical lymphocytes that expressed T-cell antigens. The patient was treated with radiotherapy that resulted in marked regression of the laryngeal tumor.[60] In 1998, Marianowski et al reported an 88-year-old man who presented with cough and change in voice quality secondary to a left aryepiglottic fold thickening. The biopsy taken from the suspected site was consistent with primary laryngeal γδ T-cell lymphoma. The patient was treated with chemoradiation following a course of steroids and antibiotics. The authors highlighted the strong association between laryngeal T-cell lymphoma and EBV.[101] In 2001, Mok et al reported a 54-year-old man who presented with an enlarged cervical mass and history of sore throat. On laryngeal examination, he had swelling of the supraglottic soft tissues. Following multiple biopsies taken from the suspected site, the lesion was diagnosed as peripheral T-cell lymphoma, Lennert lymphoma subtype. The patient was treated with chemotherapy followed by radiation therapy.[81] In 2010, Markou et al reported a 53-year-old man who presented with hoarseness secondary to right vocal fold nodular lesions.

Histopathologic and immunohistochemical examination of the biopsy specimen confirmed the coexistence of squamous cell carcinoma and T-cell lymphoma. The patient was treated with 6 sessions of CHOP chemotherapy followed by irradiation.[21] In 2012, Cui et al described a 43-year-old man who presented with dysphagia and cervical swelling of 3 months' duration. Radiologic evaluation using CT showed supraglottic and glottic mucosal swelling in addition to a subglottic tracheal fistula that led to the formation of a cervical abscess. The patient also had an esophageal diverticulum. The initial soft tissue biopsies of the neck revealed only inflammatory reactions, whereas examination of the laryngectomy specimen showed a composite lymphoma with both diffuse large B-cell lymphoma and peripheral T-cell lymphoma.[46] In 2015, Uthamalingam et al reported a 58-year-old man who presented with dysphagia and a large cervical mass that filled the left side of the neck down to the thoracic inlet. Biopsy of that mass showed atypical lymphoid cells that stained positive for CD3 and negative for CD20, CD10, CD15, CD30, and CD56, thus confirming the diagnosis of peripheral T-cell lymphoma. Following a 2-month treatment with chemotherapy, the patient developed airway obstructive symptoms that led to his death. On autopsy, the patient had a large supraglottic mass that occluded the airway and extended beyond the laryngeal compartment.[102] In the review by Broadwater et al in 2018, laryngeal T-cell lymphoma accounted for only 10% of the cases. The pathology stained positive for CD2 and CD3 and negative for CD45, CD4, CD5, CD7, CD8, and CD30, and the disease was staged as IIE.[99]

In summary, laryngeal NHL lymphomas are hard to diagnose. The clinical presentation can be misleading, as the patient often reports nonspecific symptoms of sore throat or globus sensation. Similarly, the laryngeal exam lacks any differentiating criteria. The lesion is usually submucosal but may also be polypoid or ulcerative. The supraglottis is the site affected most commonly with frequent involvement of the epiglottis and aryepiglottic folds. Subglottic lesions can occur and may cause obstructive airway symptoms. Repeated biopsies are needed often, and immunohistochemical studies are indispensable for proper diagnosis. Although the clinical presentation is confined to the site of involvement, other extranodal sites may be affected. Depending on the type of laryngeal lymphoma, the prognosis may be either good with favorable response to chemotherapy, or poor with little response to treatment.

Vocal Fold Paralysis in Patients With Non-Hodgkin Lymphoma

Vocal fold paralysis in patients with non-Hodgkin lymphoma is not uncommon. The paralysis can be secondary to compression of the recurrent laryngeal nerve along its course in the neck and chest, to lymphocytic infiltration of the vagus and/or recurrent laryngeal nerve, or to involvement of the central nervous system.

Compression of the recurrent laryngeal nerve in the neck is secondary to disease-induced enlargement of adjacent structures, such as the thyroid, esophagus or cervical lymph nodes. Malignant lymphoma of the thyroid gland represents less than 12% of thyroid malignancies,[103] with a male-to-female ratio of 1:4.[104] Elderly women are mostly affected at a mean age of 72.8 years.[104] Based on a review by Pederson et al, which included 50 cases of primary NHL of the thyroid gland, 98% of affected patients had B-phenotype, and two-thirds had history of Hashimoto disease.[104] This concurs a previous report by Heimann that alluded to the role of Hashimoto disease as a prelymphomatous condition in patients with thyroid lymphoma.[105] Affected patients usually present with compressive symptoms of the upper aerodigestive tract secondary to the rapid growth of the tumor. Luo et al reported a 68-year-old man who presented with dyspnea due to an enlarged thyroid lymphoma that coexisted with nodular goiter.[106] The most commonly reported symptoms in addition to dyspnea and stridor are dysphagia and dysphonia. Hoarseness may occur in 13% to 65% of cases, and vocal fold paralysis may be present in up to 29% of cases.[107] In a review by Klyachkin et al of 7 cases with stage I and II non-Hodgkin thyroid lymphoma, 71% had history of hoarseness and dyspnea.[108] In an investigation on the extralaryngeal causes of vocal fold paralysis using CT, Glazer et al reported thyroid lymphoma in almost 6% of patients with upper mediastinal or cervical neoplasms.[109] The suggested pathophysiology is mass compression and/or extracapsular spread with neural invasion. It is noteworthy that vocal fold paralysis in affected patients is not always secondary to tumor-induced neurolysis. In 1985, Jiu et al reported a 69-year-old woman who presented with an enlarging neck mass associated with dysphagia, dysphonia, and right vocal fold paralysis. A biopsy of the neck mass showed diffuse histiocytic lymphoma with signs of perineural lymphatic invasion. The patient was treated with external beam irradiation that led to recovery of the vocal fold paralysis. The authors alluded to the reversibility of the neural damage in cases of neural compression.[107] It is also important to note that dysphonia in patients with thyroid lymphoma is not always secondary to vocal fold paralysis. Graham reported 2 patients with thyroid lymphoma who developed hoarseness secondary to subglottic

lesions with no evidence of vocal fold paralysis.[110] Hence, the diagnosis of thyroid lymphoma requires a thorough laryngeal examination, in addition to an adequate tissue sampling and histopathologic examination. The 2 main pillars of treatment are chemotherapy and irradiation. In cases of well-localized tumors, resection of the thyroid gland is recommended.[111]

The esophagus is another extranodal structure that may be targeted in patients with NHL and may lead to vocal fold paralysis. Esophageal lymphoma is extremely rare, occurring in less than 1% of all patients with lymphoma.[112] Common risk factors include *H pylori* infection, autoimmune diseases, and viral infections.[113] There are many histologic subtypes, the most common of which are MALT lymphoma and DLBCL. Diagnostic criteria of primary esophageal lymphoma include the presence of an esophageal lesion in the absence of palpable lymph nodes or mediastinal lymphadenopathy.[114] The lesion on endoscopy is described as polypoid or nodular with ulceration and stenosis. Although the most commonly reported symptoms are dysphagia, foreign-body sensation, abdominal distension, and epigastric pain, dysphonia has also been reported.[115] In a review by Orvidas et al that included 27 patients with biopsy-proven esophageal lymphoma, 89% of whom had NHL, 22% had vocal fold paralysis, and 9 had hoarseness. Patients with proximal esophageal lesions were more likely to develop vocal symptoms in addition to dysphagia.[116] Histopathologic examination is key for diagnosis, and surgical excision is the mainstay treatment.[117] The tracheobronchial tree is an equally rare site for NHL, the involvement of which can lead to hoarseness. NHL of the tracheobronchial tree is very uncommon. In a review of 8 patients by Solomonov et al, hoarseness, cough, and dyspnea were the main symptoms. Most of the patients had aggressive lymphoma and responded well to therapy.[118]

Vocal fold paralysis also may be secondary to compression of the recurrent laryngeal nerve along its course in the chest by mediastinal and or lung masses. Mediastinal lymphadenopathy and pulmonary lesions with or without pleural effusion are common manifestations of intrathoracic NHL[119] (Figure 9–1). In a review of the radiologic findings of 61 patients with Hodgkin and non-Hodgkin lymphoma, Aquino et al reported mediastinal lymphadenopathy in 70% of the cases, with evidence of lymph node enlargement in the extrapleural space.[120] In another review of primary mediastinal tumors by Strollo et al, lymphoma and neurogenic neoplasms were described among the most common primary mediastinal tumors.[121] In a study on the usefulness of endobronchial ultrasound-guided transbronchial needle aspiration, Ko et al reported NHL in 7 out of 38 patients with mediastinal lymphadenopathy.[122] Mediastinal lymphadenopathy also may be the only sign of recurrence in patients with NHL. Rhee et al reported a 40-year-old man with nasal NK/T-cell lymphoma who developed a single mediastinal mass following full treatment with chemoradiation. The mediastinal mass was the only sign of recurrence as shown on histopathologic examination using video-assisted thoracoscopy.[123] In another study on the radiologic characteristic features of various subtypes of primary mediastinal lymphoma, Tateishi et al reported an association between vascular involvement and mediastinal DLBCL.[124] Mediastinal involvement in patients with NHL may predispose to compression of the recurrent laryngeal nerve in isolation or as part of a syndrome, such as superior vena cava syndrome (SVCS). This syndrome is caused by external compression of the su-

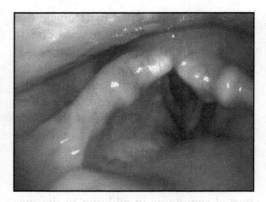

Figure 9–1. A 43-year-old male, case of non-Hodgkin lymphoma, presented to voice clinic on May 2019 with history of dysphonia and aspiration. Laryngeal endoscopy revealed left vocal fold paralysis. Further evaluation using computed tomography of the chest showed a mediastinal mass.

perior vena cava leading to a constellation of symptoms among which is hoarseness.[125] In a review on the etiology of SVCS, Cheng reported mediastinal tumors, which included lymphoma, among the most common causes aside from intravascular devices.[125] In another review on SVCS, Zimmerman et al reported NHL as the etiology in 15% of cases. Other causes included lung cancer and mediastinal infectious diseases.[126] Hoarseness in patients with SVCS often is attributed to edematous changes in the upper aerodigestive tract. Other commonly reported symptoms include dysphagia, dyspnea, and cough.[125-130] The presence of these symptoms may carry adverse effects on recurrence-free survival.[129]

Lung parenchyma is also a disease target in patients with NHL. It may or may not lead to hoarseness and/or vocal fold paralysis. Based on a large review on the clinical aspects of lung cancer, Grippi reported lymphoma in 2% to 8% of cases, with hoarseness as a manifestation of intrathoracic spread.[131] In a study by Knudsen et al on vocal fold paralysis in patients with malignancy, 1 out of 53 patients had lymphoma. The vocal fold paralysis in the patient with lymphoma was a secondary symptom and not a primary one.[132] In a review of 18 patients with primary pulmonary lymphoma by Graham et al, hoarseness was not among the main symptoms, which included cough, dyspnea, and chest pain in addition to wheezing and hemoptysis. Systemic symptoms included fatigue, weight loss, and back pain. Eleven patients out of the 18 had parenchymal tissue disease, and 7 had associated mediastinal lymphadenopathy.[133] In rare cases, NHL lymphoma may present as a chest wall mass. In 2006, Hsu et al reported 7 patients with NHL who had a chest wall mass. DLBCL was the diagnosis in 5 of the 7, and 4 patients had chest wall lymphoma as the only site of involvement.[134] These lesions are best assessed using MRI for the detection of both nodular and extranodular sites of involvement.[135] Other commonly used radiologic testing is CT. Mass-like consolidation or lobar consolidation is often described in affected patients.[136,137] It is worth noting that more than one site may be involved along the course of the recurrent laryngeal nerve.[138,139] Raufi et al reported a 49-year-old woman who presented with progressive dyspnea and cough. CT of the neck and chest revealed supraclavicular and mediastinal lymphadenopathy secondary to composite lymphoma with both T-cell and B-cell components.[139] Although the patient had no vocal fold paralysis, compression of the recurrent laryngeal nerves could have occurred.

Less common causes of vocal fold paralysis in patients with NHL are neurolymphomatosis and/or neoplastic meningitis. Neurolymphomatosis is a complication of hematologic malignancies characterized by infiltration of peripheral nerves by neurotropic lymphocytes leading to neurologic dysfunction. By definition, it is "nerve infiltration by neurotropic neoplastic cells in the setting of a known or unknown hematologic malignancy."[140] The neuropathy may manifest as paraesthesia, pain, or palsy, with pain being the most common presentation. Based on a review by Gan et al, the incidence of neurolymphomatosis in high-grade NHL can reach up to 3%.[141] Multiple cranial nerves may be affected with direct axonal destruction leading to symptoms such as decreased in hearing, vertigo, and dysphagia.[142,143] Several cases of neurolymphomatosis of the recurrent laryngeal and vagus nerves in patients with NHL have been reported in the literature. In 2012, Boasquevisque et al reported a 65-year-old man who presented with dysphonia and was found to have an increase in uptake of ^{18}F-fludeoxyglucose (F-FDG) with involvement of several peripheral nerves. The diagnosis of DLBCL and neurolymphomatosis was confirmed by biopsy and histologic examination of the right vagus nerve.[144] In 2012, Tsang et al described a 62-year-old woman diagnosed with stage IV DLBCL who presented with hoarseness and choking. Using F-FDG PET/CT, the patient was found to have neurolymphomatosis of the left vagus nerve.[145] In 2014, Yoshida et al reported a 62-year-old man who presented with change in voice quality and difficulty in swallowing. On examination, he had a deviated uvula and a decreased gag reflex. MRI showed swelling of the pineal body in addition to thickening of cranial nerves IX, X, and XI. Immunohistochemical staining of a neural biopsy confirmed the diagnosis of DLBCL. Despite the rarity of central nervous system (CNS) involvement in patients with NHL, cranial neuropathy may be a presenting sign even in the absence of headache, seizure, or gait disturbances.[146] Dixon et al reported neoplastic meningitis with involvement of multiple cranial nerves including the vagus nerve in a 74-year-old known case of DLBCL. Despite having received 6 cycles of chemotherapy, the patient developed stridor secondary to bilateral vocal fold paralysis. MRI confirmed the presence of leptomeningeal disease with enhancement of cranial nerve X, in addition to other cranial nerves.[147] Similarly, Cantalupo et al described a patient with high-grade peripheral B-cell lymphoma who presented with "Tapia syndrome," characterized by unilateral vocal fold paralysis and hypoglossal nerve injury secondary to peripheral nerve involvement by neoplastic disease.[148] In 2017, Ono et al reported 2 cases of neurolymphomatosis in patients with lymphoma. The first case was a 39-year-old patient with gastric lymphoma who presented with anorexia and abdominal pain, together with hypoesthesia of the abdominal right lower quadrant and back. The patient was staged as stage IV Burkitt lymphoma and was started on chemotherapy. Ten weeks after his presentation, he started complaining of hoarseness followed by blurring of vision of his left eye, and later dysphagia. On laryngeal examination, the patient had bilateral vocal fold paralysis. PET/CT scan revealed uptake in the left jugular vein, roots of nerves C4-C5, C5-C6, and the recurrent laryngeal nerve. On autopsy, there was marked neural invasion by lymphocytes. The second case was a 48-year-old woman diagnosed with acute-type ATL, who, following intensive chemotherapy, developed central nervous system involvement and later impaired mobility of both vocal folds that resulted in hoarseness and dyspnea. F-FDG PET showed uptake in the lower cervical plexus and recurrent laryngeal nerves, in addition to other nerves, skin, and mammary glands.[149] In 2015, Simmons et al reported a 61-year-old man who presented with dysphagia and dysphonia that was later complicated by facial weakness, decrease in hearing, and

vertiginous symptoms. On examination, he had paralysis of the right vocal fold, and repeated MRI showed a lesion in the left temporal lobe with edematous changes. Pathologic examination of that lesion revealed high-grade B-cell lymphoma, and the patient was diagnosed with primary neurolymphomatosis.[150]

In all of these reports, it is important to note that a high index of suspicion was needed to make the diagnosis of neurolymphomatosis in patients with NHL. The diagnosis is often missed because of the nonspecific clinical presentation and the difficulty of obtaining a tissue biopsy. With advances in technology, FDG-PET/CT has become a very useful diagnostic tool with a sensitivity close to 90%.[151]

Chemotherapy and Voice in Patients With Non-Hodgkin Lymphoma

Chemotherapy is the mainstay treatment for most patients with NHL. Depending on the stage of the disease and its subtype, it is often used in combination with other adjuvant therapies such as radiation or immunotherapy. Several drugs are used, the most common of which are alkylating agents, anthracyclines, and steroids. The regimen most frequently adopted is the CHOP regimen that consists of cyclophosphamide, doxorubicin, vincristine, and prednisone. Other commonly used regimens include R-CHOP where Rituximab is added, or CVP (cyclophosphamide, vincristine, and prednisone—CHOP excluding Adriamycin [doxorubicin]).[152] A review of the literature shows that the aforementioned chemotherapeutic agents may affect phonation, directly and indirectly. As a sequel to the associated systemic effects of these medications, patients with NHL undergoing chemotherapy are at risk of developing voice disorders. Among the most commonly reported side effects are nausea, vomiting, diarrhea, body fatigue, and generalized weakness. Given the importance of hydration and its strong impact on phonation, dehydration affects voice and can lead to phonatory disturbances. Similarly, the strong link of the phonatory system to general well-being explains why body fatigue and a decrease in musculoskeletal strength can affect voice negatively. A thorough discussion on the impact of chemotherapy and voice can be found in other literature, particularly in the chapter "Cancer chemotherapy: an overview and voice complications," by Mattioni et al.[153]

Chemotherapy also may have a direct affect on voice. There are a few reports in the literature on dysphonia as an adverse event related to vincristine during the course of treatment of patients with lymphoma. Vincristine is a vinca alkaloid agent frequently used in the treatment of hematologic malignancies. One of its most dire complications is neurotoxicity with axonal degeneration, leading to alteration in neural conduction.[154] Multiple cranial nerves may be affected including the vagus nerve.[155] In 1998, Burns et al described 2 cases of unilateral vocal fold palsy in patients with Hodgkin lymphoma who were on chemotherapy. One patient had full recovery following cessation of vincristine, whereas the second patient who was on vinblastine had persistent vocal fold palsy.[156] In 2007, Ahmad et al reported 3 patients with vincristine-induced bilateral vocal fold paralysis, 2 of whom had lymphoblastic leukemia, and 1 had a posterior fossa anaplastic ependymoma.[157] In 2009, Kuruvilla et al reported 4 cases of vincristine-induced recurrent left laryngeal nerve palsy. The main diagnosis was acute lymphoblastic leukemia in 2 cases, Ewing

sarcoma in 1, and rhabdo-myosarcoma of the testis in 1.[158] In 2012, Farruggia et al reported an 18-month-old diagnosed with acute lymphoblastic leukemia, who developed hoarseness and later stridor following chemotherapy with vincristine (VCR). The authors recommended reducing the dose of vincristine when resuming treatment in patients with vincristine-induced neuropathy.[159]

Vincristine-induced recurrent laryngeal nerve neurotoxicity has rarely been reported in patients with NHL. In 1999, Ryan et al described a 58-year-old woman, diagnosed with DLBCL stage IV, who developed bilateral vocal fold paralysis during her chemotherapy using CHOP regimen. The authors alluded to the need for early withdrawal of vincristine in suspected cases of drug-induced neuropathy,[160] although withdrawal of other drugs such as doxorubicin also should be considered. In 2013, Yalin et al reported a 70-year-old man diagnosed with mantle lymphoma who presented with dysphonia following the second cycle of chemotherapy (CHOP). The patient had no other symptoms, and CT of the neck and chest did not show any radiologic signs of mass or lymphadenopathy. On laryngeal examination, the patient had bilateral vocal fold paralysis. Given the known neurotoxicity of vincristine, this drug was discontinued. Four months later, the patient had full recovery from his bilateral vocal fold paralysis.[161] In 2014, Samoon et al described a 58-year-old man with DLBCL who, following 4 cycles of R-CHOP, developed hoarseness and shortness of breath. On laryngeal examination, he had bilateral vocal fold paralysis. The mobility of the vocal folds recovered, and the symptoms disappeared after cessation of chemotherapy.[162]

In summary, patients with NHL receiving vinca alkaloids should be observed for the possibility of vagus or recurrent laryngeal nerve palsy. Symptoms of hoarseness or dyspnea should prompt the physician to rule out unilateral or bilateral vocal fold paralysis. Early diagnosis of vincristine-induced or other chemotherapy-induced neuropathy and prompt cessation of therapy can lead to full recovery.

Radiotherapy in Non-Hodgkin Lymphoma and Voice

Radiotherapy is often used as a first line of therapy in patients with early stage NHL. In advanced cases, or in candidates for stem cell transplant, radiation may be used as an adjuvant to chemotherapy.[163] When external beam radiation targets the chest and neck, the mucosal lining of the upper aerodigestive tract can be affected. These adverse effects carry a substantial burden on phonation given the paramount role of the pharynx and larynx as resonators. Radiation-induced mucosal inflammation can lead to alteration in the acoustic characteristics and voice quality of affected patients.[164] Moreover, mucosal dryness subsequent to the decrease in glandular secretions can lead to abnormal laryngeal behavior with an increase in phonatory threshold pressure.[165]

Of paramount importance also is radiation-induced neurotoxicity. It is well known that chest irradiation can cause neural damage, particularly recurrent laryngeal palsy. In a review of patients who received irradiation to the neck, head, or mediastinum, Crawley and Sulica reported 10 cases of unilateral vocal fold paralysis, one of whom had T-cell lymphoma. The authors highlighted the delayed effect of irradiation and the vulnerability of the recurrent laryngeal nerve to injury despite its resilience in comparison to other motor nerves.[166] Chandran and Sataloff described a 45-year-old woman who developed hoarseness 30 years after having received chest irradiation for Hodgkin lymphoma. The patient was diagnosed with vocal fold paresis and paradoxical vocal fold movement. She was treated with thyroplasty which led to airway obstructive symptoms necessitating removal of the implant. The authors emphasized the need for judicious decisions in patients with compromised airway and the added value of laryngeal electromyography in the workup and management of these patients.[167]

References

1. National Cancer Institute. Cancer stat facts: Non-Hodgkin's lymphoma. Accessed September 26, 2019. https://seer.cancer.gov /statfacts/html/nhl.html
2. Zhang Y, Dai Y, Zheng T, Ma S. Risk factors of non-Hodgkin's lymphoma. *Expert Opin Med Diagn.* 2011;5(6):539–550.
3. Patel P, Hanson DL, Sullivan PS, et al. Incidence of types of cancer among HIV-infected persons compared with the general population in the United States, 1992–2003. *Ann Intern Med.* 2008;148(10):728–736.
4. Larsson SC, Wolk A. Body mass index and risk of non-Hodgkin's lymphoma: a meta-analysis of prospective studies. *Eur J Cancer.* 2011;47(16):2422–2430.
5. Shankland KR, Armitage JO, Hancock BW. Non-Hodgkin lymphoma. *Lancet.* 2012;380 (9844):848–857.
6. Wang TF, Bartlett NL. Lymphomas of the head and neck. In: Flint PW, Haughey BH, Lund VJ, et al, eds. *Cummings' Otolaryngology-Head and Neck Surgery.* 6th ed. Philadelphia, PA: Elsevier; 2015:1805–1815.
7. Hong SA, Tajudeen BA, Choi S, Husain IA. Epidemiology and prognostic indicators in laryngeal lymphoma: A population-based analysis. *Laryngoscope.* 2018;128(9): 2044–2049.

8. Kim KH, Kim RB, Woo SH. Individual participant data meta-analysis of primary laryngeal lymphoma: Focusing on the clinical characteristics and prognosis. *Laryngoscope*. 2015;125(12):2741–2748.

9. American Cancer Society. Cancer Statistics Center. Non-Hodgkin lymphoma. Accessed October 1, 2019. https://www.cancer.org /cancer/non-hodgkin-lymphoma/about /key-statistics.html

10. Arican A, Dincol D, Akbulut H, et al. Clinicopathologic features and prognostic factors of primary extranodal non-Hodgkin's lymphoma in Turkey. *Am J Clin Oncol*. 1999;22(6):587–592.

11. Hermans R, Horvath M, De Schrijver T, Lemahieu SF, Baert AL. Extranodal non-Hodgkin lymphoma of the head and neck. *J Belge Radiol*. 1994;77(2):72–77.

12. Urquhart A, Berg R. Hodgkin's and non-Hodgkin's lymphoma of the head and neck. *Laryngoscope*. 2001;111(9):1565–1569.

13. Jacobs C, Hoppe RT. Non-Hodgkin's lymphomas of head and neck extranodal sites. *Int J Radiat Oncol Biol Phys*. 1985;11(2): 357–364.

14. Hatta C, Ogasawara H, Okita J, Kubota A, Ishida M, Sakagami M. Non-Hodgkin's malignant lymphoma of the sinonasal tract—treatment outcome for 53 patients according to REAL classification. *Auris Nasus Larynx*. 2001;28(1):55–60.

15. Yoon YH, Park WY, Choi YJ, Cho KS. Synchronous, primary, diffuse, large B-cell lymphomas involving the ethmoid sinus and epiglottis: a rare clinical entity. *Laryngoscope*. 2013;123(3):702–704.

16. Elisei AM, Norgard MJ, Durant JR, Kelly DR. Unusual manifestations of non-Hodgkin's lymphoma. *Cancer*. 1979;44(1): 269–272.

17. Ogasawara H, Kimura J, Morisaki Y, Kumoi T. Malignant lymphoma in unusual areas of the head and neck: parapharyngeal space and temporal fossa. *Auris Nasus Larynx*. 1985;12(2):125–133.

18. Weber AL, Rahemtullah A, Ferry JA. Hodgkin and non-Hodgkin lymphoma of the head and neck: clinical, pathologic, and imaging evaluation. *Neuroimaging Clin N Am*. 2003;13(3):371–392.

19. Horny HP, Kaiserling E. Involvement of the larynx by hemopoietic neoplasms. An investigation of autopsy cases and review of the literature. *Pathol Res Pract*. 1995;191(2): 130–138.

20. Zhao P, Zhou Y, Li J. Primary laryngeal lymphoma in China: a retrospective study of the last 25 years. *J Laryngol Otol*. 2019;133(9): 792–795.

21. Markou K, Goudakos J, Constantinidis J, Kostopoulos I, Vital V, Nikolaou A. Primary laryngeal lymphoma: report of 3 cases and review of the literature. *Head Neck*. 2010;32(4):541–549.

22. Korst RJ. Primary lymphoma of the subglottic airway in a patient with Sjogren's syndrome mimicking high laryngotracheal stenosis. *Ann Thorac Surg*. 2007;84(5):1756–1758.

23. Patiar S, Ramsden JD, Freeland AP. B-cell lymphoma of the larynx in a patient with rheumatoid arthritis. *J Laryngol Otol*. 2005;119(8):646–648.

24. Franzen A, Kurrer MO. Malignant lymphoma of the larynx: a case report and review of the literature. *Laryngorhinootologie*. 2000;79(10):579–583.

25. Anderson HA, Maisel RH, Cantrell RW. Isolated laryngeal lymphoma. *Laryngoscope*. 1976;86(8):1251–1257.

26. Cavalot AL, Preti G, Vione N, Nazionale G, Palonta F, Fadda GI. Isolated primary non-Hodgkin's malignant lymphoma of the larynx. *J Laryngol Otol*. 2001;115(4):324–326.

27. Kawaida M, Fukuda H, Shiotani A, Nakagawa H, Kohno N, Nakamura A. Isolated non-Hodgkin's malignant lymphoma of the larynx presenting as a large pedunculated tumor. *ORL J Otorhinolaryngol Relat Spec*. 1996;58(3):171–174.

28. Ferlito A, Rinaldo A, Devaney KO, Devaney SL, Milroy CM. Impact of phenotype on treatment and prognosis of laryngeal malignancies. *J Laryngol Otol*. 1998;112(8):710–714.

29. Zapparoli M, Trolese AR, Remo A, Sina S, Bonetti A, Micheletto C. Subglottic malt-lymphoma of the larynx: an unusual

presentation of chronic cough. *Int J Immunopathol Pharmacol.* 2014;27(3):461–465.

30. Rahman B, Bilal J, Sipra QU, Riaz IB. All that wheezes is not asthma: a case of diffuse large B-cell lymphoma of the larynx. *Case Rep Oncol Med.* 2017;2017:7072615.

31. Word R, Urquhart AC, Ejercito VS. Primary laryngeal lymphoma: case report. *Ear Nose Throat J.* 2006;85(2):109–111.

32. Kania RE, Hartl DM, Badoual C, Le Maignan C, Brasnu DF. Primary mucosa-associated lymphoid tissue (MALT) lymphoma of the larynx. *Head Neck.* 2005; 27(3):258–262.

33. Cheng CJ, Chen PR, Liu MC, Kuo MS, Hsu YH. Primary malignant lymphoma of mucosa-associated lymphoid tissue of larynx. *Otolaryngol Head Neck Surg.* 1999;121(5):661–662.

34. National Comprehensive Cancer Network. NCCN Guidelines for treatment of cancer by site, 2016. Accessed October 2, 2019. https://www.nccn.org/professionals/physi cian_gls/default.aspx#cll

35. Lee DY, Kang K, Jung H, et al. Extranodal involvement of diffuse large B-cell lymphoma in the head and neck: An indicator of good prognosis. *Auris Nasus Larynx.* 2019;46(1):114–121.

36. DeSanto LW. Weiland LH. Malignant lymphoma of the larynx. *Laryngoscope.* 1970;80(6):966–978.

37. Wang CC. Malignant lymphoma of the larynx. *Laryngoscope.* 1972;82(1):97–100.

38. Ferlito A, Carbone A, Volpe R. Diagnosis and assessment of non-Hodgkin's malignant lymphomas of the larynx. *ORL J Otorhinolaryngol Relat Spec.* 1981:43(2):61–78.

39. Mackenty JE, Faulkner ER. Malignant disease of the larynx: rare types, premalignant conditions and conditions simulating malignancy. *Arch Otolaryngol.* 1934; 20(3):297–328.

40. Mills WH, Domiguez R, McCall JW. Simultaneous carcinoma and malignant lymphoma of the larynx: case report and review of literature. *Laryngoscope.* 1947;57(7): 491–500.

41. Morgan K, MAcLennan KA, Narula A, Bradley PJ, Morgan DA. Non-Hodgkin's

lymphoma of the larynx (stage IE). *Cancer.* 1989;64(5):1123–1127.

42. Ohta N, Suzuki H, Fukase S, Ksajima N, Aoyagi M. Primary non-Hodgkin's lymphoma of the larynx (Stage IE) diagnosed by gene rearrangement. *J Laryngol Otol.* 2001;115(7):596–599.

43. Nayak JV, Cook JR, Molina JT, et al. Primary lymphoma of the larynx: new diagnostic and therapeutic approaches. *ORL J Otorhinolaryngol Relat Spec.* 2003;65(6):321–326.

44. Agada FO, Mistry D, Grace AR, Coatesworth AP. Large B-cell non-Hodgkin's lymphoma presenting as a laryngeal cyst. *J Laryngol Otol.* 2005;119(8):658–660.

45. Roca B, Vidal-Tegedor B, Moya M. Primary non-Hodgkin lymphoma of the larynx. *South Med J.* 2005;98(3):388–389.

46. Cui W, Fan F, Zhang D, Garnett D, Tilzer L. Primary composite lymphoma of the larynx, composed of diffuse large B-cell lymphoma and peripheral T-cell lymphoma, not otherwise specified, presenting as left subglottic tracheal fistula, esophageal diverticulum, and neck abscess. *Ann Clin Lab Sci.* 2012;42(1):73–80.

47. Revanappa MM, Sattur AP, Naikmasur VG, Thakur AR. Disseminated non-Hodgkin's lymphoma presenting as bilateral salivary gland enlargement: a case report. *Imaging Sci Dent.* 2013;43(1):59–62.

48. Akhtar S, Rana TA, Aldei A, Maghfoor I, Almutawa AM. Upper aero-digestive tract lymphomas presenting as polypoidal/pedunculated lesions: case report and review of literature. *Head Neck Pathol.* 2014;8(3): 317–321.

49. Sharma V, Gupta S, Patel M, Dora T, Sancheti S. Diffuse large B cell lymphoma of larynx. *J Assoc Physicians India.* 2018;66(5):91–93.

50. Horny HP, Ferlito A, Carbone A. Laryngeal lymphoma derived from mucosa-associated lymphoid tissue. *Ann Otol Rhinol Laryngol.* 1996;105(7):577–583.

51. Isaacson PG, Norton AJ, eds. *Extranodal lymphomas.* Edinburgh, Scotland: Churchill Livingstone; 1994.

52. Isaacson P, Wright DH. Malignant lymphoma of mucosa-associated lymphoid tissue. *Cancer*. 1983;52(8):1410–1416.

53. Zinzani PL, Magagnoli M, Galieni P, et al. Nongastrointestinal low-grade mucosa-associated lymphoid tissue lymphoma: analysis of 75 patients. *J Clin Oncol*. 1999;17(4):1254.

54. Fung EK, Neuhauser TS, Thompson LD. Hodgkin-like transformation of a marginal zone B-cell lymphoma of the larynx. *Ann Diagn Pathol*. 2002;6(1):61–66.

55. Wotherspoon AC, Ortiz-Hidalgo C, Falzon MR, Isaacson PG. *Helicobacter pylori*-associated gastritis and primary B-cell gastric lymphoma. *Lancet*. 1991;338(8776): 1175–1176.

56. Tsang RW, Gospodarowicz MK, Pintilie M, et al. Stage I and II MALT lymphoma: results of treatment with radiotherapy. *Int J Radiat Oncol Biol Phys*. 2001; 50(5):1258–1264.

57. Diebold J, Audouin J, Viry B, Ghandour C, Betti P, D'Ornano G. Primary lymphoplasmacytic lymphoma of the larynx: a rare localization of MALT-type lymphoma. *Ann Otol Rhinol Laryngol*. 1990;99(7):577–580.

58. Kobayashi H, Nemoto Y, Namiki K, Nakazawa K, Mukai M. Primary malignant lymphoma of the trachea and subglottic region. *Intern Med*. 1992;31(5):655–658.

59. Hisashi K, Komune S, Inoue H, Komiyama S, Sugimoto T, Miyoshi M. Coexistence of MALT-type lymphoma and squamous cell carcinoma of the larynx. *J Laryngol Otol*. 1994;108(11):995–997.

60. Kato S, Sakura M, Takooda S, Sakurai M, Izumo T. Primary non-Hodgkin's lymphoma of the larynx. *J Laryngol Otol*. 1997; 111(6):571–574.

61. de Bree R, Mahieu HF, Ossenkoppele GJ, van der Valk P. Malignant lymphoma of mucosa-associated lymphoid tissue in the larynx. *Eur Arch Otorhinolaryngol*. 1998;255 (7):368–370.

62. Usui N, Nikaido T, Katori M, Takei Y, Kasama K, Jaffe ES. MALT lymphoma of the larynx. *Rinsho ketsueki*. 2000;41(7): 601–606.

63. Puig Garces P, Martínez Beneito P, Piles Galdon A, Serrano Badia E, Pérez Garriques T. Subglottic MALT-type lymphoma: unusual location. *Acta Otorrinolaringol Esp*. 2002;53(9):693–696.

64. Caletti G, Togliani T, Fusaroli P, et al. Consecutive regression of concurrent laryngeal and gastric MALT lymphoma after anti–*Helicobacter pylori* therapy. *Gastroenterology*. 2003;124(2):537–543.

65. Kuhnt T, Wollschläger B, Bloching M, Krause U, Dunst J. Extranodal non-Hodgkin's lymphoma of MALT-type stage I. A case report. *Strahlenther Onkol*. 2003;179(6):396–400.

66. Dabaja BS, Ha CS, Wilder RB, et al. Importance of esophagogastroduodenoscopy in the evaluation of non-gastrointestinal mucosa-associated lymphoid tissue lymphoma. *Cancer*. 2003;9(4):321–324.

67. Aiyer RG, Soni G, Chougule S, Unnikrishnan, Nagpal T. Extranodal non-Hodgkin's lymphoma of larynx. *Indian J Otolaryngol Head Neck Surg*. 2004;56(4):298–300.

68. Andratschke M, Stelter K, Ihrler S, Hagedorn H. Subglottic tracheal stenosis as primary manifestation of a marginal zone B-cell lymphoma of the larynx. *In Vivo*. 2005;19(3):547–550.

69. Steffen A, Jafari C, Merz H, Galle J, Berger G. Subglottic MALT lymphoma of the larynx—more attention to the glottis. *In Vivo*. 2007;21(4):695–698.

70. Arndt S, Veelken H, Schmitt-Gräff A, Aschendorff A, Maier W, Richter B. Multifocal extranodal mucosa-associated lymphoid tissue lymphoma affecting the larynx. *Ann Otol Rhinol Laryngol*. 2007;116(4):257–261.

71. Kuo JR, Hou YY, Chu ST, Chien CC. Subglottic stenosis induced by extranodal mucosa-associated lymphoid tissue lymphoma. *J Chin Med Assoc*. 2011;74(3):144–147.

72. Zhao K, Luo YZ, Zhou SH, et al. ^{18}F-fluorodeoxyglucose positron emission tomography/computed tomography findings in mucosa-associated lymphoid tissue lymphoma of the larynx: a case report and literature review. *J Int Med Res*. 2012;40(3): 1192–1206.

73. Yilmaz M, Ibrahimov M, Mamanov M, Rasidov R, Oktem F. Primary marginal zone B-cell lymphoma of the larynx. *J Craniofac Surg.* 2012;23(1):e1–2.

74. Bielinski C, Luu HS, Mau T. Mucosa-associated lymphoid tissue (MALT) lymphoma presenting as subglottic stenosis: single-agent treatment using rituximab. *Otolaryngol Head Neck Surg.* 2014;150(2): 334–335.

75. González-Murillo EA, Castro-Rodríguez A, Sánchez-Venegas JC, Pena-Ruelas CI. Subglottic MALT lymphoma of the larynx in a patient with rheumatoid arthritis. *Acta Otorrinolaringol Esp.* 2014;5(65):317–319.

76. Hua J, Iwaki Y, Inoue M, Takiguchi Y, Ota Y, Hagihara M. Mucosa-associated lymphoid tissue lymphoma of the larynx. *Rinsho ketsueki.* 2014;55(3):340–344.

77. Liu M, Liu B, Liu B, et al. Mucosa-associated lymphoid tissue lymphoma of the larynx: a case report and literature review. *Medicine.* 2015;94(17):e788.

78. Chan JK, Sin VC, Wong KF, et al. Non-nasal lymphoma expressing the natural killer cell marker CD56: a clinicopathologic study of 49 cases of an uncommon aggressive neoplasm. *Blood.* 1997;89(12):4501–4513.

79. Jaffe ES, Chan JK, Su IJ, et al. Report of the workshop on nasal and related extranodal angiocentric T/natural killer cell lymphomas. Definitions, differential diagnosis, and epidemiology. *Am J Surg Pathol.* 1996;20(1):103–111.

80. Nakamura S, Katoh E, Koshikawa T, et al. Clinicopathologic study of nasal T/NK-cell lymphoma among the Japanese. *Pathol Int.* 1997;47(1):38–53.

81. Mok JS, Pak MW, Chan KF, Chow J, Hasselt CA. Unusual T- and T/NK-cell non-Hodgkin's lymphoma of the larynx: a diagnostic challenge for clinicians and pathologists. *Head Neck.* 2001;23(8):625–628.

82. Tardío JC, Moreno A, Pérez C, Hernández-Rivas JA, López-Carreira M. Primary laryngeal T/NK-cell lymphoma, nasal-type: an unusual location for an aggressive subtype of extranodal lymphoma. *Eur Arch Otorhinolaryngol.* 2008;265(6):705–708.

83. Monobe H, Nakashima M, Tominaga K. Primary laryngeal natural killer/T-cell lymphoma—report of a rare case. *Head Neck.* 2008;30(11):1527–1530.

84. Friedmann D, Troob SH, Suurna MV, Liu C. Primary natural killer T cell lymphoma of the supraglottis. *Otolaryngol Head Neck Surg.* 2011;145(2 Suppl):P196.

85. de la Rosa Astacio F, Barbera Durbán R, Vaca González M, Cobeta Marco I. Laryngotracheal NK/T lymphoma: clinical case. *Acta Otorrinolaringol Esp.* 2011; 62(1):71–73.

86. Hirai T, Fukushima N, Nakashimo Y, Katagiri Y, Kubota K, Ishibashi T. A case of epiglottic NK/T cell malignant lymphoma. *Nihon Jibiinkoka Gakkai Kaiho.* 2011;114(10):814–819.

87. Cikojević D, Glunčić I, Pešutić-Pisac V, Klančnik M, Čolović Z. Primary laryngeal NK/T-cell non-Hodgkin lymphoma: a case report. *Ear Nose Throat J.* 2012;91(7):E10–E12.

88. Uri N, Schindler Y, Quitt M, Valkovsky O, Barzilai G. Primary NK/T-cell lymphoma of the larynx. *Ear Nose Throat J.* 2012;91(5): 206–207.

89. Zhou ML, Zhao K, Zhou SH, Wang QY, Zheng ZJ, Lu ZJ. Role of PET/CT in the diagnosis, staging, and follow-up of a nasal-type natural killer T-cell lymphoma in the larynx: a case report and literature review. *Int J Clin Exp Med.* 2014;7(11):4483–4491.

90. Köybaşı S, Seyhan S, Biçer YÖ, Üner A, Yeşilırmak A. Nasal type natural killer T-cell lymphoma involving naso-oropharynx and larynx. *Kulak burun bogaz ihtis derg.* 2014;24(6):364–367.

91. Zhu SY, Yuan Y, Liu K, et al. Primary NK/T-cell lymphoma of the larynx: Report of 2 cases and review of the English-, Japanese-, and Chinese-language literature. *Ear Nose Throat J.* 2016;95(4–5):E1–8.

92. Gungor A, Pennington L, Sankararaman S, Zaid-Kaylani S, Jeroudi MA. A 14-year-old boy with extranodal natural killer cell lymphoma of the nose, nasopharynx, larynx, and trachea in remission 6 years after pri-

mary diagnosis. A longitudinal case report. *Am J Otolaryngol.* 2016;37(6):563–566.

93. Meleca JB, Hanick A, Lamarre E, Bryson PC. Post-treatment sequelae and management of primary laryngeal NK/T-cell lymphoma: a case report. *Am J Otolaryngol.* 2018;39(6): 781–784.

94. Xiang CX, Chen ZH, Zhao S, et al. Laryngeal extranodal nasal-type natural killer/T-cell lymphoma. *Am J Surg Pathol.* 2019;43(7): 995–1004.

95. Shankland KR, Armitage JO, Hancock BW. Non-Hodgkin lymphoma. *Lancet.* 2012;380 (9844):848–857.

96. Budhy TI, Soenarto SD, Yaacob HB, Ngeow WC. Changing incidence of oral and max-illofacial tumours in East Java, Indonesia, 1987–1992. Part 2: malignant tumours. *Br J Oral Maxillofac Surg.* 2001;39(6):460–464.

97. Parkins GE, Armah GA, Tettey Y. Orofacial tumours and tumour-like lesions in Ghana: a 6-year prospective study. *Br J Oral Maxillofac Surg.* 2009;47(7):550–554.

98. Walter C, Ziebart T, Sagheb K, Rahimi-Nedjat RK, Manz A, Hess G. Malignant lymphomas in the head and neck region—a retrospective, single-center study over 41 years. *Int J Med Sci.* 2015;12(2):141–145.

99. Broadwater DR, Peker D. Systemic Non-Hodgkin T cell lymphomas presenting in the head and neck region: an institutional experience of a rare entity. *Head Neck Pathol.* 2018;12(4):481–487.

100. Smith MS, Browne JD, Teot LA. A case of primary laryngeal T-cell lymphoma in a patient with acquired immunodeficiency syndrome. *Am J Otolaryngol.* 1996;17(5): 332–334.

101. Marianowski R, Wassef M, Amanou L, Herman P, Tran-Ba-Huy P. Primary T-cell non-Hodgkin lymphoma of the larynx with subsequent cutaneous involvement. *Arch Otolaryngol Head Neck Surg.* 1998; 124(9):1037–1040.

102. Uthamalingam P, Bal A, Malhotra P, Rabin-dranath E. Primary laryngeal peripheral T-cell lymphoma—an autopsy report with review of literature. *J Cancer Res Ther.* 2015; 11(3):647.

103. Grimley RP, Oates GD. The natural history of thyroid lymphomas. *Br J Surg.* 1980;67(7):175–177.

104. Pedersen RK, Pedersen NT. Primary non-Hodgkin's lymphoma of the thyroid gland: a population based study. *Histopathology.* 1996;28(1):25–32.

105. Heimann R. Primary malignant lymphomas of the thyroid. A brief review. *Acta Otorhinolaryngol Belg.* 1987;41(5):727–735.

106. Luo B, Chen JM, Liu J, et al. A case of intra-vascular large B cell lymphoma presenting as nodular goiter. *Diagn Pathol.* 2017;12 (1):64.

107. Jiu JB, Sobol SM, Grozea PN. Vocal cord paralysis and recovery with thyroid lymphoma. *Laryngoscope.* 1985;95(1):57–59.

108. Klyachkin ML, Schwartz RW, Cibull M, et al. Thyroid lymphoma: is there a role for surgery? *Am Surg.* 1998;64(3):234–238.

109. Glazer HS, Aronberg DJ, Lee JK, Sagel SS. Extralaryngeal causes of vocal cord paralysis: CT evaluation. *Am J Roentgenol.* 1983;141(3): 527–531.

110. Graham CP Jr. Hoarseness associated with lymphoma of the thyroid gland. *South Med J.* 1982;75(12):1566–1567.

111. Ansell SM, Grant CS, Habermann TM. Primary thyroid lymphoma. *Semin Oncol.* 1999;26(3):316–323.

112. Rosenberg SA, Diamond HD, Jaslow-itz B, Craver LF. Lymphosarcoma: a review of 1269 cases. *Medicine (Baltimore).* 1961;40:31–84.

113. Muller AM, Ihorst G, Mertelsmann R, Engel-hardt M. Epidemiology of non-Hodgkin's lymphoma (NHL): trends, geographic distribution, and etiology. *Ann Hematol.* 2005; 84(1):1–12

114. Ye ZY, Cao QH, Liu F, et al. Primary esophageal extranasal NK/T cell lymphoma with biphasic morphology: a case report and literature review. *Medicine (Baltimore).* 2015;94(28):e1151.

115. Zhu Q, Xu B, Xu K, Li J, Jin XL. Primary non-Hodgkin's lymphoma in the esophagus. *J Dig Dis.* 2008;9:241–244.

116. Orvidas LJ, McCaffrey TV, Lewis JE, Kurtin PJ, Habermann TM. Lymphoma involving

the esophagus. *Ann Otol Rhinol Laryngol.* 1994;103(11):843–848.

117. Peng JC, Zhong L, Ran ZH. Primary lymphomas in the gastrointestinal tract. *J Dig Dis.* 2015;16(4):169–176.

118. Solomonov A, Zuckerman T, Goralnik L, Ben-Arieh Y, Rowe JM, Yigla M. Non-Hodgkin's lymphoma presenting as an endobronchial tumor: report of eight cases and literature review. *Am J Hematol.* 2008;83(5):416–419.

119. Celikoglu F, Teirstein AS, Krellenstein DJ, Strauchen JA. Pleural effusion in non-Hodgkin's lymphoma. *Chest.* 1992;101(5): 1357–1360.

120. Aquino SL, Chen MY, Kuo WT, Chiles C. The CT appearance of pleural and extrapleural disease in lymphoma. *Clin Radiol.* 1999;54(10):647–650.

121. Strollo DC, Rosado-de-Christenson LM, Jett JR. Primary mediastinal tumors: part ll. Tumors of the middle and posterior mediastinum. *Chest.* 1997;112(5):1344–1357.

122. Ko HM, da Cunha Santos G, Darling G, et al. Diagnosis and subclassification of lymphomas and non-neoplastic lesions involving mediastinal lymph nodes using endobronchial ultrasound-guided trans-bronchial needle aspiration. *Diagn Cytopathol.* 2013;41(12):1023–1030.

123. Rhee KH, Hong SC, An JM, et al. Mediastinal single nodal relapse of a nasal NK/T cell lymphoma. *Korean J Intern Med.* 2007; 22(3):201–205.

124. Tateishi U, Müller NL, Johkoh T, et al. Primary mediastinal lymphoma: characteristic features of the various histological subtypes on CT. *J Comput Assist Tomogr.* 2004;28(6):782–789.

125. Cheng S. Superior vena cava syndrome: a contemporary review of a historic disease. *Cardiol Rev.* 2009;17(1):16–23.

126. Zimmerman S, Davis M. Rapid fire: superior vena cava syndrome. *Emerg Med Clin North Am.* 2018;36(3):577–584.

127. Lochridge SK, Knibbe WP, Doty DB. Obstruction of the superior vena cava. *Surgery.* 1979;85(1):14–24.

128. Nogeire C, Mincer F, Botstein C. Long survival in patients with bronchogenic carcinoma complicated by superior vena cava obstruction. *Chest.* 1979;75(3):325–329.

129. Perez-Soler R, McLaughlin P, Velaquez WS, et al. Clinical features and results of management of superior vena cava syndrome secondary to lymphoma. *J Clin Oncol.* 1984;2(4):260–266.

130. Wilson LD, Detterbeck FC, Yahalom J. Superior vena cava syndrome with malignant causes. *N Engl J Med.* 2007;356(18): 1862–1869.

131. Grippi MA. Clinical aspects of lung cancer. *Semin Roentgenol.* 1990;25(1):12–24.

132. Knudsen R, Gaunsbaek MQ, Schultz JH, Nilsson AC, Madsen JS, Asgari N. Vocal cord paralysis as primary and secondary results of malignancy. A prospective descriptive study. *Laryngoscope Investig Otolaryngol.* 2019;4(2):241–245.

133. Graham BB, Mathisen DJ, Mark EJ, Takvorian RW. Primary pulmonary lymphoma. *Ann Thorac Surg.* 2005;80(4):1248–1253.

134. Hsu PK, Hsu HS, Li AF, et al. Non-Hodgkin's lymphoma presenting as a large chest wall mass. *Ann Thorac Surg.* 2006;81(4):1214–1218.

135. Bergin CJ, Healy MV, Zincone GE, Castellino RA. MR evaluation of chest wall involvement in malignant lymphoma. *J Comput Assist Tomogr.* 1990;14(6):928–932.

136. McCulloch GL, Sinnatamby R, Stewart S, Goddard M, Flower CD. High-resolution computed tomographic appearance of MALT-oma of the lung. *Eur Radiol.* 1998;8(9): 1669–1673.

137. Ooi GC, Chim CS, Lie AK, Tsang KW. Computed tomography features of primary pulmonary non-Hodgkin's lymphoma. *Clin Radiol.* 1999;54(7):438–443.

138. Havas T, Lowinger D, Priestley J. Unilateral vocal fold paralysis: causes, options and outcomes. *Aust N Z J Surg.* 1999;69(7): 509–513.

139. Raufi A, Jerkins J, Lyou Y, Jeyakumar D. A patient with supraclavicular lymphade-

nopathy and anterior mediastinal mass presenting as a rare case of composite lymphoma: a case report and literature review. *Case Rep Oncol.* 2016;9(3):854–860.

140. Grisariu S, Avni B, Batchelor TT, et al. Neurolymphomatosis: an international primary CNS lymphoma collaborative group report. *Blood.* 2010;115(24):5005–5011.

141. Gan HK, Azad A, Cher L, Mitchell PL. Neurolymphomatosis: diagnosis, management, and outcomes in patients treated with rituximab. *Neuro Oncol.* 2010;12(2): 212–215.

142. Blioskas S, Tsaligopoulos M, Kyriafinis G, et al. Bilateral secondary neurolymphomatosis of the internal auditory canal nerves: a case report. *Am J Otolaryngol.* 2013;34(5): 556–558.

143. Sakai N, Ito-Yamashita T, Takahashi G, et al. Primary neurolymphomatosis of the lower cranial nerves presenting as dysphagia and hoarseness: a case report. *J Neuro Surg Rep.* 2014;75(1):e62–e66.

144. Boasquevisque GS, Guidoni J, Moreira de Souza LA, et al. Bilateral vagus nerve neurolymphomatosis diagnosed using PET/CT and diffusion-weighted MRI. *Clin Nucl Med.* 2012;37(9):e225–e228.

145. Tsang HH, Lee EY, Anthony MP, Khong PL. 18F-FDG PET/CT diagnosis of vagus nerve neurolymphomatosis. *Clin Nucl Med.* 2012; 37(9):897–898.

146. Yoshida T, Tezuka Y, Hirosawa T, et al. Pineal malignant B-cell lymphoma with lower cranial nerve involvement. *Intern Med.* 2014;53(11):1205–1208.

147. Dixon PR, Alsaffar H, Symons SP, Enepekides D, Higgins KM. Neoplastic meningitis presenting with dysphagia and bilateral vocal cord paralysis. *Laryngoscope.* 2014;124(8):1912–1914.

148. Cantalupo G, Spagnoli C, Cerasti D, Piccolo B, Crisi G, Pisani F. Tapia's syndrome secondary to laterocervical localization of diffuse large cell lymphoma. *Brain Dev.* 2014;36(6):548–550.

149. Ono Y, Kazuma Y, Ochi Y, Matsuoka R, Imai Y, Ishikawa T. Two cases of neuro-

lymphomatosis with fatal bilateral vocal cord paralysis that were diagnosed with 18F-fluorodeoxyglucose positron emission tomography (FDG PET)/CT. *Intern Med.* 2017;56(10):1193–1198.

150. Simmons DB, Bursaw AW. Lymphoma presenting as acute-onset dysphagia. *Case Rep Neurol Med.* 2015;2015:745121.

151. Zhou WL, Wu HB, Weng CS, et al. Usefulness of 18F-FDG PET/CT in the detection of neurolymphomatosis. *Nucl Med Commun.* 2014;35(11):1107–1111.

152. American Cancer Society. Chemotherapy for Non-Hodgkin's lymphoma. Updated August 1, 2018. Accessed October 2, 2019. https://www.cancer.org/cancer/non-hodgkin-lymphoma/treating/chemotherapy.html

153. Mattioni J, Opperman DA, Solimando DA, Sataloff RT. Cancer chemotherapy: an overview and voice implications. In: Sataloff RT. *Professional Voice: The Science and Art of Clinical Care*, 4th ed. San Diego, CA: Plural Publishing; 2017:1137–1140.

154. Oakes SG, Santone KS, Powis G. Effect of some anticancer drugs on the surface membrane electrical properties of differentiated murine neuroblastoma cells. *J Natl Cancer Inst.* 1987;79:155–161.

155. Bay A, Yilmaz C, Yilmaz N, Oner AF. Vincristine induced cranial polyneuropathy. *Indian J Pediatr.* 2006;73(6):531–533.

156. Burns BV, Shotton JC. Vocal fold palsy following vinca alkaloid treatment. *J Laryngol Otol.* 1998;112(5):485–487.

157. Ahmed A, Williams D, Nicholson J. Vincristine-induced bilateral vocal cord paralysis in children. *Pediatr Blood Cancer.* 2007;48(2):248.

158. Kuruvilla G, Perry S, Wilson B, El-Hakim H. The natural history of vincristine-induced laryngeal paralysis in children. *Arch Otolaryngol Head Neck Surg.* 2009;135(1):101–105.

159. Farruggia P, Tropia S, Cannella S, Bruno G, Oddo G, D'Angelo P. Vocal cord palsy after vincristine treatment in a child and the inefficacy of glutamic acid in the prevention

of relapse: a case report. *J Med Case Rep*. 2012;6(1):128.

160. Ryan SP, DelPrete SA, Weinstein PW, et al. Low-dose vincristine-associated bilateral vocal cord paralysis. *Conn Med*. 1999; 63(10):583–584.

161. Yalin SF, Trabulus S, Yalin AS, Yalin GY, Ongoren S, Altiparmak MR. Vocal cord paralysis during the treatment of mantle cell lymphoma with vincristine. *Int J Clin Pharm*. 2013;35(3):306–308.

162. Samoon Z, Shabbir-Moosajee M. Vincristine-induced vocal cord palsy and successful re-treatment in patient with diffuse large B cell lymphoma: a case report. *BMC Res Notes*. 2014;7:318.

163. American Cancer Society. Radiation therapy for Non-Hodgkin's lymphoma. Updated August 26, 2019. Accessed October 2, 2019. https://www.cancer.org/cancer/non-hodgkin-lymphoma/treating/radiation-therapy.html

164. Sagiroglu S, Kurtul N. The effect of supraclavicular radiotherapy on Acoustic Voice Quality Index (AVQI), spectral amplitude and perturbation values. *J Voice*. 2019. doi:10.1016/j.jvoice.2019.01.003

165. Fung K, Yoo J, Leeper HA, et al. Effects of head and neck radiation therapy on vocal function. *J Otolaryngol*. 2001;30(3): 133–139.

166. Crawley BK, Sulica L. Vocal fold paralysis as a delayed consequence of neck and chest radiotherapy. *Otolaryngol Head Neck Surg*. 2015;153(2):239–243.

167. Chandran SK, Sataloff RT. Treatment of postradiation laryngeal compromise. *Ear Nose Throat J*. 2010;89(2):58–59.

10

Renal Carcinoma and Voice

Abdul-Latif Hamdan, Robert Thayer Sataloff, and Mary J. Hawkshaw

Epidemiology and Risk Factors

Renal carcinoma is one of the most common cancers in men and women. The estimated number of newly diagnosed cases in the United States in 2019 is 73 820.[1] The incidence has risen over the last 2 decades, more so in elderly persons (70 to 79 years), at an average of 3.4% per year.[2] The increase in incidence has been attributed partially to the widespread screening for malignancies using radiologic imaging such as ultrasound and computed tomography (CT).[3,4] In a study by Wernli et al, renal carcinoma was the most common malignancy noted on CT colonography in patients undergoing screening for colon cancer.[5] It is the most lethal malignancy of the urologic system, with a poor overall prognosis and 5-year survival. The mortality rate is decreasing, particularly in Western countries due to early diagnosis and advances in therapy.[2] Nevertheless, renal carcinoma is still among the leading causes of cancer-related death worldwide with an estimated 14 770 mortalities in the United States in 2019.[1]

Renal carcinoma is a silent disease. Incidental diagnosis is made in 50% of cases, and only a minority of patients present with the clinical triad of flank pain, mass, and hematuria.[6,7] The disease progresses with diverse symptoms and signs including anemia, leukemoid reactions, polyneuritis, and hypercalcemia.[8] Several risk factors have been identified among which are male gender, older age, smoking, hypertension, increased body mass index (BMI), and increased exposure to carcinogens.[9–12] History of smoking has been confirmed as a dose-dependent risk factor for renal carcinoma.[13] In a large meta-analysis that included 8032 cases, smokers had a relative risk of 1.38 in comparison to nonsmokers.[10] Similarly, an increase in BMI and waist-to-hip ratio has been linked to renal carcinoma. Obesity has been associated with a higher prevalence and a relative risk of 1.8.[14–16] Hypertension increases the long-term risk of renal carcinoma in men as well. In a review of the medical records of 759 men with renal cell carcinoma (RCC), Chow et al reported a direct association between high blood pressure and the risk of developing RCC, which increased at the sixth year of follow-up.[17] Other significant risk factors include Von Hippel-Lindau disease, decrease in glomerular filtration rate, end-stage renal disease, renal transplant recipients,[18–22] in addition to genetic predisposition.[23,24]

Several tests are recommended for screening for renal carcinoma, the most common of which are serum and/or urinary biomarkers.[2] The serum and urinary biomarkers used frequently are aquaporin 1 (AQP1) and Perilipin 2 (PLIN2). The specificity and sensitivity of these biomarkers have been reported as high as 100% and 92%, respectively. A less commonly used biomarker with comparable diagnostic yield is the composite 3-marker assay using nicotinamide N-methyltransfarase, L-plastin, and nonmetastatic cell 1 protein.[25] Another useful screening modality is ultrasound, which is effective in detecting renal lesions between 10 and 35 mm in size in 82% of cases.[26,27] Commonly used diagnostic ultrasound criteria include the rounded shape and solid echogenicity of the renal mass. CT is a less commonly used screening modality with a relatively low diagnostic yield. In a study by Fenton et al, the pooled prevalence of asymptomatic renal cancer using screening CT was 0.21% of cases, with a range between 0.14% and 0.28%.[28] The diagnosis of renal carcinoma relied heavily on tissue histopathologic examination, which is requested prior to the initiation of any form of therapy. Percutaneous needle biopsy is considered highly effective for providing a tissue specimen and in supporting treatment decisions in patients with both benign and malignant renal masses.[29] It also has been proven to differentiate cystic masses adequately from lymphomas and other malignancies.[30,31] In rare cases, a partial or radical nephrectomy is needed to provide an adequate tissue specimen.[31] Based on histopathologic examination, RCC is the most common type of renal carcinoma accounting for 70% to 85% of cases. There is a high predilection for men, with the male-to-female ratio being 1.7:1. Among RCC, clear cell RCC is the most frequent, occurring in 87.7% of cases.[32,33] It is important to note that histologic features such as clear cells or papillary structures may be present in more than one type of RCC. Given the mosaic morphology, 4% of RCC cases are not assigned any specific category.[34,35]

Renal carcinoma is known for its tendency to metastasize. Given the diversity in its metastatic spread and its clinical presentation, renal carcinoma is known as the "great imitator."[36(p847)] Metastatic disease is identified in 23% to 40% of cases at the time of diagnosis, with multiple metastasis being more frequent in younger patients compared to elderly persons.[36-39] Any organ in the body may be a target for renal carcinoma metastasis. The organs most commonly affected are the lungs and bones in 50% and 49% of cases, respectively.[40,41] Less frequently involved sites are the liver, skin, adrenal glands, soft tissues, and pleura. Metastasis of renal carcinoma to the head and neck has been discussed thoroughly in the literature. Based on numerous reports, the prevalence is around 15% of cases.[8,42,43] Various structures may be affected, most common of which are the paranasal sinuses, pharynx, tongue, temporal bone, eye, mandible, and salivary glands.[44-51] The clinical presentation varies in relation to the site of metastasis, and often leads to localized symptoms such as epistaxis, facial pain, tinnitus, and soft tissue swelling.[44,52] In 2017, Serra et al reported a 79-year-old woman who presented with epistaxis and recurrent rhinorrhea 10 years following left nephrectomy for RCC. The patient was diagnosed with nasal metastasis from her primary tumor.[53] In a review of 644 patients who underwent parotidectomies, Franzen et al reported 39 metastatic cases, 1 of whom had RCC. The patient was a 74-year-old woman who presented with painless swelling of the left parotid gland 6 years following a nephrectomy. The authors highlighted that primary tumors below the clavicle metastasizing to the head and neck region may present with confusing symptoms and signs.[54]

Metastasis of renal carcinoma to the larynx has been discussed in the literature. This chapter reviews the impact of renal carcinoma on the phonatory apparatus. Cases of metastasis to the larynx and structures contiguous to the larynx are summarized. Treatment-induced dysphonia, particularly in patients on targeted therapy, is also reviewed. This information is valuable for otolaryngologists and physicians in the workup of and treatment of voice patients with a history of renal carcinoma and dysphonia.

Disease-Induced Dysphonia in Patients With Renal Carcinoma

Laryngeal Metastasis in Patients With Renal Carcinoma

Renal carcinoma is the second most common tumor metastasizing to the larynx, second to melanoma. It is followed by lung cancer, breast cancer, and prostate cancer.[36] Review of the literature through 1956 shows only 4 cases of renal carcinoma metastasizing to the larynx, reported by Turner in 1924, Oppikoder in 1932, Maxwell in 1942, and Tamura et al in 1956.[55–58] In 1966, Fields reported a 61-year-old woman who presented with hoarseness and choking 1 year after being diagnosed with and treated for adenocarcinoma of the right kidney. On laryngeal examination, she had a whitish subglottic lesion, the pathology of which was identical to the primary renal carcinoma.[59] In 1973, Myamoto and Helmus reported a 79-year-old man who developed laryngeal metastasis 17 years after being diagnosed with hypernephroma for which he had undergone left nephrectomy. The presenting symptoms of dysphagia, dysphonia,

and aspiration were attributed to a right aryepiglottic fold lesion. Histopathologic examination of that lesion revealed metastatic hypernephroma.[8] In 1987, Maung et al highlighted the indolent course of laryngeal metastatic renal carcinoma in a case report and emphasized the favorable outcome of surgical intervention.[60] That same year, Ferlito et al described a 73-year-old man who presented with a history of hoarseness. On laryngeal examination, he had a polypoid subglottic lesion biopsy that confirmed the presence of glycogen content. Further investigation revealed a right kidney tumor with focal vascular invasion consistent with RCC. The authors highlighted the importance of detecting submucosal lesions on laryngeal examination and the need for histochemical staining in order to establish the diagnosis of metastatic carcinoma.[61] In 1992, Greenberg et al described hoarseness as the presenting symptom of laryngeal metastasis in a 55-year-old man. Laryngeal examination and CT showed an isolated subglottic lesion, and biopsy revealed clear cell carcinoma. Further imaging of the abdomen revealed a renal mass that was later shown to be identical in pathology to that of the larynx.[39] In 1993, Mochimatsu et al reported 7 cases of primary tumors metastasizing to the head and neck region, among which were 3 cases of primary RCC. The metastatic sites in the head and neck were the paranasal sinuses (4 cases), tonsils (1 case), parotid (1 case), and larynx (1 case). The patient with laryngeal metastasis was a 64-year-old man with no prior history of malignancy who presented with foreign-body sensation in the throat. On laryngeal examination, he had a right arytenoid mass biopsy, results of which were consistent with metastatic clear cell carcinoma.[62] That same year, Marlowe et al described a 54-year-old man who presented with hoarseness and dysphagia of 1 month's duration. On laryngeal examination, he had edema and fullness of the right vocal fold. Radiologic imaging of the neck performed a month later showed a laryngeal vascular lesion with destruction of the thyroid lamina. Histologic examination of that lesion revealed an endocrine pattern, and electron microscopic analysis indicated metastatic clear cell adenocarcinoma.[63] In 1995, Hittel and Born reported a 42-year-old woman who developed an anterior commissure lesion 6 years after being diagnosed with a right kidney hypernephroma. The authors emphasized the need for a high index of suspicion in the workup of patients with laryngeal submucosal masses and history of renal cancer, and the need to perform immunohistochemical staining for the resected tissue.[64] In 1996, Issing et al described a 73-year-old woman who presented with a false vocal fold lesion on the right 6 years after being diagnosed with and treated for a hypernephroma. The patient underwent suspension microlaryngoscopy and laser excision of the lesion that showed metastatic RCC. The authors alluded to the unpredictable behavior of these tumors and the need for adequate therapy given the long survival rates of many affected patients.[65] In 2000, Dee et al reported a 48-year-old man who presented with dysphonia 7 years following left radical nephrectomy for clear cell carcinoma. On laryngeal examination, the patient had a polypoid supraglottic mass consistent with the metastatic renal tumor on histologic examination.[66] In 2000, Navarro et al described 3 cases of metastatic renal carcinoma to the head and neck region, among which was a patient with laryngeal metastasis who presented with hemoptysis and hoarseness. Laryngeal examination and CT of the neck revealed a vascular lesion of the right ventricle with involvement of the ipsilateral vocal fold. A biopsy taken from that lesion showed metastatic clear

cell carcinoma. Further evaluation of the abdomen showed a right kidney tumor.[67] In 2004, Rossini et al reported a 54-year-old man who presented with dysphagia and foreign-body sensation in the throat 3 years after being diagnosed with and treated for RCC. On laryngeal examination, he had an epiglottic vascular lesion reaching the laryngeal ventricle and left false vocal fold. The lesion was excised *en bloc* using carbon dioxide laser, and histopathologic examination showed metastatic RCC.[68] In 2006, Stodulski et al described the clinical presentation of 4 patients with RCC metastasis to the head and neck, among whom was a patient with laryngeal metastasis. The authors highlighted the clinical presentation of these lesions and their relatively poor prognosis.[69] In 2012, Katsube et al reported a 79-year-old man who presented with dysphonia as the first symptom of laryngeal RCC metastasis. The authors emphasized the need to consider laryngeal lesions as being metastatic even in patients with a long history of renal cancer that had been successfully treated.[70] In 2012, Mehdi et al reported a 57-year-old man who developed laryngeal metastasis from renal clear cell carcinoma 9 years after being treated with surgery and adjuvant radiotherapy. The patient had a right pyriform fossa vascular and ulcerative lesion abutting the right true vocal fold and causing dysphonia. Biopsy of the lesion stained positive for cytokeratin (CK), vimentin, and epithelial membrane antigen (EMA). The patient was diagnosed with metastatic RCC.[71] That same year, Sarkis et al described a 70-year-old man diagnosed with renal carcinoma, who presented with dyspnea, dysphonia, and stridor. On laryngeal examination, he had a left pedunculated ventricular lesion. The patient underwent excision of the lesion under suspension microlaryngoscopy using the CO_2 laser. The pathology was consistent with metastatic renal carcinoma.[72]

The previous reports show that metastasis of renal carcinoma to the larynx may occur in isolation or with other metastatic lesions. The laryngeal metastasis is often silent, and the symptoms may precede or follow the diagnosis of the primary tumor by up to 31 years.[73] The symptoms may mimic those reported by patients with primary laryngeal neoplasms. Affected patients complain of dysphonia, dyspnea, foreign-body sensation, and/or hemoptysis. On laryngeal examination, the lesion is often vascular, is lobulated, and has normal overlying mucosa. The supraglottis is the site affected most commonly, and a high index of suspicion is needed to make the diagnosis. The lesions show strong contrast enhancement and flow voids on MRI.[74] Histopathologic staining for lipid and glycogen, and immunohistochemical positivity for specific markers such as vimentin, CD-10, and epithelial membrane antigen are helpful in differentiating metastatic lesions from primary laryngeal neoplasia.[36] When present, laryngeal metastasis is an ominous sign. Although the prognosis is considered poor, surgical resection is offered to patients with solitary metastasis with the hope of prolonging life.[39,75] In patients with metastatic disease, systemic therapy in the form of targeted therapy or immunotherapy is recommended.[76–79]

Metastasis to Structures Contiguous With the Larynx

Renal carcinoma can affect voice by metastasizing to structures contiguous with the larynx. A commonly reported metastatic target is the thyroid gland.[8] Metastasis of renal carcinoma to the thyroid gland is not surprising given the rich blood supply of the thyroid reaching up to 560 mL/100 g tissue/minute.[80] Metastasis to the thyroid

gland from distant primaries has been reported in 1.9% to 26.4% of cases.[81,82] The large disparity in prevalence is attributed to the type of study conducted, autopsy versus clinical, and to the methodology used.[83–86] A thorough review of the literature shows numerous reports of renal carcinoma with thyroid metastasis. In 1981, Ericson et al described 10 patients with thyroid gland metastasis, 7 of whom had RCC as a primary tumor. Eight patients complained of a lump sensation in the neck, and 1 patient presented with stridor secondary to bilateral vocal fold paralysis. The diagnosis was confirmed using fine-needle aspiration (FNA) in 5 out of 9 patients, 3 of whom had renal carcinoma.[87] In a review of the clinical and pathologic features of metastatic neoplasia to the thyroid gland, Czech et al reported renal carcinoma as the most frequent primary tumor, followed by breast adenocarcinoma. The authors emphasized the usefulness of FNA in the workup and diagnosis of patients with suspected thyroid nodules.[88] In 1985, McCabe et al reported 17 patients with metastatic thyroid neoplasms, 2 of whom had renal carcinoma as a primary tumor. The main symptom in all cases was a neck mass, in addition to dysphonia in one patient and dysphagia in 2.[89] In 1991, Hudson et al reported a 61-year-old woman with bilateral clear cell renal carcinoma who presented with a painless neck mass 13 months after her diagnosis with kidney tumors. The patient underwent neck exploration and left hemithyroidectomy that revealed metastatic renal disease. The patient recovered, and no other metastatic site was detected on follow-up.[90] That same year, Hallbauer et al emphasized the added value of FNA biopsy in the preoperative planning for patients with a thyroid mass, and the role of cytochemical analysis in the workup of metastatic lesions.[91] In 1994, Niiyama et al reported a 72-year-old patient with

RCC who presented with nodular goiter 3 months following left radical nephrectomy. A left lobectomy was performed, and histologic examination showed the presence of metastatic renal carcinoma. The authors pointed to the possibility of thyroid metastasis even in the absence of distant metastasis to other organs.[92] In 1995, Rosen et al described a patient with renal carcinoma among 11 patients with secondary malignancy of the thyroid gland. The authors emphasized the role of FNA and biopsy and its high diagnostic yield (90%) in cases of thyroid metastatic disease.[93] In 1996, Pagano et al reviewed usual and unusual clinical metastasis of RCC in the English literature. The lungs and bones were the most common usual metastatic sites in 50% and 49% of cases, respectively, whereas thyroid metastasis was described as an unusual endocrine metastatic site in only 4 cases. The scarcity of thyroid metastasis was attributed to the indolent course of metastasis and the asymptomatic presentation of affected patients.[38] In 1997, Nakhjavani et al reported the kidney as the primary tumor site in one-third of patients with metastatic thyroid disease. The review included 43 patients, all of whom were diagnosed by FNA cytology. It is worth noting that the mean time between the diagnosis of the primary neoplasia and thyroid metastasis was 106 months.[94] In 1999, Palazzo et al reported 4 patients with RCC metastasizing to the thyroid gland, all of whom had neck swelling that was treated surgically by hemithyroidectomy or total thyroidectomy. Two of the 4 patients complained also of dysphonia.[95] In 1999, Chen et al reported the clinical presentation of 10 patients with metastatic thyroid disease. Five patients of the 10 had RCC as a primary neoplasm, 1 of whom had metastasis to both lobes of the thyroid gland. Two of the 10 patients had dysphonia and dyspnea on presentation. The time between

the initial treatment of the primary neoplasia and the performance of thyroidectomy reached 19.5 years.[96] In 2004, Kihara et al described an 87-year-old woman diagnosed with RCC, who presented with history of dysphagia and a right neck mass. To alleviate her symptoms, the patient underwent right hemithyroidectomy that showed complete replacement of the right thyroid lobe by tumor. Tissue staining was positive for LeuM1 and vimentin, consistent with metastatic primary renal carcinoma.[97] In 2007, Papi et al reviewed the clinical and pathologic features of 36 cases of thyroid metastasis and evaluated the role of surgery in the management of these cases. The kidneys, lung, esophagus, and breast were the main sites of primary tumor.[98] The authors concluded that thyroid metastasis is a poor prognostic sign and that thyroidectomy has a limited role in affected patients.[98] In 2012, Katsube et al reported a 61-year-old woman who developed thyroid gland metastasis 2½ years after being treated for RCC. The patient was managed successfully with surgical resection of her thyroid metastatic lesion.[70] In that same year, Demir et al reported 2 patients with RCC who developed thyroid metastatic disease many years after the diagnosis of their primary tumor. The first patient presented with hoarseness and dyspnea secondary to an enlarging thyroid mass that invaded the right side of the laryngeal framework and resulted in subglottic stenosis. The second patient presented with dyspnea and neck edema with circumferential narrowing of the trachea. In both cases, the diagnosis of thyroid metastatic disease was confirmed using immunohistochemical staining for vimentin, CD-10, and epithelial membrane antigen.[99] In 2016, Gheorghiu et al described an 82-year-old woman who presented with a thyroid mass 16 years after having a nephrectomy for a clear cell carcinoma. Ultrasonography showed a 9.9-cm macronodular right lobe that necessitated a near-total thyroidectomy. The pathology was consistent with metastatic RCC. It is noteworthy that the patient was asymptomatic with no compressive symptoms or dysphonia.[100]

In summary, metastasis of renal carcinoma to the thyroid gland is not uncommon. It may occur many years after successful treatment of the primary tumor. Patients may be asymptomatic or complain of compressive symptoms with or without dysphonia. The metastatic lesion is often masked by an enlarged goiter or mistaken for thyroid adenomatous changes. FNA and biopsy with adequate tissue staining are crucial for proper diagnosis.[101] In cases of isolated thyroid metastasis, surgery is the treatment of choice with the aim of curing the disease.

The esophagus is another metastatic site contiguous with the larynx. There are many reports in the literature of metastatic disease to the esophagus, preceding or following the diagnosis of renal carcinoma. The symptoms reported most commonly are dysphagia and weight loss.[102–104] Dysphonia has not been described in affected patients, although it should not be overlooked as a symptom of advanced esophageal metastatic disease secondary to either neoplastic invasion or compression of the recurrent laryngeal nerve. This statement holds true also in patients with RCC and metastasis to the supraclavicular area. In a review of the distribution of infraclavicular primary tumors in patients with metastasis to the supraclavicular area, Sagheb et al reported renal carcinoma in 8 out of 73 cases. Supraclavicular metastasis was the presenting sign in 2 of the 8 described cases. The diagnosis of metastatic disease preceded the diagnosis of the primary renal carcinoma in 1 patient. The most common presenting symptoms were swelling, pain, and paraesthesia.[105] Renal carcinoma also can cause dysphonia by metastasizing to various structures along the vocal tract. Disease metastasis to the base of tongue and palatine tonsils can lead to change in voice quality by altering vocal tract resonance. In 2000, Navarro et al described a 62-year-old man who presented with pleuritic and chest pain. CT of the chest showed multiple lung nodules, enlarged mediastinal lymph nodes, and a left supraclavicular mass. Head and neck examination revealed a base of tongue lesion, the biopsy of which demonstrated RCC. The patient was treated with chemotherapy followed by interstitial radiation.[67] Massaccesi et al described a 76-year-old patient with RCC who developed metastasis to the palatine tonsil 3 years following a nephrectomy. The patient had bone metastasis at multiple sites that was treated by palliative radiation therapy prior to his presentation. Incisional biopsy from the tonsillar lesion revealed metastasis clear cell RCC.[106]

Depression and Anxiety in Patients With Renal Cell Carcinoma

Depression and anxiety are common in patients with cancer. In a study by Thekdi et al on 287 patients with RCC, near half of the patients scored above the scale cut-offs for depression. The authors reported a strong association between depression, post-traumatic stress syndrome (PTSS), and cancer-related symptoms. Moreover, patients with comorbid depression and PTSS suffered excessive fatigue and sleep disturbances.[107] There is also growing evidence in the literature to suggest that depression and anxiety are not only psychological burdens in patients with cancer but also are poor prognostic factors with adverse effect on disease progression and overall survival.[108,109] In a study by Cohen et al on the predictive role of depressive symptoms, the authors proved that depression is an important predictor of survival. Circadian rhythm alterations and genomic pathways also were assessed using genome transcriptional profile in 217 patients with RCC.[110] These findings are in agreement with the well-known, stress-induced tumor angiogenesis. This phenomenon is mediated via the cAMP-PKA pathway, the activation of which has been shown to promote tumor growth.[111] These findings lead us to conclude that psychosocial screening for depression and stress-related disorders is essential in patients with RCC, and that the integration of psychological care is paramount in the standard care of these patients.[112] Measurements of several inflammatory markers such as C-reactive protein (CRP) may prove useful in predicting stress and depressive symptoms in affected patients.[113] Otolaryngologists should be aware of these concerns since they may diagnose RCC in patients with dysphonia long after treatment of the primary tumor. Referral for further evaluation is appropriate but might be missed if not initiated by the otolaryngologist.

The previous reports have important clinical implications on voice given the well-known association between psychological stress, depression, and phonation. Holmqvist et al investigated the effect of stress reaction on voice using a questionnaire and reported a significant association between vocal symptoms and stress symptoms, especially in women. The study was conducted on 1728 subjects, and 10 symptoms related to stress and voice were used. Muscle tension in the throat correlated with all stress symptoms.[114] The impact of psychological stress on voice has also been substantiated by numerous studies showing acoustic alterations in affected patients. Weeks et al reported an increase in the fundamental frequency during the performance of social

threat tasks and highlighted the importance of vocal pitch as an indicator of social anxiety disorders with gender-specific differentiation.[115] Similarly, Mundt et al, in their investigation on vocal acoustic biomarkers of depression, reported changes in the prosodic features of speech with prolongation of speech pauses. The study was conducted on 105 patients with major depression, and speech samples were collected using an automated telephone system. Moreover, the aforementioned changes in speech pattern improved following treatment.[116] Another important acoustic parameter that is affected markedly by depression is jitter, the cycle-to-cycle variation in fundamental frequency. Ozdas et al reported jitter to be a significant discriminator between patients with psychological distress who were near-suicidal in comparison to nondepressed subjects.[117]

In summary, given the high prevalence of depressive symptoms in patients with renal carcinoma, and given the impact of psychological burden on voice, physicians should be aware that patients with renal carcinoma and depression probably are at increased risk of having dysphonia. This conclusion remains hypothetical. Future studies looking at the prevalence of dysphonia in patients with renal carcinoma and depression versus patients with renal carcinoma and no depression is needed.

Therapy-Induced Dysphonia in Patients With Renal Carcinoma

RCC is a very morbid condition. Almost one-third of affected patients have metastatic disease at the time of presentation.[37,38] This high metastatic rate presents a major challenge that is hard to overcome with surgery alone, be it simple, partial, or radical nephrectomy. In patients with advanced disease, other forms of adjuvant therapies are needed. These include external beam radiotherapy, arterial embolization before or after surgery, and systemic therapy in the form of immunotherapy and/or antiangiogenic targeted therapy. Given the well-known hypervascularity of renal carcinoma, patients with metastatic disease usually are treated in a sequential manner with antiangiogenic medications, namely, inhibitors of the vascular endothelial growth factor (VEGF) pathway, and of the mammalian target of rapamycin pathway. The approved tyrosine kinase inhibitors that target the VEGF pathway or axis are sorafenib, lenvatinib, and cabozantinib, in addition to sunitinib and axitinib.[118] Although targeted therapy has improved the 5-year survival in patients with advanced metastatic disease, the improvement came at a cost. Dysphonia has been reported as an adverse event in up to 30% of patients treated with antiangiogenic therapy.[119] The etiology of dysphonia in affected patients is not well understood. Suggested mechanisms include edema of the vocal folds and/or ischemia of the overlying mucosal cover.[119] Other known adverse effects of antiangiogenic therapy that might impact voice are related to the gastrointestinal system. Diarrhea, vomiting, and nausea are reported frequently as adverse events, similar to those reported in chemotherapy. In a study on the overall survival of patients with advanced RCC treated with tyrosine kinase inhibitors (cabozantinib) versus inhibitor of mTOR (everolimus), the major side effects reported in the former group were diarrhea, anemia, and hypomagnesaemia in 13%, 6%, and 5% of cases, respectively.[120] In another study looking at the efficacy of third-line targeted therapy in patients with advanced RCC who failed prior VEGF inhibitor therapy, dovitinib, a tyrosine-kinase that inhibits VEGF

and fibroblast growth factor pathways, was associated with diarrhea in 20% of cases.[121] Similarly, in a study on the effect of lenvatinib combined with everolimus in the treatment of metastatic RCC, 20% of patients suffered from diarrhea.[122] Given the paramount role of hydration in phonation, it is reasonable to conclude that the aforementioned gastrointestinal side effects associated with targeted therapy and/or chemotherapy have an adverse impact on voice.[123] In addition, patients with diarrhea often cannot tighten abdominal muscles firmly and consistently, thereby undermining "support," the power source of the voice. This can lead to dysphonia associated with compensatory hyperfunction of neck muscles. More details on chemotherapy and voice can be found in the literature.[124]

Another important treatment-induced side effect that is often underrated in patients with advanced RCC is fatigue. Fatigue is defined as "a distressing, persistent, and subjective sense of tiredness related to cancer or cancer treatment that is not proportional to recent activity or usual functioning."[125] It is a common adverse event of chemotherapy and/or targeted therapy,[119,126] with potentially a dire impact on voice.[127] According to a study by Larkin et al, 1 out of 2 patients with RCC undergoing treatment reports various grades of fatigue, and 1 out of 3 suffers from high-grade fatigue.[128] This is in agreement with a study by Curt based on 2 large national surveys on fatigue in cancer patients, which further confirms that fatigue is a long-lasting burden with a strong impact on quality of life of patients undergoing chemotherapy.[129] In a study by Motzer et al on the efficacy of everolimus, an inhibitor of the mammalian target of rapamycin, 1 out of 5 patients experienced mild to moderate fatigue as an adverse event to treatment. The study was conducted on 410 patients who had progression of metastatic RCC despite treatment with VEGF inhibitors.[130] In another study comparing sorafenib, a VEGF pathway inhibitor, with dovitinib, fatigue was an adverse event in 8% and 10% of the cases, respectively.[121] The pathophysiology of fatigue related to cancer treatment is multifaceted. In addition to the disturbance in muscle metabolism and function, and to the alterations in serotonin and cytokine production, there is myelosuppression and thyroid dysfunction, all of which may exacerbate the subjective symptom of fatigue experienced by patients.[131–133] Given the seriousness of fatigue as a complaint in patients with RCC on therapy, the National Comprehensive Cancer Network advocated 4 strategies for the management of cancer-related fatigue, be it disease or treatment induced. The first and second strategies are based on patients' counselling, education, and self-monitoring for the purpose of energy conservation. The third strategy focuses on energy restoration through activity enhancement, improvement in sleeping pattern, and psychosocial engagement. The use of medications such as psychostimulants is reserved as a last strategic tool.[128] The fatigue especially, but also its treatment, may affect voice.

The previous reports lead us to conclude that fatigue is a common adverse event of therapy in patients with renal cancer. The associated muscle weakness can negatively impact voice given that the larynx is a musculoskeletal structure. In professional voice users, this may be detrimental and can lead to physical, emotional, and financial burdens.

References

1. American Cancer Society. Cancer Facts and Figures 2019. Updated 2019. Accessed October 15, 2019. https://www.cancer.org /research/cancer-facts-statistics/all-cancer -facts-figures/cancer-facts-figures-2019.html

2. Rossi SH, Klatte T, Usher-Smith J, Stewart GD. Epidemiology and screening for renal cancer. *World J Urol*. 2018;36(9): 1341–1353.

3. Hock LM, Lynch J, Balaji KC. Increasing incidence of all stages of kidney cancer in the last 2 decades in the United States: an analysis of surveillance, epidemiology and end results program data. *J Urol*. 2002; 167(1):57–60.

4. Lightfoot N, Conlon M, Kreiger N, et al. Impact of noninvasive imaging on increased incidental detection of renal cell carcinoma. *Eur Urol*. 2000;37(5):521–527.

5. Wernli KJ, Rutter CM, Dachman AH, Zafar HM. Suspected extracolonic neoplasms detected on CT colonography: literature review and possible outcomes. *Acad Radiol*. 2013;20(6):667–674.

6. Welch HG, Skinner JS, Schroeck FR, Zhou W, Black WC. Regional variation of computed tomographic imaging in the United States and the risk of nephrectomy. *JAMA Intern Med*. 2018;178(2):221–227.

7. Ochsner MG. Renal cell carcinoma: five year follow-up study of 70 cases. *J Urol*. 1965;93: 361–363.

8. Miyamoto R, Helmus C. Hypernephroma metastatic to the head and neck. *Laryngoscope*. 1973;83(6):898–905.

9. Lotan Y, Karam JA, Shariat SF, et al. Renal-cell carcinoma risk estimates based on participants in the prostate, lung, colorectal, and ovarian cancer screening trial and national lung screening trial. *Urol Oncol*. 2016;34(4):167.e9–16.

10. Hunt JD, van der Hel OL, McMillan GP, Boffetta P, Brennan P. Renal cell carcinoma in relation to cigarette smoking: meta-analysis of 24 studies. *Int J Cancer*. 2005;114(1):101–108.

11. Ljungberg B, Bensalah K, Canfield S, et al. EAU guidelines on renal cell carcinoma: 2014 update. *Eur Urol*. 2015;67(5):913–924.

12. Starke N, Singla N, Haddad A, Lotan Y. Long-term outcomes in a high-risk bladder cancer screening cohort. *BJU Int*. 2016; 117(4):611–617.

13. Theis RP, Dolwick Grieb SM, Burr D, Siddiqui T, Asal NR. Smoking, environmental tobacco smoke, and risk of renal cell cancer: a population-based case-control study. *BMC Cancer*. 2008;8:387.

14. Renehan AG, Tyson M, Egger M, Heller RF, Zwahlen M. Body-mass index and incidence of cancer: a systematic review and meta-analysis of prospective observational studies. *Lancet*. 2008;371(9612):569–578.

15. Adams KF, Leitzmann MF, Albanes D, et al. Body size and renal cell cancer incidence in a large US cohort study. *Am J Epidemiol*. 2008;168(3):268–277.

16. Luo J, Margolis KL, Adami HO, et al. Body size, weight cycling, and risk of renal cell carcinoma among postmenopausal women: the Women's Health Initiative (United States). *Am J Epidemiol*. 2007;166(7):752–759.

17. Chow WH, Gridley G, Fraumeni JF Jr, Jarvholm B. Obesity, hypertension, and the risk of kidney cancer in men. *N Engl J Med*. 2000;343(18):1305–1311.

18. Binderup ML, Bisgaard ML, Harbud V, et al. Von Hippel-Lindau disease (vHL). National clinical guideline for diagnosis and surveillance in Denmark. 3rd ed. *Dan Med J*. 2013;60(12):B4763.

19. Wong G, Howard K, Webster AC, Chapman JR, Craig JC. Screening for renal cancer in recipients of kidney transplants. *Nephrol Dial Transplant*. 2011;26(5):1729–1739.

20. Kalble T, Lucan M, Nicita G, et al. EAU guidelines on renal transplantation. *Eur Urol*. 2005;47(2):156–166.

21. Clark MA, Shikanov S, Raman JD, et al. Chronic kidney disease before and after partial nephrectomy. *J Urol*. 2011;185(1):43–48.

22. Lowrance WT, Ordoñez J, Udaltsova N, Russo P, Go AS. CKD and the risk of incident cancer. *J Am Soc Nephrol*. 2014;25(10):2327–2334.

23. Nielsen SM, Rhodes L, Bianco I, et al. Von Hippel-Lindau disease: genetics and role of genetic counseling in a multiple neoplasia syndrome. *J Clin Oncol*. 2016; 34(18):2172–2181.

24. Gudbjartsson T, Jónasdóttir TJ, Thoroddsen A, et al. A population-based familial aggregation analysis indicates genetic contribution in a majority of renal cell carcinomas. *Int J Cancer*. 2002;100(4):476–479.

25. Su Kim D, Choi YD, Moon M, et al. Composite three-marker assay for early detection of kidney cancer. *Cancer Epidemiol Biomarkers Prev*. 2013;22(3):390–398.

26. Riccabona M, Szolar D, Preidler K, et al. Renal masses—evaluation by amplitude coded colour Doppler sonography and multiphasic contrast-enhanced CT. *Acta Radiol*. 1999; 40(4):457–461.

27. Jamis-Dow CA, Choyke PL, Jennings SB, Linehan WM, Thakore KN, Walther MM. Small (≤3-cm) renal masses: detection with CT versus US and pathologic correlation. *Radiology*. 1996;198(3):785–788.

28. Fenton JJ, Weiss NS. Screening computed tomography: will it result in overdiagnosis of renal carcinoma? *Cancer*. 2004;100(5): 986–990.

29. Campbell SC, Novick AC, Belldegrun A, et al. Guideline for management of the clinical T1 renal mass. *J Urol*. 2009;182(4): 1271–1279.

30. Ahmad AE, Finelli A, Jewett MAS. Surveillance of small renal masses. *Urology*. 2016;98:8–13.

31. Marconi L, Dabestani S, Lam TB, et al. Systematic review and meta-analysis of diagnostic accuracy of percutaneous renal tumour biopsy. *Eur Urol*. 2016;69(4):660–673.

32. Shingarev R, Jaimes EA. Renal cell carcinoma: new insights and challenges for a clinician scientist. *Am J Physiol Renal Physiol*. 2017;313:F145–F154.

33. Patard JJ, Leray E, Rioux-Leclercq N, et al. Prognostic value of histologic subtypes in renal cell carcinoma: a multicenter experience. *J Clin Oncol*. 2005;23(12):2763–2771.

34. Moch H. An overview of renal cell cancer: pathology and genetics. *Semin Cancer Biol*. 2013;23(1):3–9.

35. Algaba F, Akaza H, López-Beltrán A, et al. Current pathology keys of renal cell carcinoma. *Eur Urol.* 2011;60(4):634–643.

36. Ferlito A, Caruso G, Recher G. Secondary laryngeal tumors. Report of seven cases with review of the literature. *Arch Otolaryngol Head Neck Surg.* 1988;114(6):635–639.

37. Saitoh H. Distant metastasis of renal adenocarcinoma. *Cancer.* 1981;48(6):1487–1491.

38. Pagano S, Franzoso F, Ruggeri P. Renal cell carcinoma metastases. Review of unusual clinical metastases, metastatic modes and patterns and comparison between clinical and autopsy metastatic series. *Scand J Urol Nephrol.* 1996;30(3):165–172.

39. Greenberg RE, Cooper J, Krigel RL, Richter RM, Kessler H, Petersen RO. Hoarseness; a unique clinical presentation for renal cell carcinoma. *Urology.* 1992;40(2):159–161.

40. Hsiang-Che H, Chang KP, Ming Chen T, Kwai-Fong W, Ueng SH. Renal cell carcinoma metastases in the head and neck. *Chang Gung Med J.* 2006;29(4 Suppl):59–65.

41. Wong JA, Rendon RA. Progression to metastatic disease from a small renal cell carcinoma prospectively followed with an active surveillance protocol. *Can Urol Assoc J.* 2007;1(2):120–122.

42. Som PM, Norton KI, Shugar JM, et al. Metastatic hypernephroma to the head and neck. *AJNR Am J Neuroradiol.* 1987;8(6): 1103–1106.

43. Boles R, Cerny J. Head and neck metastases from renal cell carcinoma. *Mich Med.* 1971; 70(16):616–618.

44. Bernstein JM, Montgomery WW, Balogh K Jr. Metastatic tumors to the maxilla, nose and paranasal sinuses. *Laryngoscope.* 1966; 76(4):621–650.

45. Sabo R, Sela M, Sabo G, Herskovitz P, Feinmesser R. Metastatic hypernephroma to the head and neck: unusual case reports and review of the literature. *J Otolaryngol.* 2001;30(3):140–144.

46. MacKenzie DW, Waugh TR. Cystadenoma pseudo-papilliferum malignum of the kidney with metastasis in the tongue. *Urology.* 1927;18(4):331–346.

47. McNattin RF, Dean AL. A case of renal adenocarcinoma with unusual manifestations. *Amer J Cancer.* 1931;15:1570–1576.

48. Del Carmen BV, Korbitz BC. Oral metastasis from hypernephroma. *J Am Geriatr Soc.* 1970;18(9):743–746.

49. Schuknecht HF, Allam AF, Murakami Y. Pathology of secondary malignant tumors of the temporal bone. *Am Otol Rhinol Laryngol.* 1968;77(1):5–22.

50. Willis RA ed. *The Spread of tumors in the human body.* London, UK: Butterworths. 1952;296.

51. Amdur J, Leopold IH. Metastatic hypernephroma to the orbit. Report of a case and review of the literature. *Am J Ophthalmol.* 1959;48:386–388.

52. Curry NS, Schabel SI, Betsill WL Jr. Small renal neoplasms diagnostic imaging, pathologic features and clinical course. *Radiology.* 1986;158(1):113–117.

53. Serra A, Caltabiano R, Giorlandino A, et al. Nasal metastasis as the first manifestation of a metachronous bilateral renal cell carcinoma. *Pathologica.* 2017;109(4): 421–425.

54. Franzen AM, Günzel T, Lieder A. Parotid gland metastases of distant primary tumours: a diagnostic challenge. *Auris Nasus Larynx.* 2016;43(2):187–191.

55. Turner AL. Metastatic malignant tumor of the larynx secondary to adenocarcinoma of the right kidney. *J Laryngol Otol.* 1924;39: 181–194.

56. Oppikoder E. Metastasis of renal hypernephroma in upper respiratory tract and ear. *Arch f Ohren-Nasen-u Kehlkopf.* 1932;129: 271–292.

57. Maxwell JH. *Metastatic hypernephroma of the larynx.* Univ Hosp Med Bull Ann Arbor Mich. 1942.

58. Tamura H, Nakamoto M, Ein Fall, von Grawitz. Tumor mit metastase in kehlkopf. Monatsschr. *Ohrenheilkd Laryngorhinol.* 1956;354–357.

59. Fields JA. Renal carcinoma metastasis to the larynx. *Laryngoscope.* 1966;76(1):99– 101.

60. Maung R, Burke RC, Hwang WS. Metastatic renal carcinoma to larynx. *J Otolaryngol.* 1987;16(1):16–18.

61. Ferlito A, Pesavento G, Meli S, Recher G, Visoná A. Metastasis to the larynx revealing a renal cell carcinoma. *J Laryngol Otol.* 1987;101(8):843–850.

62. Mochimatsu I, Tsukuda M, Furukawa S, Sawaki S. Tumours metastasizing to the head and neck—a report of seven cases. *J Laryngol Otol.* 1993;107(12):1171–1173.

63. Marlowe SD, Swartz JD, Koenigsberg R, Zwillenberg S, Marlowe FI, Looby C. Metastatic hypernephroma to the larynx: an unusual presentation. *Neuroradiology.* 1993; 35(3):242–243.

64. Hittel JP, Born IA. Unusual metastatic site of a kidney carcinoma. A case report with review of the literature. *Laryngorhinootologie.* 1995;74(10):642–644.

65. Issing PR, Heermann R, Ernst A, Kuske M, Lenarz T. Distant metastasis of renal cell carcinomas to the head-neck area. *Laryngorhinootologie.* 1996;75(3):171–174.

66. Dee SL, Eshghi M, Otto CS. Laryngeal metastasis 7 years after radical nephrectomy. *Arch Pathol Lab Med.* 2000;124(12): 1833–1834.

67. Navarro F, Vicente J, Villanueva MJ, Sánchez A, Provencio M, España P. Metastatic renal cell carcinoma to the head and neck area. *Tumori.* 2000;86(1):88–90.

68. Rossini M, Bolzoni A, Piazza C, Peretti G. Renal cell carcinoma metastatic to the larynx. *Otolaryngol Head Neck Surg.* 2004;131 (6):1029–1030.

69. Stodulski D, Stankiewicz C, Skorek A. Renal cell carcinoma metastases to the head and neck. *Otolaryngologia polska.* 2006;60 (6):893–899.

70. Katsube Y, Tsukahara K, Nakamura K, et al. Treatment experience of the metastatic renal cell carcinomas to the head and neck region in our department. *Nihon Jibiinkoka Gakkai kaiho.* 2012;115(10):917–920.

71. Mehdi I, Satayapal N, Abdul Aziz MI. Renal cell carcinoma metastasizing to larynx: a case report. *Gulf J Oncolog.* 2012;(11):70–74.

72. Sarkis P, Bou-Malhab F, Mouaccadieh L. Solitary laryngeal metastasis from renal cell carcinoma of the kidney: clinical case and review of the literature. *Prog Urol.* 2012;22 (5):307–309.

73. Kradjian RM, Bennington JL. Renal carcinoma recurrent 31 years after nephrectomy. *Arch Surg.* 1965;90:192–195.

74. Becker M, Moulin G, Kurt AM, et al. Nonsquamous cell neoplasms of the larynx: radiologic-pathologic correlation. *Radiographics.* 1998;18(5):1189–1209.

75. Jonas D, Weber W, Beckert H, et al. Surgery of the primary tumor of metastasizing renal carcinoma. *Urol Int.* 1984;39(2):110–113.

76. Zhang X, Shen P, Yao J, Chen N, Liu J, Zeng H. Sunitinib rechallenge with dose escalation in progressive metastatic renal cell carcinoma: a case report and literature review. *Medicine (Baltimore).* 2018;97(31):e11565.

77. Tannir NM, Pal SK, Atkins MB. Second-line treatment landscape for renal cell carcinoma: a comprehensive review. *Oncologist.* 2018;23(5):540–555.

78. Wei C, Wang S, Ye Z, Chen Z. Efficacy of targeted therapy for advanced renal cell carcinoma: a systematic review and meta-analysis of randomized controlled trials. *Int Braz J Urol.* 2018;44(2):219–237.

79. Unverzagt S, Moldenhauer I, Nothacker M, et al. Immunotherapy for metastatic renal cell carcinoma. *Cochrane Database Syst Rev.* 2017;(5):CD011673.

80. Willis, RA. Metastatic tumors in the thyroid gland. *Am J Pathol.* 1931;7(3):187–208.

81. Abrahms HL, Spiro R, Goldstein N. Metastases in carcinoma: analysis of 1,000 autopsy cases. *Cancer.* 1950;3(1):74–85.

82. Brierre JT Jr, Dickinson LG. Clinically unsuspected thyroid disease. *GP.* 1964;30: 94–98.

83. Berge T, Lundberg S. Cancer in Malmo 1958–1969: an autopsy study. *Acta Pathol Microbiol Scand Suppl.* 1977;(260):1–235.

84. Shimaoka K, Sokal JE, Pickren JW. Metastatic neoplasms in the thyroid gland. Pathological and clinical findings. *Cancer.* 1962; 15:557–565.

85. Silverberg SG, Vidone RA. Metastatic tumors in the thyroid. *Pacific Med Surg.* 1966;74: 175–180.

86. Mortensen J, Woolner LB, Bennett WA. Secondary malignant tumors of the thyroid gland. *Cancer.* 1956;9(2):306–309.

87. Ericsson M, Biörklund A, Cederquist E, Ingemansson S, Åkerman M. Surgical treatment of metastatic disease in the thyroid gland. *J Surg Oncol.* 1981;17(1):15–23.

88. Czech JM, Lichtor TR, Carney JA, van Heerden JA. Neoplasms metastatic to the thyroid gland. *Surg Gynecol Obstet.* 1982; 155(4):503–505.

89. McCabe DP, Farrar WB, Petkov TM, Finkelmeier W, O'Dwyer P, James A. Clinical and pathologic correlations in disease metastatic to the thyroid gland. *Am J Surg.* 1985;150(4):519–523.

90. Hudson MA, Kavoussi LR, Catalona WJ. Bilateral renal cell carcinoma with metastasis to thyroid. *Urology.* 1991;37(2):145–148.

91. Halbauer M, Kardum-Skelin I, Vranesić D, Crepinko I. Aspiration cytology of renal-cell carcinoma metastatic to the thyroid. *Acta Cytologica.* 1991;35(4):443–446.

92. Niiyama H, Yamaguchi K, Nagai E, Furukawa K, Torisu M, Tanaka M. Thyroid gland metastasis from renal cell carcinoma masquerading as nodular goitre. *Aust N Z J Surg.* 1994;64(4):286–288.

93. Rosen IB, Walfish PG, Bain J, Bedard YC. Secondary malignancy of the thyroid gland and its management. *Ann Surg Oncol.* 1995; 2(3):252–256.

94. Nakhjavani MK, Gharib H, Goellner JR, van Heerden JA. Metastasis to the thyroid gland: a report of 43 cases. *Cancer.* 1997; 79(3):574–578.

95. Palazzo FF, Bradpiece HA, Morgan MW. Renal cell carcinoma metastasizing to the thyroid gland. *Scand J Urol Nephrol.* 1999; 33(3):202–204.

96. Chen H, Nicol TL, Udelsman R. Clinically significant, isolated metastatic disease to the thyroid gland. *World J Surg.* 1999;23(2): 177–181.

97. Kihara M, Yokomise H, Yamauchi A. Metastasis of renal cell carcinoma to the thyroid gland 19 years after nephrectomy: a case report. *Auris Nasus Larynx.* 2004;31 (1):95–100.

98. Papi G, Fadda G, Corsello SM, et al. Metastases to the thyroid gland: prevalence, clinicopathological aspects and prognosis: a 10-year experience. *Clin Endocrinol.* 2007; 66(4):565–571.

99. Demir L, Erten C, Somali I, et al. Metastases of renal cell carcinoma to the larynx and thyroid: two case reports on metastasis developing years after nephrectomy. *Can Urol Assoc J.* 2012;6(5):E209–212.

100. Gheorghiu ML, Iorgulescu R, Vrabie CD, Tupea CC, Ursu HI. Thyroid metastasis from clear cell carcinoma of the kidney 16 years after nephrectomy. *Acta Endocrinol.* 2016;12(1):80–84.

101. Pusztaszeri M, Wang H, Cibas ES, et al. Fine-needle aspiration biopsy of secondary neoplasms of the thyroid gland: a multi-institutional study of 62 cases. *Cancer Cytopathol.* 2015;123(1):19–29.

102. Izumo W, Ota M, Narumiya K, Shirai Y, Kudo K, Yamamoto M. Esophageal metastasis of renal cancer 10 years after nephrectomy. *Esophagus.* 2015;12(1):91–94.

103. Ali S, Atiquzzaman B, Krall K, Kumar R, Liu B, Hebert-Magee S. Not your usual suspect: clear cell renal cell carcinoma presenting as ulcerative esophagitis. *Cureus.* 2018; 10(6):e2821.

104. Padda MS, Si WM. Rare presentation of renal cell cancer as dysphagia: a case report. *J Med Case Rep.* 2019;13(1):89.

105. Sagheb K, Manz A, Albrich SB, Taylor KJ, Hess G, Walter C. Supraclavicular metastases from distant primary solid tumours: a retrospective study of 41 years. *J Maxillofac Oral Surg.* 2017;16(2):152–157.

106. Massaccesi M, Morganti AG, Serafini G, et al. Late tonsil metastases from renal cell cancer: a case report. *Tumori.* 2009;95(4): 521–524.

107. Thekdi SM, Milbury K, Spelman A, et al. Posttraumatic stress and depressive symptoms in renal cell carcinoma: association with quality of life and utility of single-

item distress screening. *Psychooncology.* 2015;24(11):1477–1484.

108. Satin JR, Linden W, Phillips MJ. Depression as a predictor of disease progression and mortality in cancer patients: a meta-analysis. *Cancer.* 2009;115(22):5349–5361.

109. Giese-Davis J, Collie K, Rancourt KM, Neri E, Kraemer HC, Spiegel D. Decrease in depression symptoms is associated with longer survival in patients with metastatic breast cancer: a secondary analysis. *J Clin Oncol.* 2011;29(4):413–420.

110. Cohen L, Cole SW, Sood AK, et al. Depressive symptoms and cortisol rhythmicity predict survival in patients with renal cell carcinoma: role of inflammatory signaling. *PloS One.* 2012;7(8):e42324.

111. Thaker PH, Han LY, Kamat AA, et al. Chronic stress promotes tumor growth and angiogenesis in a mouse model of ovarian carcinoma. *Nat Med.* 2006;12(8):939–944.

112. Holland J, Weiss T. The new standard of quality cancer care: integrating the psychosocial aspects in routine cancer from diagnosis through survivorship. *Cancer J.* 2008;14(6):425–428.

113. Eraly SA, Nievergelt CM, Maihofer AX, et al. Assessment of plasma C-reactive protein as a biomarker of posttraumatic stress disorder risk. *JAMA Psychiatry.* 2014;71(4):423–431.

114. Holmqvist S, Santtila P, Lindström E, Sala E, Simberg S. The association between possible stress markers and vocal symptoms. *J Voice.* 2013;27(6):787.e1–787.e10.

115. Weeks JW, Lee CY, Reilly AR, et al. "The Sound of Fear": assessing vocal fundamental frequency as a physiological indicator of social anxiety disorder. *J Anxiety Disord.* 2012;26(8):811–822.

116. Mundt JC, Vogel AP, Feltner DE, Lenderking WR. Vocal acoustic biomarkers of depression severity and treatment response. *Biol Psychiatry.* 2012;72(7):580–587.

117. Ozdas A, Shiavi RG, Silverman SE, Silverman MK, Wilkes DM. Investigation of vocal jitter and glottal flow spectrum as possible cues for depression and near-term suicidal risk. *IEEE Trans Biomed Eng.* 2004;51(9):1530–1540.

118. Hsieh JJ, Purdue MP, Signoretti S, et al. Renal cell carcinoma. *Nat Rev Dis Primers.* 2017;3:17009.

119. Saavedra E, Hollebecque A, Soria JC, Hartl DM. Dysphonia induced by antiangiogenic compounds. *Invest New Drugs.* 2014;32(4):774–782.

120. Choueiri TK, Escudier B, Powles T, et al. Cabozantinib versus everolimus in advanced renal cell carcinoma (METEOR): final results from a randomised, open-label, phase 3 trial. *Lancet Oncol.* 2016;17(7):917–927.

121. Motzer RJ, Porta C, Vogelzang NJ, et al. Dovitinib versus sorafenib for third-line targeted treatment of patients with metastatic renal cell carcinoma: an open-label, randomised phase 3 trial. *Lancet Oncol.* 2014;15(3):286–296.

122. Motzer RJ, Hutson TE, Glen H, et al. Lenvatinib, everolimus, and the combination in patients with metastatic renal cell carcinoma: a randomised, phase 2, open-label, multicentre trial. *Lancet Oncol.* 2015;16(15):1473–1482.

123. Solomon NP, DiMattia MS. Effects of a vocally fatiguing task and systemic hydration on phonation threshold pressure. *J Voice.* 2000;14(3):341–362

124. Sataloff RT, Castell DO, Katz PO, Sataloff DM, Hawkshaw MJ. Reflux and other gastroenterologic conditions that may affect the voice. In Sataloff RT. *Professional Voice: The Science and Art of Clinical Care.* San Diego, CA: Plural Publishing; 2017:907–998.

125. Cancer-related fatigue. Version 1, 2009. NCCN Clinical Practice Guidelines in Oncology. National Comprehensive Cancer Network. Accessed October, 15, 2019. https://www.nccn.org/store/login/login.aspx?ReturnURL=https://www.nccn.org/professionals/physician_gls/pdf/fatigue.pdf

126. Osorio JC, Motzer RJ, Voss MH. Optimizing treatment approaches in advanced renal cancer. *Oncology.* 2017;31(12):919–926, 928–930.

127. Hamdan AL, Sataloff RT, Hawkshaw MJ. Sleep, body fatigue, and voice. In: Hamdan AL, Sataloff RT, Hawkshaw M, eds. *Laryngeal Manifestations of Systemic Diseases*. San Diego, CA: Plural Publishing; 2018:83–86.

128. Larkin JM, Pyle LM, Gore ME. Fatigue in renal cell carcinoma: the hidden burden of current targeted therapies. *Oncologist*. 2010;15(11):1135–1146.

129. Curt GA. The impact of fatigue on patients with cancer: Overview of fatigue 1 and 2. *Oncologist*. 2000;5(Suppl 2):9–12.

130. Motzer RJ, Escudier B, Oudard S, et al. Efficacy of everolimus in advanced renal cell carcinoma: a double-blind, randomised, placebo-controlled phase III trial. *Lancet*. 2008;372(9637):449–456.

131. Montoya L. Managing hematologic toxicities in the oncology patient. *J Infus Nurs*. 2007;30(3):168–172.

132. Malik UR, Makower DF, Wadler S. Interferon-mediated fatigue. *Cancer*. 2001; 92(6 Suppl):1664–1668.

133. Torino F, Corsello SM, Longo R, Barnabel A, Gasparini G. Hypothyroidism related to tyrosine kinase inhibitors: an emerging toxic effect of targeted therapy. *Nat Rev Clin Oncol*. 2009;6(4):219–228.

11

Gastric Cancer and Voice

Abdul-Latif Hamdan, Robert Thayer Sataloff, and Mary J. Hawkshaw

Epidemiology and Risk Factors

Carcinoma of the stomach is the fifth most common cancer in the world.[1] The estimated number of newly diagnosed cases worldwide in 2019 was 27 510.[2] It is more common in elderly persons above the age of 70 years, and men are more affected than women.[2] The prevalence is higher in overpopulated and low socioeconomic countries such as in parts of Asia and South America, in comparison to countries in North America and North Europe.[3–5] In Eastern countries, the prevalence is on the rise partially due to the aging population and partially due to improved screening.[6,7] Gastric carcinoma has a poor prognosis as only 1 of 4 patients is diagnosed at an early stage.[8] The 5-year survival is low worldwide and does not exceed 31% across all stages.[2] In the United States, it ranges between 5% in patients with distant metastasis and 67% in patients with localized disease. It is the third leading cause of cancer-related deaths worldwide, and it accounts for 1 of 12 cancer-related mortalities.[9] The total number of gastric-cancer deaths in 2019 was 783 000 worldwide, with 11 140 mortalities reported in the United States. The death rates have decreased over the last 3 decades, especially in Japan, because of aggressive screening and early diagnosis.[2,10]

The etiology of gastric cancer is multifactorial. Infectious agents, most importantly *Helicobacter pylori*, have been strongly implicated. Patients who are seropositive for *H pylori* are 3 times more likely to develop gastric cancer in comparison to those who are seronegative.[11,12] The etiologic role of *H pylori* is not surprising given the well-known association between *H pylori* infection and many inflammatory and neoplastic gastric pathologies, the most common of which is mucosa-associated lymphoid tissue (MALT) lymphoma. Infection with *H pylori* results in the release of reactive oxygen species that lead to DNA hypermethylation and mutations along the course of the disease.[13] Based on a large review by Lu and Li, eradication of *H pylori* is a strategic step toward the prevention of gastric carcinoma, the success of which varies among affected individuals.[14] Another infectious agent that contributes to the development of gastric cancer, but to a lesser extent, is Epstein-Barr virus (EBV).[15] In a meta-analysis that included 15 952 patients with gastric carcinoma, the pooled prevalence of EBV infection was estimated as 8.7%, with men being twice more affected than women. The prevalence of EBV infection was higher in cardial and/or antral tumors, and in gastric remnants following gastrectomy.[16] Gastric cancer also has been linked to genetic polymorphism and to the expression of inflammatory mediators, such as tumor necrosis factor-α. Inflammatory mediators induce an exaggerated suppression of gastric acidity, which acts as a trigger for the precancerous cascade that starts with atrophic gastritis and ends with gastric cancer.[17-19] In 2006, Camargo et al performed a meta-analysis looking at the link between polymorphism of interleukin-1β and its receptor antagonist genes, and gastric cancer. The authors reported a strong association between the 2 in Caucasians and not in Asians. The association was more significant in the noncardial type of cancer.[17]

Environmental risk factors and dietary habits also play crucial roles in the pathogenesis of gastric carcinoma. The etiologic role of alcohol intake and smoking has been supported by some and refuted by others. Increased exposure of the gastric mucosa to acetaldehyde, an intermediate in alcohol fermentation and a key carcinogenic compound present in tobacco smoke, has been shown to enhance the formation of cancer.[20] However, in a large case-control study that included 915 patients with gastric cancer, Gao et al reported only a minor role for smoking and alcohol intake in cancer of the upper gastrointestinal system.[21] A high intake of salt and processed meat also has been identified as a contributing factor to the development of gastric cancer.[4,22] In a study by Jooseens et al looking at the etiologic role of dietary salt in a large cohort of patients from 24 countries, the authors reported a moderate correlation between gastric carcinoma mortality and the intake of sodium in both men and women (0.70 and 0.74, respectively). When combined with nitrate, the adjusted ratios increased to 0.77

and 0.63 in men and women, respectively.[23] Similarly, in an investigation by Gonzalez et al on the role of dietary intake of meat in gastric carcinogenesis, the authors demonstrated a significant association between noncardial cancer and the intake of total meat, red meat, and processed meat, with hazard ratios of 3.52, 1.73, and 2.45, respectively. The association was more significant in patients with H pylori infection, in comparison to those with no H pylori infection. The study included 521 457 patients from 10 different European countries.[22] In addition, genetic predisposition is an important host factor in patients with gastric carcinoma. In a meta-analysis by Loh et al that included 203 studies and in which 225 polymorphisms across 95 genes were assessed, the authors reported a significant association between gastric carcinoma and 37 polymorphisms across 27 genes in Asians. There also was a significant association between gastric carcinoma and 12 polymorphisms across 11 genes in Caucasians.[18]

There are different classifications of gastric carcinoma. Based on their morphologic appearance, tumors are stratified as polypoid, ulcerative with or without well-defined borders, or infiltrative. Tumors also are classified based on their cell of origin, tumor mutations, tissue markers, and the presence or absence of intercellular junctions.[24-26] Other classifications are based on tumor anatomical location, as cardial versus distal types, degree of invasion, mucosal, submucosal, and with or without advanced lymph node metastasis. In terms of location, gastric cancer occurs most commonly in the upper third of the stomach in association with adenocarcinoma of the lower esophagus.[27,28] It is less frequent in the lower and mid-third of the stomach, and spans the entire stomach in less than 7% of cases.[27] Recent reports indicate an increase in the prevalence of proximal tu-

mors probably due to the rising incidence of gastroesophageal reflux disease.[29] Affected patients may be asymptomatic until the late stages of the disease. Early symptoms include dyspepsia and nausea, whereas late symptoms include abdominal pain, vomiting, hematemesis, anemia, and weight loss. Only 20% of patients are diagnosed at an early stage of the disease, with differences in the clinicopathologic picture being noted between age groups.[24] In a study by Manuel in 2018, diffuse infiltrative cancer and less differentiated cancer were more common in the younger group in comparison to the older group (70% versus 33.7%, respectively, and 63.4% versus 33.1%, respectively).[30] In a large study looking at the impact of age on the clinical presentation of patients with gastric carcinoma, Waddah et al reported that young patients were more likely to present with advanced disease and distant metastasis. However, their adjusted, stage-stratified relative survival was more favorable.[31] The contention that younger patients have a worse prognosis because of the advanced stage of the disease at the time of diagnosis remains controversial.[30,31] In a large study by Santoro et al that included 508 patients with gastric cancer, younger patients were found to have more advanced disease but similar prognosis when matched with older patients according to stage of disease.[32] However, in a large review of 3818 patients with gastric cancer, by Isobe et al, the 5-year survival was worse in the younger group in comparison to the older group. Depth of invasion and high local and distant metastatic rates were 2 of the reasons suggested for the worse 5-year survival.[33] Another potential cause for the worse prognosis is perineural invasion as reported by Zhou et al in their review of the clinicopathologic features of gastric carcinoma in young patients.[34]

In view of the high morbidity of gastric cancer and its detrimental effect on the body, the possible mechanisms by which gastric carcinoma can cause dysphonia warrant consideration. A review of the literature on gastric-cancer–induced weight loss and fatigue and their impact on voice as well as of the association between targeted therapy and dysphonia guides voice clinicians called on to care for patients with this potentially devastating disease.

Disease-Induced Dysphonia in Patients With Gastric Carcinoma

Metastasis of Gastric Carcinoma to the Head and Neck and Its Impact on Voice

Gastric carcinoma can metastasize to various sites in the body. The metastasis is either hematogenous or through the lymphatic route. The sites affected most commonly are the visceral lymph nodes, peritoneum, omentum, liver, and lungs.[35,36] The head and neck are rarely affected, with infrequent involvement of the cervical lymph nodes, skin, salivary glands, and tonsils. Bhatia et al investigated the frequency of abnormal cervical lymph nodes using ultrasound with or without fine-needle aspiration in 223 patients with gastric carcinoma. The authors reported a prevalence of 6%, 50% of whom had metastatic disease.[37] Rajeshwari et al reported a patient with gastric malignancy and cutaneous metastasis in the neck, highlighting the importance of early diagnosis of these lesions in the management of visceral primary malignancies.[38] Similarly, Gunduz et al described a patient with gastric adenocarcinoma who presented with multiple cutaneous lesions in the head and neck, and they stressed the relatively high frequency (10%) of skin metastasis in patients with visceral malignancies.[39] Emanuelli et al reported 11 patients with parotid cancer from distant primary tumors, one of whom had gastric carcinoma. The authors emphasized the role of immunohistochemistry in the diagnosis of metastatic lesions.[40] The tonsils are also a common metastatic target in patients with gastric carcinoma.[41,42] In their review of the literature, Gallo et al highlighted the commonality in the clinical picture of patients with gastric cancer and tonsillar metastasis, and that of patients with infectious or lymphoproliferative diseases.[42] A less frequently affected metastatic site in patients with gastric carcinoma is the internal auditory canal. Kim et al reported the first case of internal auditory canal metastasis secondary to leptomeningeal carcinomatosis in a patient with gastric carcinoma. The patient had vertigo, facial palsy, and hearing loss.[43]

There are no reports in the literature of gastric carcinoma metastasis to the larynx. Nevertheless, metastasis of gastric carcinoma to structures contiguous with the larynx and along the vocal tract puts the phonatory system in jeopardy. Future research looking at the vocal characteristics of patients with gastric carcinoma and metastasis to the tonsils, salivary glands, and/or cervical lymph nodes with possible compression or invasion of the recurrent laryngeal nerve is warranted.

Gastric Carcinoma-Induced Weight Loss and Its Impact on Voice

Weight loss is a common problem in patients with gastric carcinoma. A study by Andreyav et al showed that 85% of patients with gastric carcinoma have weight loss, and 1 out of 3 suffers a weight loss that exceeds 10%.[44] In a study by Manuel et al

on the clinical characteristics of 207 patients with distal gastric carcinoma, weight loss and gastric pain were the main symptoms. Younger patients had a higher rate of advanced-stage disease and a lower 5-year survival rate.[31] These results are in agreement with the study of Seker et al on the clinicopathologic features of 133 patients with gastric carcinoma. The authors reported weight loss and abdominal pain in 51.2% and 67.0% of cases, respectively.[45] In another review by Liu et al which included 2163 patients with gastric carcinoma undergoing curative gastrectomy, 70.3% had weight loss less than 3 kg, and 29.7% had weight loss more than 3 kg. Moreover, elevated prognostic nutritional index and preoperative weight loss were associated with anemia.[46]

Cancer-induced weight loss may affect the voice by altering the shape and configuration of the vocal tract, particularly in overweight and obese patients. Numerous studies have shown that subjects with high body mass index have excessive fat deposition in the lateral palatopharyngeal walls, base of tongue, and submental area.[47-49] A decrease in weight may reduce the concentration of these fat depositions, leading to an alteration in the configuration of the vocal tract and subsequently to a change in the position and distribution of formant frequencies.[50] Moreover, a decrease in weight may reduce laryngeal resistance by decreasing tissue bulk in the vocal tract. Solomon et al, in their study on weight loss and voice, reported an association between phonatory threshold pressure and body mass index. Weight-loss–induced reduction in laryngeal resistance can result in a decrease in the pressure needed to set the vocal folds into association.[51] Weight loss also may impact phonation through its effect on the respiratory system. Impairment in breathing capacity secondary to decreased diaphragmatic contraction, or to lung compression or invasion, jeopardizes the power supply of phonation. Similarly, weight-loss–induced alteration in sex hormones levels may adversely impact voice, given that the larynx is a hormone target. The impact is mediated through the well-known proliferative and rheologic effects of estrogen and testosterone on the vocal folds. A more detailed discussion on the impact of weight loss on voice can be found in the book *Obesity and Voice.*[52]

When weight loss is severe enough to interfere with daily bodily functions, it is often referred to as cachexia. Cachexia by definition is a syndrome that refers to loss of skeletal muscle mass that leads to dysfunction in daily activities. The process of weight loss is progressive and may or may not be accompanied by loss of fat tissue.[53] Affected patients suffer from nausea, generalized pain, dysgeusia, fatigue, and poor appetite. These symptoms not only impact disease survival and complication rate in patients with gastric carcinoma, but they also impair the function of many systems in the body, including the phonatory system.[54-56] Voice is linked strongly to general well-being. Preservation of lean body mass is important for the daily function of any musculoskeletal structure in the body including the larynx. A decrease in muscle mass and function can be detrimental to phonation, especially in professional voice users who rely on physical fitness for optimal voice performance. To that end, the monitoring of inflammatory markers such as C-reactive protein and others is helpful for early identification of cancer cachexia. Body composition analysis using dual-energy x-ray absorptiometry, computed tomography, or bioimpedance, also may assist following up affected patients.[57-59] Once detected, cancer-induced decrease in muscle mass should alert the physician to the increased risk of dysphonia in affected

patients, and to the urgent need to restore muscle mass. Restoration of muscle mass can be achieved through enhancement of dietary habits and nutrition, and by reversing metabolic abnormalities through pharmacologic interventions.

Gastric-Cancer–Induced Fatigue and Its Impact on Voice

Cancer-related fatigue is a well-recognized condition leading patients to experience a need to rest. It is thought of as a protective response to avoid excessive exertion, even though the desire to rest may not be commensurate with the preceding amount of effort exerted. Fatigue is a common complaint in patients with cancer with an estimated prevalence of 70% to 100%.[60] This sensation has been investigated thoroughly in the literature in attempts to mitigate this symptom and provide preventive measures. The pathophysiology of fatigue has been based primarily on hematologic and endocrine variations reported commonly in affected patients.[61,62] In a review by Ryan et al, several mechanisms were proposed among which are alterations in muscle function, dysregulation in 5-HT neurotransmitter, and activation of vagal afferent pathways.[63] Patients with gastric carcinoma are more subject to fatigue given the marked weight loss secondary to gastrointestinal obstruction and the decrease in caloric intake.[31,44] The associated decrease in muscle function and strength also is compounded by the presence of metabolic alterations and comorbidities such as vitamin B12 and vitamin D deficiencies. In a study by Zou et al that included 203 patients with gastric cancer, 91.6% of cases reported fatigue as clinically relevant. Less than half of those affected had no prior chemotherapy or history of mental or cognitive impairment. Of interest in this study was the negative association between resilience and cancer-related fatigue. Resilience, defined as "a process or capacity that maintains an individual's physical and psychological well-being,"[64] explained the variation in the manifestation of cancer-related fatigue among cancer patients. Other important factors that mediated the relationship between fatigue and patients with gastric cancer were symptoms of dyspnea, dyspepsia, change in bowel habits, and exercise. Park et al reported a significant association between these symptoms and fatigue in a survey that included 42 patients with fatigue and 157 patients without fatigue.[65]

When present, fatigue carries a significant burden on quality of life of affected patients. Emotional, physical, and functional components are all affected. Given the strong link between phonation and body fatigue, more so in professional voice users, patients with gastric carcinoma suffering from fatigue are almost certainly more prone to develop vocal symptoms. This conclusion remains hypothetical, and future studies in this field are needed.

Depression in Patients With Gastric Carcinoma and Its Impact on Voice

Emotional disturbances are common in patients with cancer, the most prevalent of which is a mixture of depression and anxiety.[66] In a cross-sectional study by Brintzenhofe-Szoc et al looking at cancer-specific prevalence of anxiety and depression, higher rates were observed in patients with gastric and pancreatic cancer in comparison to those with breast cancer. Overall, anxiety and depression symptoms were observed in 24% and 18.3% of cases, respectively. The study included 8265 cancer patients, and the prevalence of anxiety and depression was retrieved using the Brief Symptom Inventory.[67] Hu et al conducted a retrospective study looking at the incidence of depressive disorders in 28 753 patients with gastric cancer in comparison to 28 753 matched controls.[68] The results indicated a higher cumulative incidence in the study group versus the control group. The difference between the 2 groups was attributed to the high emotional stress experienced by gastric cancer patients who were often diagnosed at a late stage of the disease. The psychological distress experienced by patients with gastric cancer varies with the anatomical location of the tumor and knowledge of cancer diagnosis. Bergquist et al reported a higher rate of depression in patients with gastroesophageal junction cancer versus those with distal gastric cancer.[69] Similarly, Tavoli et al reported higher scores for anxiety and depression in patients who knew about their diagnosis versus those who did not. The study was conducted on 142 patients with gastrointestinal cancer, 30% of whom had gastric carcinoma. Using the Hospital Anxiety and Depression Scale, the odds ratios for anxiety and depression were 2.7 and 2.8, respectively.[70] The ability to cope with stress in patients with gastric cancer seems to be linked to brain-derived neurotrophic factors (BDNFs). In a study by Koh et al that included 91 patients with gastric cancer, the authors demonstrated an association between the style of coping with cancer measured using the mini-Mental Adjustment to Cancer Scale, and polymorphism in BDNF Val66Met. The authors also alluded to the predictive role of genotyping in the coping style adopted.[71] What is more worrisome is the adverse effect of depression on survival rate in affected patients. In a large study by Yu et al investigating the link between depression and survival rate, the authors reported a significantly elevated mortality risk hazard ratio

(HR = 3.34) in a group of 300 patients with gastric cancer.[72]

This leads us to conclude that patients with gastric carcinoma are at a higher risk of developing depression and anxiety along the course of the disease. Given the strong link between psychogenic stress and voice,[73] a higher prevalence of dysphonia in patients with gastric cancer is predicted. Future studies investigating phonatory disturbances in patients with gastric carcinoma and psychological burdens versus patients with gastric carcinoma and no psychological burdens are needed.

Treatment-Induced Dysphonia in Patients With Gastric Carcinoma

Surgery-Induced Dysphonia in Patients With Gastric Carcinoma

Surgery is the mainstay treatment of gastric carcinoma. The type of gastrectomy and lymph node dissection vary with the location of the tumor, its extent, and the stage of the disease. Proximal gastrectomy is performed for patients with tumors in the upper half of the stomach, whereas distal gastrectomy is performed for patients with tumors located in the distal half of the stomach. Total gastrectomy is usually advocated in patients with advanced gastric carcinoma.[74,75] Three main approaches for gastrectomy have been described, each with its own advantages and disadvantages. These include the open, laparoscopic, and endoscopic approaches. The open and laparoscopic approaches frequently are performed in patients in whom radical surgery with extended lymph node dissection is recommended, with shorter recovery and better quality of life being reported in patients who undergo the laparoscopic approach.[75–78] Endoscopic mucosal resection and endoscopic submucosal dissection are recommended for patients with lesions confined to the mucosa and/or submucosa. The scope of application of endoscopic mucosal resection and endoscopic submucosal dissection expanded over the last decade to include more patients with a wider spectrum of disease. Irrespective of the type of surgery performed or approach used, the postoperative period of patients undergoing gastrectomy is invariably turbulent. Patients have a marked reduction in quality of life in several ways. In a study by Lim et al looking at the quality of life and nutrition in surviving gastric-cancer patients, the authors reported lower quality of life in those who survived for less than 1 year, as well as those who survived for more than 1 year. The authors emphasized the importance of nutrition in gastrectomy patients and the need to intervene early in order to enhance the quality of life of affected patients.[79] In another study on the quality of life of patients undergoing laparoscopic-assisted distal gastrectomy in comparison to open distal subtotal gastrectomy, Sou Lee et al reported worsening of physical, emotional, and social functioning in both groups of patients. Change in dietary habits, early satiety, loss of appetite, and fatigue were some of the adverse events experienced in the short and prolonged postoperative period. The study included 80 patients who were assessed during a period that extended from a few months postoperatively through 5 years.[80] Clearly, gastrectomy patients suffer malnutrition that leads to weight loss and fatigue. Given the strong link between phonation and general well-being, gastrectomy patients who experience weight loss and fatigue are at high risk of developing vocal symptoms.

Reflux is another important comorbidity commonly encountered in patients undergoing surgery for gastric carcinoma. In a study by Karanicolas et al looking at the quality of life in patients who underwent partial gastrectomy versus complete gastrectomy, the former group had a higher prevalence of reflux. Moreover, patients who underwent proximal gastrectomy had more reflux than those who had distal gastrectomy (70% versus 35%).[81] In a prospective study by Avery et al on 58 patients with gastric carcinoma who underwent gastrectomy, the authors reported a decline in the functional aspect of quality of life. Reflux and dysphagia were among the common symptoms at baseline and at 6 months following treatment, in those who survived for more than 2 years, as well as in those who died in less than 2 years. Moreover, there was an increase in nausea and vomiting in both groups postoperatively. In conclusion, the authors emphasized the need to share with patients the adverse effects of surgery and the means to address those effects.[82] Similarly, Huang et al investigated the impact of clinical stage of gastric carcinoma and the type of gastrectomy on quality of life in a cross-sectional study that included 51 disease-free gastric adenocarcinoma patients. The prevalence of reflux disease increased following surgery in both early and late stages of the disease, with a higher percentage reported in the total gastrectomy group in comparison to the subtotal gastrectomy group (17% versus 13%).[83]

These reports are in agreement with numerous studies on reflux in gastrectomy patients. There is mounting evidence in the literature to support the high prevalence of gastroesophageal reflux disease (GERD) following bariatric surgery, particularly sleeve resection. The symptoms reported most commonly reported are heartburn, vomiting, and regurgitation. The progression of GERD or its *de novo* occurrence in patients following partial gastrectomy has been attributed to alterations in the angle of His and/or to disruption of the lower esophageal sphincter.[84–88] As a result, gastrectomy patients are more likely to have retrograde flow of gastric contents into the laryngopharyngeal complex. The loss of an important anatomical reflux barrier can lead to inflammatory changes in the laryngeal mucosa, which in turn can lead to dysphonia. A thorough discussion on GERD and laryngopharyngeal reflux disease can be found in *Professional Voice: The Science and Art of Clinical Care*.[89]

Chemotherapy-Induced Dysphonia in Patients With Gastric Carcinoma

Chemotherapy in the form of cisplatin and fluoropyrimidine-based drugs is prescribed commonly as adjuvant or first-line therapy in patients with advanced gastric carcinoma.[75] This is in view of the fact that half of patients who undergo radical gastrectomy recur either locally or distantly despite the performance of extended lymph node dissection. Frequently reported side effects of chemotherapy are nausea, vomiting, and diarrhea, all of which often lead to dehydration and thickening of mucus. These emetic effects are encountered commonly with the use of cisplatin and more so with the use of a combination of emetogenic drugs in the management of gastric carcinoma.[90] Another adverse event of particular interest is chemotherapy-induced fatigue. Curt et al performed a study that looked at the prevalence of fatigue in 379 patients with cancer and reported the prevalence of daily fatigue in 30% of the cases, the majority of whom had to change their daily activities and routine. Moreover, 75% of those who were employed had to change their job because of the limitations in activity.[91] Based on national surveys by the same author looking at the impact of fatigue on patients with cancer, 76% experienced fatigue monthly, and the duration of the bouts extended to 2 weeks in almost one-third of the cases. The sensation of fatigue was reported as more intrusive and persistent than other side effects of chemotherapy. In almost half of the patients, fatigue had a marked and significant impact on quality of life.[91]

The previously discussed chemotherapy adverse events have a negative impact on voice. The associated systemic dehydration secondary to vomiting and diarrhea can lead to vocal changes given the paramount role of hydration in phonation. With thickening of laryngeal mucus, there is increased friction of the vocal folds during phonation, which may lead to vocal fold injury and pathology. Moreover, the acidic and nonacidic content of the refluxate material during vomiting may induce further laryngeal injury. Similarly, chemotherapy-induced fatigue can adversely impact voice, especially in professional voice users. A thorough discussion of chemotherapy and voice can be found in *Professional Voice: The Science and Art of Clinical Care.*[90]

Targeted Therapy-Induced Dysphonia in Patients With Gastric Carcinoma

Despite the efficacy of chemotherapy in patients with gastric carcinoma,[92,93] second-line targeted therapy is being advocated for patients with drug resistance. The fast evolution in molecular biology has not only improved the understanding of the variation in behavior of different gastric tumors, but also has spurred the identification of predictive factors and individualized treatment mo-

dalities. Both monoclonal antibodies such as bevacizumab or aflibercept (Regeneron Pharmaceuticals, New York) and tyrosine kinase inhibitors are now used to target genetic and epigenetic mutations in patients with metastatic gastric carcinoma.[94] This systemic therapy is recommended as an adjuvant therapy either perioperatively or postoperatively in patients with advanced gastric cancer who failed surgery and/or chemotherapy. Numerous adverse events to antiangiogenic therapy are described in the literature, among which is dysphonia. In 2010, Hartl et al reported 5 patients who developed dysphonia and abnormal Voice Handicap Index scores following treatment with antiangiogenic medications. All 5 cases were found to have whitish vocal fold mucosal lesions and a decrease in mucosal waves attributed to drug-induced ischemic changes.[95] In 2012, the same authors described a 46-year-old woman with metastatic adenocarcinoma who failed chemotherapy and was started on paclitaxel-bevacizumab. Three weeks following the start of monoclonal antibody therapy, the patient developed hoarseness with intermittent aphonia. On laryngeal examination, she had whitish plaques on her vocal folds with sparing of the anterior commissure. Microlaryngoscopy revealed disappearance of the mucosal lining at the middle two-thirds of the vocal folds. Histologic examination of a vocal fold biopsy taken showed signs of necrosis with surrounding inflammatory changes.[96] In 2014, Caruso et al described a 60-year-old woman with metastatic colon carcinoma who presented with dysphonia 1 week following the start of bevacizumab, an anti-vascular endothelial growth factor (anti-VEGF). On laryngeal examination, the patient had symmetrical whitish vocal fold mucosal lesions.[97] The patient failed antifungal treatment, and the lesions were attributed to a reduction in blood supply to the vocal folds' capillaries.[97,98] In a review by

Erika et al on side effects of antiangiogenic therapy, dysphonia was described among other systemic side effects. The frequency of dysphonia ranged from 7% to 37% with the use of anti-VEGF compounds, and from 0% to 33% with the use of small molecule tyrosine-kinase inhibitors. The lowest frequency was observed using sunitinib (Pfizer Inc., New York) and the highest using aflibercept. Dysphonia was attributed to the presence of vocal fold edematous changes, dehydration, and/or mucosal necrosis.[99] This latter is commensurate with the well-known antiangiogenic action of these drugs, which prevents the formation of new vessels within and around the tumor. In 2019, Melo et al reported a case of transient hoarseness following treatment with ramucirumab. A 73-year-old man diagnosed with gastric adenocarcinoma presented with dysphonia following a third cycle of chemotherapy that included ramucirumab, a VEGF inhibitor. On laryngeal examination, the patient had scarring of both vocal folds. Given the potential causality between treatment and the laryngeal findings, ramucirumab was discontinued while keeping paclitaxel therapy. On follow-up, there was complete regression of the vocal fold lesions with recovery of the voice.[100] Although most of the reported side effects are cardiovascular in nature,[101,102] a change in voice quality following antiangiogenic treatment should alert the physician to the possibility of drug-induced vocal fold pathology.

References

1. Bray F, Ferlay J, Soerjomataram I, Siegel RL, Torre LA, Jemal A. Global cancer statistics 2018: GLOBOCAN estimates of incidence and mortality worldwide for 36 cancers in 185 countries. *CA Cancer J Clin.* 2018;68(6):394–424.

2. American Cancer Society. Key Statistics about Stomach Cancer. Accessed November 5, 2019. https://www.cancer.org/cancer/stomach-cancer/about/key-statistics.html

3. Zeb A, Rasool A, Nasreen S. Occupation and cancer incidence in district Dir (NWFP), Pakistan, 2000–2004. *Asian Pac J Cancer Prev.* 2006;7(3):483–484.

4. Zhong C, Li NK, Bi JW, Wang BC. Sodium intake, salt taste and gastric cancer risk according to *Helicobacter pylori* infection, smoking, histological type and tumor site in China. *Asian Pac J Cancer Prev.* 2012;13(6):2481–2484.

5. Torre LA, Bray F, Siegel RL, Ferlay J, Lortet-Tieulent J, Jemal A. Global cancer statistics, 2012. *CA Cancer J Clin.* 2015;65(2):87–108.

6. Balakrishnan M, George R, Sharma A, Graham DY. Changing trends in stomach cancer throughout the world. *Curr Gastroenterol Rep.* 2017;19(8):36.

7. Lin L, Yan L, Liu Y, Yuan F, Li H, Ni J. Incidence and death in 29 cancer groups in 2017 and trend analysis from 1990 to 2017 from the Global Burden of Disease Study. *J Hematol Oncol.* 2019;12(1):96.

8. Foo M, Leong T. Adjuvant therapy for gastric cancer: current and future directions. *World J Gastroenterol.* 2014;20(38):13718–13727.

9. Rawla P, Barsouk A. Epidemiology of gastric cancer: global trends, risk factors and prevention. *Prz Gastroenterol.* 2019;14(1):26–38.

10. Sugano K. Screening of gastric cancer in Asia. *Best Prac Res Clin Gastroenterol.* 2015;29(6):895–905.

11. World Cancer Research Fund/American Institute for Cancer Research (WCRF/AIRC). Continuous Update Project Expert Report 2018. Diet, nutrition, physical activity and stomach cancer. Accessed November 5, 2019. http://dietandcancerreport.org

12. Mukaisho K, Nakayama T, Hagiwara T, Hattori T, Sugihara H. Two distinct etiologies

of gastric cardia adenocarcinoma: interactions among pH, *Helicobacter pylori*, and bile acids. *Front Microbiol.* 2015;6:412.

13. Schneider BG, Peng DF, Camargo MC, et al. Promoter DNA hypermethylation in gastric biopsies from subjects at high and low risk for gastric cancer. *Int J Cancer.* 2010;127(11):2588–2597.

14. Lu B, Li M. *Helicobacter pylori* eradication for preventing gastric cancer. *World J Gastroenterol.* 2014;20(19):5660–5665.

15. Burgess DE, Woodman CB, Flavell KJ, et al. Low prevalence of Epstein-Barr virus in incident gastric adenocarcinomas from the United Kingdom. *Br J Cancer.* 2002;86(5):702–704.

16. Murphy G, Pfeiffer R, Camargo MC, Rabkin CS. Meta-analysis shows that prevalence of Epstein–Barr virus-positive gastric cancer differs based on sex and anatomic location. *Gastroenterology.* 2009;137(3):824–833.

17. Camargo MC, Mera R, Correa P, et al. Interleukin-1β and interleukin-1 receptor antagonist gene polymorphisms and gastric cancer: a meta-analysis. *Cancer Epidemiol Biomarkers Prev.* 2006;15(9):1674–1687.

18. Loh M, Koh KX, Yeo BH, et al. Meta-analysis of genetic polymorphisms and gastric cancer risk: variability in associations according to race. *Eur J Cancer.* 2009;45(14):2562–2568.

19. Persson C, Canedo P, Machado JC, El-Omar EM, Forman D. Polymorphisms in inflammatory response genes and their association with gastric cancer: a HuGE systematic review and meta-analysis. *Am J Epidemiol.* 2011;173(3):259–270.

20. Salaspuro M. Interactions of alcohol and tobacco in gastrointestinal cancer. *J Gastroenterol Hepatol.* 2012;27(2):135–139.

21. Gao Y, Hu N, Han XY, et al. Risk factors for esophageal and gastric cancers in Shanxi province, China: A case-control study. *Cancer Epidemiol.* 2011;35(6):e91–e99.

22. Gonzalez CA, Jakszyn P, Pera G, et al. Meat intake and risk of stomach and esophageal adenocarcinoma within the European Pro-spective Investigation into Cancer and Nutrition (EPIC). *J Natl Cancer Inst.* 2006;98(5):345–354.

23. Joossens JV, Hill MJ, Elliott P, et al. Dietary salt, nitrate and stomach cancer mortality in 24 countries. European cancer prevention (ECP) and the INTERSALT Cooperative Research Group. *Int J Epidemiol.* 1996;25(3):494–504.

24. Correa P. Gastric cancer: overview. *Gastroenterol Clin North Am.* 2013;42(2):211–217.

25. Lauren P. The two histological main types of gastric carcinoma: diffuse and so-called intestinal-type carcinoma. An attempt at a histo-clinical classification. *Acta Pathol Microbiol Scand.* 1965;64:31–49.

26. Waldum HL, Fossmark R. Types of gastric carcinomas. *Int J Mol Sci.* 2018;19(12):4109.

27. Durrani AA, Yaqoob N, Abbasi S, Siddiq M, Moin S. Pattern of upper gastrointestinal malignancies in Northern Punjab. *Pak J Med Sci.* 2009;25(2):302–307.

28. Roder M. The epidemiology of gastric cancer. *Gastric Cancer.* 2002;5(1):5–11.

29. Edge SB, Byrd DR, Compton CC, eds. *AJCC Cancer Staging Manual.* New York, NY: Springer-Verlag; 2009.

30. Braga-Neto MB, Carneiro JG, de Castro Barbosa AM, et al. Clinical characteristics of distal gastric cancer in young adults from Northeastern Brazil. *BMC Cancer.* 2018;18(1):131.

31. Al-Refaie WB, Hu CY, Pisters PW, Chang GJ. Gastric adenocarcinoma in young patients: a population-based appraisal. *Ann Surg Oncol.* 2011;18(10):2800–2807.

32. Santoro R, Carboni F, Lepiane P, Ettorre GM, Santoro E. Clinicopathological features and prognosis of gastric cancer in young European adults. *Br J Surg.* 2007;94(6):737–742.

33. Isobe T, Hashimoto K, Kizaki J, et al. Characteristics and prognosis of gastric cancer in young patients. *Oncol Rep.* 2013;30(1):43–49.

34. Zhou F, Shi J, Fang C, Zou X, Huang Q. Gastric carcinomas in young (younger than 40 years) Chinese patients: clinicopathology,

family history, and postresection survival. *Medicine*. 2016;95(9):e2873.

35. Ben Kridis W, Marrekchi G, Mzali R, Daoud J, Khanfir A. Prognostic factors in metastatic gastric carcinoma. *Exp Oncol*. 2019;41(2): 173–175.

36. Tan HL, Chia CS, Tan GHC, et al. Metastatic gastric cancer: does the site of metastasis make a difference? *Asia Pac J Clin Oncol*. 2019;15(1):10–17.

37. Bhatia KS, Griffith JF, Ahuja AT. Stomach cancer: prevalence and significance of neck nodal metastases on sonography. *Eur Radiol*. 2009;19(8):1968–1972.

38. Rajeshwari M, Sakthivel P, Sikka K, Jain D. "Carcinoma en cuirasse" in the neck: extremely unusual initial presentation of gastric cancer. *BMJ Case Rep*. 2019;12(4): e228418.

39. Gündüz Ö, Emeksiz MC, Atasoy P, Kidir M, Yalçin S, Demirkan S. Signet-ring cells in the skin: a case of late-onset cutaneous metastasis of gastric carcinoma and a brief review of histological approach. *Dermatol Reports*. 2017;8(1):6819.

40. Emanuelli E, Ciorba A, Borsetto D, et al. Metastasis to parotid gland from non Head and Neck tumors. *J BUON*. 2018;23(1): 163–166.

41. Sun YC, Liaw CC, Liao CT, Lee KF. Gastric adenocarcinoma with tonsil and submaxillary gland metastases: case report. *Changgeng Yi Xue Za Zhi*. 1999;22(1):143–146.

42. Gallo A, Pescarmona E, Crupi J, Corsetti GL, De Vincentiis M. Bilateral tonsillar metastasis of gastric adenocarcinoma. *Head Neck*. 1992;14(1):55–57.

43. Kim CH, Shin JE, Roh HG, Lee JS, Yoon SY. Sudden hearing loss due to internal auditory canal metastasis of Her2-positive gastric cancer: a case report. *Oncol Lett*. 2014;8(1):394–396.

44. Andreyev HJ, Norman AR, Oates J, Cunningham D. Why do patients with weight loss have a worse outcome when undergoing chemotherapy for gastrointestinal malignancies? *Eur J Cancer*. 1998;34(4): 503–509.

45. Seker M, Aksoy S, Ozdemir NY, Uncu D, Zengin N. Clinicopathologic features of gastric cancer in young patients. *Saudi J Gastroenterol*. 2013;19(6):258–261.

46. Liu X, Qiu H, Huang Y, et al. Impact of preoperative anemia on outcomes in patients undergoing curative resection for gastric cancer: a single-institution retrospective analysis of 2163 Chinese patients. *Cancer Med*. 2018;7(2):360–369.

47. Horner RL, Mohiaddin RH, Lowell DG, et al. Sites and sizes of fat deposits around the pharynx in obese patients with obstructive sleep apnoea and weight matched controls. *Eur Respir J*. 1989;2(7):613–622.

48. Shelton KE, Woodson H, Gay S, Suratt PM. Pharyngeal fat in obstructive sleep apnea. *Am Rev Respir Dis*. 1993;148(2):462–466.

49. Mortimore IL, Marshall I, Wraith PK, Sellar RJ, Douglas NJ. Neck and total body fat deposition in nonobese and obese patients with sleep apnea compared with that in control subjects. *Am J Respir Crit Care Med*. 1998;157(1):280–283.

50. Sataloff RT. Vocal tract resonance. In: Sataloff RT. *Professional Voice: The Science and Art of Clinical Care*. 4th ed. San Diego, CA: Plural Publishing; 2017:309–328.

51. Solomon NP, Helou LB, Dietrich-Burns K, Stojadinovic A. Do obesity and weight loss affect vocal function? *Semin Speech Lang*. 2011;32(1):31–42.

52. Hamdan AL, Sataloff RT, Hawkshaw MJ. Effect of weight loss on voice. In: Hamdan AL, Sataloff RT, Hawkshaw MJ, eds. *Obesity and Voice*. San Diego, CA: Plural Publishing; 2019:369–382.

53. Del Fabbro E. Current and future care of patients with the cancer anorexia-cachexia syndrome. *Am Soc Clin Oncol Educ Book*. 2015:e229–e237.

54. Bachmann J, Heiligensetzer M, Krakowski-Roosen H, Buchler MW, Friess H, Martignoni ME. Cachexia worsens prognosis in patients with resectable pancreatic cancer. *J Gastrointest Surg*. 2008;12(7):1193–1201.

55. Hauser CA, Stockler MR, Tattersall MH. Prognostic factors in patients with recently diagnosed incurable cancer: a systematic

review. *Support Care Cancer*. 2006;14(10): 999–1011.

56. Quinten C, Coens C, Mauer M, et al. Baseline quality of life as a prognostic indicator of survival: a meta-analysis of individual patient data from EORTC clinical trials. *Lancet Oncol*. 2009;10(9):865–871.

57. Di Sebastiano KM, Mourtzakis M. A critical evaluation of body composition modalities used to assess adipose and skeletal muscle tissue in cancer. *Appl Physiol Nutr Metab*. 2012;37(5):811–821.

58. Del Fabbro E, Parsons H, Warneke CL, et al. The relationship between body composition and response to neoadjuvant chemotherapy in women with operable breast cancer. *Oncologist*. 2012;17(10):1240–1245.

59. Crawford GB, Robinson JA, Hunt RW, Piller NB, Esterman A. Estimating survival in patients with cancer receiving palliative care: is analysis of body composition using bioimpedance helpful? *J Palliat Med*. 2009;12(11):1009–1014.

60. National Comprehensive Cancer Network. NCCN Clinical Practice Guidelines in Oncology. Cancer-related Fatigue. Version 1. 2009. Accessed November 5, 2019. http://www.nccn.org/professionals/physician_gls/PDF/fatigue.pdf

61. Montoya L. Managing hematologic toxicities in the oncology patient. *J Infus Nurs*. 2007;30(3):168–172.

62. Torino F, Corsello SM, Longo R, Bernabei A, Gasparini G. Hypothyroidism related to tyrosine kinase inhibitors: an emerging toxic effect of targeted therapy. *Nat Rev Clin Oncol*. 2009;6(4):219–228.

63. Ryan JL, Carroll JK, Ryan EP, Mustian KM, Fiscella K, Morrow GR. Mechanisms of cancer-related fatigue. *Oncologist*. 2007; 12(1):22–34.

64. Zou G, Li Y, Xu R, Li P. Resilience and positive affect contribute to lower cancer-related fatigue among Chinese patients with gastric cancer. *J Clin Nurs*. 2018;27(7–8): e1412–e1418.

65. Park W, Lee JK, Kim CR, Shin JY. Factors associated with fatigue in Korean gastric can-

cer survivors. *Korean J Fam Med*. 2015;36(6): 328–334.

66. Smith HR. Depression in cancer patients: pathogenesis, implications and treatment (Review). *Oncol Lett*. 2015;9(4):1509–1514.

67. Brintzenhofe-Szoc KM, Levin TT, Li Y, Kissane DW, Zabora JR. Mixed anxiety/depression symptoms in a large cancer cohort: prevalence by cancer type. *Psychosomatics*. 2009;50(4):383–391.

68. Hu LY, Liu CJ, Yeh CM, et al. Depressive disorders among patients with gastric cancer in Taiwan: a nationwide population-based study. *BMC Psychiatry*. 2018;18(1):272.

69. Bergquist H, Ruth M, Hammerlid E. Psychiatric morbidity among patients with cancer of the esophagus or the gastro-esophageal junction: a prospective, longitudinal evaluation. *Dis Esophagus*. 2007;20(6):523–529.

70. Tavoli A, Mohagheghi MA, Montazeri A, Roshan R, Tavoli Z, Omidvari S. Anxiety and depression in patients with gastrointestinal cancer: does knowledge of cancer diagnosis matter? *BMC Gastroenterol*. 2007;7:28.

71. Koh MJ, Jeung HC, Namkoong K, Chung HC, Kang JI. Influence of the BDNF Val-66Met polymorphism on coping response to stress in patients with advanced gastric cancer. *J Psychosom Res*. 2014;77(1):76–80.

72. Yu H, Wang Y, Ge X, Wu X, Mao X. Depression and survival in Chinese patients with gastric cancer: a prospective study. *Asian Pac J Cancer Prev*. 2012;13(1):391–394.

73. Rosen DC, Heuer RJ, Sasso DA, Sataloff RT. Psychological aspects of voice disorders. In: Sataloff RT. *Professional Voice: The Science and Art of Clinical Care*. 4th ed. San Diego, CA: Plural Publishing; 2017:705–736.

74. Santoro R, Ettorre GM, Santoro E. Subtotal gastrectomy for gastric cancer. *World J Gastroenterol*. 2014;20(38):13667–13680.

75. Orditura M, Galizia G, Sforza V, et al. Treatment of gastric cancer. *World J Gastroenterol*. 2014;20(7):1635–1649.

76. Ohtani H, Tamamori Y, Noguchi K, et al. A meta-analysis of randomized controlled trials that compared laparoscopy-assisted and open distal gastrectomy for

early gastric cancer. *J Gastrointest Surg.* 2010;14(6):958–964.

77. Adachi Y, Suematsu T, Shiraishi N, et al. Quality of life after laparoscopy-assisted Billroth I gastrectomy. *Ann Surg.* 1999;229 (1):49–54.

78. Kim YW, Baik YH, Yun YH, et al. Improved quality of life outcomes after laparoscopy-assisted distal gastrectomy for early gastric cancer: results of a prospective random-ized clinical trial. *Ann Surg.* 2008;248(5): 721–727.

79. Lim HS, Cho GS, Park YH, Kim SK. Comparison of quality of life and nutri-tional status in gastric cancer patients undergoing gastrectomies. *Clin Nutr Res.* 2015;4(3):153–159.

80. Lee SS, Ryu SW, Kim IH, Sohn SS. Qual-ity of life beyond the early postoperative period after laparoscopy-assisted distal gastrectomy: the level of patient expecta-tion as the essence of quality of life. *Gastric Cancer.* 2012;15(3):299–304.

81. Karanicolas PJ, Graham D, Gönen M, Strong VE, Brennan MF, Coit DG. Qual-ity of life after gastrectomy for adenocar-cinoma: a prospective cohort study. *Ann Surgery.* 2013;257(6):1039–1046.

82. Avery K, Hughes R, McNair A, Alderson D, Barham P, Blazeby J. Health-related qual-ity of life and survival in the 2 years after surgery for gastric cancer. *Eur J Surg Oncol.* 2010;36(2):148–154.

83. Huang CC, Lien HH, Wang PC, Yang JC, Cheng CY, Huang CS. Quality of life in disease-free gastric adenocarcinoma sur-vivors: impacts of clinical stages and re-constructive surgical procedures. *Dig Surg.* 2007;24(1):59–65.

84. El Labban S, Safadi B, Olabi A. The effect of Roux-en-Y gastric bypass and sleeve gas-trectomy surgery on dietary intake, food preferences, and gastrointestinal symptoms in post-surgical morbidly obese Lebanese subjects: a cross-sectional pilot study. *Obes Surg.* 2015;25(12):2393–2399.

85. Savarino E, Marabotto E, Savarino V. Effects of bariatric surgery on the esophagus. *Curr Opin Gastroenterol.* 2018;34(4):243–248.

86. Genco A, Soricelli E, Casella G, et al. Gastroesophageal reflux disease and Bar-rett's esophagus after laparoscopic sleeve gastrectomy: a possible, underestimated long-term complication. *Surg Obes Relat Dis.* 2017;13(4):568–574.

87. Mandeville Y, Van Looveren R, Vancoil-lie PJ, et al. Moderating the enthusiasm of sleeve gastrectomy: up to fifty percent of reflux symptoms after ten years in a consecutive series of one hundred lapa-roscopic sleeve gastrectomies. *Obes Surg.* 2017;27(7):1797–1803.

88. Nadaleto BF, Herbella FA, Patti MG. Gas-troesophageal reflux disease in the obese: pathophysiology and treatment. *Surgery.* 2016;159(2):475–486.

89. Sataloff RT, Castell DO, Katz PO, Sataloff RT, Sataloff DM, Hawkshaw MJ. Reflux and other gastroenterologic conditions that may affect the voice. In: Sataloff RT. *Professional Voice: The Science and Art of Clinical Care.* 4th ed. San Diego, CA: Plural Publishing; 2017:907–998.

90. Mattioni J, Opperman DA, Solimadno Jr DA, Sataloff RT. Chemotherapy: an over-view and voice implications. In: Sataloff RT. *Professional Voice: The Science and Art of Clinical Care.* 4th ed. San Diego, CA: Plural Publishing; 2017:1137–1140.

91. Curt GA, Breitbart W, Cella D, et al. Im-pact of cancer-related fatigue on the lives of patients: new findings from the Fatigue Coalition. *Oncologist.* 2000;5(5):353–360.

92. Wagner AD, Grothe W, Haerting J, Kleber G, Grothery A, Fleig W. Chemotherapy in advanced gastric cancer: a systematic review and meta-analysis based on aggre-gate data. *J Clin Oncol.* 2006;24(18):2903–2909.

93. Kang JH, Lee SI, Lim DH, et al. Salvage chemotherapy for pretreated gastric can-cer: a randomized phase III trial compar-ing chemotherapy plus best supportive care with best supportive care alone. *J Clin Oncol.* 2012;30(13):1513–1518.

94. Jácome AA, Coutinho AK, Lima EM, An-drade AC, dos Santos JS. Personalized med-icine in gastric cancer: where are we and

where are we going? *World J Gastroenterol.* 2016;22(3):1160–1171.

95. Hartl DM, Ferté C, Loriot Y, et al. Dysphonia induced by vascular endothelium growth factor/vascular endothelium growth factor receptor inhibitors. *Invest New Drugs.* 2010;28(6):884–886.

96. Hartl DM, Bahleda R, Hollebecque A, Bosq J, Massard C, Soria JC. Bevacizumab-induced laryngeal necrosis. *Ann Oncol.* 2012;23(1): 276–278.

97. Caruso AM, Meyer TK, Allen CT. Hoarseness after metastatic colon cancer treatment. *JAMA Otolaryngol Head Neck Surg.* 2014;140(9):881–882.

98. Shord SS, Bressler LR, Tierney LA, Cuellar S, George A. Understanding and managing the possible adverse effects associated with bevacizumab. *Am J Health Syst Pharm.* 2009;66(11):999–1013.

99. Saavedra E, Hollebecque A, Soria JC, Hartl DM. Dysphonia induced by anti-angiogenic compounds. *Invest New Drugs.* 2014;32(4): 774–782.

100. Melo ÉG, Silveira PA, Mello CA. Transient vocal fold lesion and hoarseness associated with the use of ramucirumab: case report. *Eur Ann Otorhinolaryngol Head Neck Dis.* 2019;136(4):317–319.

101. Chen HX, Cleck JN. Adverse effects of anti-cancer agents that target the VEGF pathway. *Nat Rev Clin Oncol.* 2009;6(8):465–477.

102. Schmidinger M, Bellmunt J. Plethora of agents, plethora of targets, plethora of side effects in metastatic renal cell carcinoma. *Cancer Treat Rev.* 2010;36(5):416–424.

12

Liver Cancer and Voice

Abdul-Latif Hamdan, Robert Thayer Sataloff, and Mary J. Hawkshaw

Epidemiology and Clinical Presentation

Liver cancer is the fourth most common cancer in the world, with more than 800 000 newly diagnosed cases yearly worldwide.[1] More than 85% of new cases occur in Eastern Asia, including China and Mongolia, Southeast Asia, and Eastern Africa.[2,3] A much lower prevalence is observed in developed countries except in Japan, Italy, and France.[3] In the United States, there were an estimated 42 030 newly diagnosed cases in 2019.[1] Liver cancer affects both genders in their fifth to sixth decades of life.[4] Men are affected more than women, with a male-to-female ratio of 2:1 worldwide.[5] In the United States, the estimated prevalence in men in 2019 was 29 480 in comparison to 12 550 in women.[1] The overall 5-year survival rate of liver cancer is low. It is still considered as the third most common cause of cancer-related death in the world, accounting for more than 700 000 deaths yearly. There were an estimated 31 780 deaths in 2019, stratified as 21 600 men and 10 180 women.[1]

Based on several histopathologic characteristics, different types of primary liver cancer have been described in the literature. The most common types are hepatocellular carcinoma (HCC) and cholangiocarcinoma, accounting for 75% to 80% and 10% to 20% of all cases, respectively. Less commonly described tumors include angiosarcoma and hemangiosarcoma, originating from the intrahepatic vascular lining. Liver cancer also may be secondary (ie, the result of distant metastasis). The most common sites of primary tumors metastasizing to the liver are the lungs, breast, colon, and pancreas.[6]

Several risk factors for liver cancer have been mentioned in the literature, the most important of which is infection with hepatitis C or hepatitis B.[4] Hepatitis C infection increases the risk of liver cancer with an odds ratio of 39.89%, and a population attributable fraction of 22.4%.[7] Similarly, infection with hepatitis B increases the risk of hepatocellular carcinoma with an odds ratio of 11.17%.[7,8] The risk is compounded when there is exposure to additional factors such as food toxins (eg, aflatoxin), commonly present in Sub-Saharan Africa and East Asia,[9–12] or arsenic, a well-known carcinogenic environmental element.[13,14] Alcohol consumption is another prominent risk factor in liver cancer.[15,16] In a large meta-analysis on alcohol intake and cancer risk, Bagnardi et al reported a moderate association between alcohol consumption and incidence of liver cancer.[16] In a review by

Turati et al, the relative risk of alcohol consumption (more than 6 drinks per day) was 1.22 in comparison to those who do not drink alcohol.[17] Similarly, nonalcoholic fatty liver disease (NAFLD) has been associated with liver cancer.[18] Based on a large epidemiologic study by Younossi et al, which included 8 515 431 patients, the incidence of hepatocellular carcinoma in patients with NAFLD was estimated as 0.44 per 1000 person-years.[18] This may reflect the strong link between obesity, overweight, and liver cancer, with a marked increased risk observed in obese subjects.[19] Smoking is also a well-known significant risk factor for liver cancer. In a large meta-analysis by Lee et al that included 98 studies, the relative risk of liver cancer in smokers was estimated as 1.51,[20] with a dose-response relationship for both duration and extent of smoking.[21] Dietary habits also have been linked to the prevalence of liver cancer.[22–26] Consumption of fatty foods increases the risk of liver cancer, whereas the consumption of white meat, fish, vegetables, and dairy products has been shown to have a reverse relationship with the prevalence of HCC. Hormonal factors, dietary iron intake, and hemochromatosis are additional variables that affect the prevalence of liver cirrhosis and hepatocellular carcinoma.[27] Diabetes and unprotected sex also may increase the risk of liver cancer.

The clinical presentation of patients with liver cancer varies markedly. Affected patients may be asymptomatic until late stages of the disease, or they may present with acute symptoms of abdominal pain, obstructive jaundice, nausea, and vomiting. The history may reveal weight loss and excessive generalized fatigue.[28] The laryngological manifestations of liver cancer are reported uncommonly and often are masked by the systemic complaints of the patient and the associated comorbidities of the disease. This chapter reviews the current literature on voice changes in patients with liver cancer, with emphasis on the etiologic role of extrahepatic metastasis. Treatment-induced dysphonia also is discussed. Proper knowledge of the association between liver cancer and voice is important for laryngologists and other physicians involved in the care of affected patients.

Dysphonia in Patients With Liver Cancer and Extrahepatic Metastasis

Extrahepatic metastasis in patients with liver cancer is not uncommon. In a radiologic review using computed tomography (CT), Katyal et al showed extrahepatic metastasis in 148 of 413 patients with HCC.[29] In a retrospective review of the clinical features of 482 patients with HCC, Natsuizaka et al reported extrahepatic metastasis in 13.5% of cases.[30] Similarly, in an autopsy study associating morphological features of HCC with distant metastasis, extrahepatic lesions were reported in almost two-thirds of cases (64%).[31] Several determinants of metastasis were described in the literature in attempts to identify high-risk patients. The predictors most commonly reported were the morphological features of the tumor, the stage of the disease, and the presence or absence of intrahepatic vascular invasion. In 1987, in an autopsy review of 98 patients with HCC, Sawabe et al described an association between extrahepatic metastasis and vascular invasion of the hepatic and portal vein. The infiltrative type of HCC had a higher rate of pulmonary metastasis in comparison to the expansive type of HCC.[31] In a radiologic investigation on the association between tumor stage and the frequency of HCC metastasis, advanced stage of the disease (stages III and IVA) was identified in the majority of patients with metastasis (86%).[29] These results were supported by another study on the clinical features of 482 patients with HCC, which also proved that advanced stage of disease and vessel invasion were associated significantly with extrahepatic metastasis.[30]

The diagnosis of extrahepatic metastasis in patients with liver cancer is based on radiologic signs and on histologic criteria. The advances in radiology undoubtedly have enhanced the diagnosis as well as the management of patients with metastatic HCC. Biphasic CT with arterial phase enhancement has been shown to differentiate metastatic lesions from benign masses,[29] while magnetic resonance imaging (MRI) with gadolinium enhancement have helped to delineate the anatomical extent of metastasis, with high sensitivity for metastatic vascular lesions.[32] ^{18}F-Fludeoxyglucose (FDG) positron emission tomography (PET) has also been shown to be useful not only in detecting distant metastasis and in staging of the disease, but also in selecting treatment strategies and in predicting outcome and overall prognosis.[33] In a study on 104 patients with HCC, Cho et al showed an association between the ratio of maximal tumor standardized uptake value (SUV) to the mean mediastinum SUV, tumor size, node metastasis, and stage of the disease. The authors demonstrated that patients with high TSU max/MSU mean ratio had higher mortality rate and recurrence rate following treatment by transarterial chemoembolization.[34] The type of liver cancer is determined usually by histopathologic examination and staining. Pathologic markers such as the presence of acidophilic cells, Mallory bodies, and bile are highly indicative of liver carcinoma. Immunohistochemistry is also very helpful in differentiating metastatic HCC from other metastatic tumors. Hepatocyte paraffin 1 expression, as well as hepatocytes cytokeratin 8 and 18, are highly specific for HCC.[3,35]

Extrahepatic metastasis in patients with HCC affects various organs, the most common of which are the abdominal lymph nodes, lungs, bones, and adrenal glands. Based on an autopsy study looking at determinants of extrahepatic metastasis in nearly one hundred patients with HCC, lung metastasis accounted for 62% of metastatic cases.[31] Similarly, Katyal et al reported lung metastasis in 55% of cases, followed by abdominal lymph nodes and bone metastasis in 41% and 28% of cases, respectively.[29] Other sites affected less commonly are the kidneys, brain, ovaries, muscles, and skin.[30,36,37] Lee et al reported a 43-year-old woman who presented with an ovarian mass 2 years following treatment of HCC. The hypermetabolic rate of the mass on PET was suggestive of recurrence of her primary tumor. The patient underwent surgical exploration and right salpingo-oophorectomy, which confirmed metastatic HCC.[36] Similarly, D'Antonio et al described a 54-year-old woman with a history of HCC and liver transplant, who presented with a suspicious renal mass. A left nephrectomy was performed. Immunohistochemistry of the resected kidney revealed renal metastasis.[38] Michalaki et al described a case of HCC metastasizing to muscular structures around the humerus and emphasized the need to consider soft tissue masses in the differential diagnosis of metastatic diseases. The authors also highlighted the added value of immunohistochemical staining in differentiating metastatic HCC from other lesions.[39] Tunc et al reported a 55-year-old man diagnosed previously with hepatitis, who presented with right-sided numbness and weakness. A CT image of the head showed multiple enhancing lesions. Radiologic imaging of the abdomen and pelvis revealed a hepatic hypodense mass, biopsy of which confirmed the diagnosis of HCC.[40]

Metastasis of liver cancer to the mediastinum and/or head and neck structures is rare. The mode of spread is mostly hematogenous with retrograde flow of venous blood from the abdomen upward secondary to an increase in intra-abdominal pressure.[41] An alternative mode of spread is through the lymphatic system. The route is usually either through a sequential spread along the regional lymph nodes of the abdomen, mediastinum, and neck, or through a skip pattern with involvement of cervical lymph nodes in isolation. The skip pattern has been attributed partially to disease-induced alteration in and/or occlusion of lymphatic channels.[42]

In the following section, the authors review the prevalence of extrahepatic metastasis of HCC in the mediastinum, head and neck, and larynx, and their impact on voice.

Dysphonia in Patients With Liver Cancer and Metastasis to the Head and Neck

Metastasis of liver cancer to the head and neck is not very common. The most reported metastatic sites are the oral cavity, nasopharynx, and cervical lymph nodes.

Liver Cancer Metastasis to the Oral Cavity

Malignant lesions in the oral cavity are either primary or metastatic in origin. Metastasis usually occurs via entrapment and deposition of malignant cells within chronically inflamed tissues.[43] The most commonly described distant primaries metastasizing to the oral cavity are lung cancer, renal cancer, and lymphoma. Metastatic HCC to the oral cavity is rare.[44-47] In 2004, Pires et al described a 60-year-old man with HCC and metastasis to the gingiva of the lower jaw. The patient had additional extrahepatic metastatic sites

in the knees, skin, and scalp. The authors highlighted the apparent increased risk of oral metastasis in patients with HCC and systemic dissemination.[45] In 2004, Eugenio et al reported a 70-year-old man who presented with multiple polypoid lesions of the gingiva and alveolar crest. Immunohistochemical staining of a biopsy taken from that lesion was positive for α1-antichymotrypsin, hepatocyte antigen, and cytokeratin. Following a metastatic workup, the patient was diagnosed with primary carcinoma of the liver for which he received transarterial chemoembolization.[46] In 2008, Li et al reported a 55-year-old man, diagnosed previously with HCC, who presented with pain, tenderness, and swelling of the lower jaw. CT showed evidence of a mandibular fracture surrounded by a mass, biopsy of which was consistent with metastatic HCC.[47] In 2013, Greenstein et al described a 68-year-old man known to have hepatitis B and HCC who presented with a hemorrhagic, multilobulated, gingival mass of the upper jaw. Radiologic images of the maxilla showed evidence of bone erosion. A biopsy of the lesion and histopathologic examination confirmed the presence of metastatic HCC.[44]

In all of these cases, the main presenting symptoms were oral fullness, bleeding, and pain. A change in voice quality was not reported but could have been a presenting symptom given the anatomical alteration in the oral cavity induced by the growing metastatic lesion. Dysphonia might have been masked by the overwhelming oral bleeding and pain. The oral cavity is one of the main resonators of the phonatory apparatus, distortion of which may affect the position and dispersion of formant frequencies, particularly the first and second formants.[48] Moreover, the restriction in jaw movement, as in cases of metastatic lesions to the mandible body or condyle, may jeopardize the ability to have a widely open oral cavity, an important requisite in professional voice users. Space, depth, and volume are important determinants of voice quality and projection, the limitation of which by metastatic disease may adversely affect vocal performance.[49]

Liver Cancer Metastasis to the Nasopharynx

Metastatic lesions in the nasopharynx from various distant neoplasias in the body are not uncommon. These lesions are often overlooked in view of the nondifferentiating symptoms and signs in affected patients. A high index of suspicion is needed in order to make the proper diagnosis, as many cases are misdiagnosed and treated for sinusitis. Only 3 case reports have been reported in the literature. In 2013, Abhay et al reported a 70-year-old man with no prior medical history who presented with nasal obstruction and bleeding of a few weeks' duration. Nasopharyngoscopy and biopsy showed moderately differentiated adenocarcinoma. Immunohistochemistry was negative for CK20 and positive for Hepar-1 and AFP. PET-CT was ordered and confirmed the presence of a hypodense lesion in the liver, with signs of cirrhosis and portal hypertension. The radiologic signs were highly suggestive of liver carcinoma, but the patient did not agree to pursue any further intervention.[50] In 2015, Guo and Wang reported a 50-year-old man, diagnosed previously with hepatitis B and HCC, who presented with headache, impaired vision, blepharoptosis, and difficulty in swallowing. PET-CT showed bone erosion at the base of skull, very suggestive of a neoplastic lesion. A biopsy confirmed the diagnosis of metastatic HCC, for which the patient was treated successfully by radiation therapy. The authors highlighted the short time between the diagnosis of the primary HCC and nasopharyngeal metastasis (2 months)

and the lack of other metastatic lesions.[51] Li-Li et al reported a case of nasopharyngeal metastatic HCC following liver transplantation. The patient was a 45-year-old man, with history of hepatitis B and liver cirrhosis, who presented with symptoms of headache, dysphagia, and dysphonia. MRI of the base of the skull revealed signs of bone destruction suggestive of a neoplastic process. Histologic examination of a biopsy confirmed the presence of a metastatic liver lesion. The patient was treated with radiotherapy with marked improvement in his symptoms. The authors highlighted the etiologic role of Epstein–Barr virus (EBV) in the pathophysiology of metastatic nasopharyngeal lesions, and the pathogenic role of chronic inflammation in tumorigenesis.[52] Moreover, they emphasized the higher risk of metastasis in patients with large hepatic lesions and/or poor histopathologic grading, similar to what has been reported by Jonas et al in their study on the predictive role of histopathologic grading and vascular invasion in patients with liver carcinoma undergoing liver transplantation.[53]

In the 3 described cases of metastatic HCC to the nasopharynx, dysphonia was a presenting symptom in one patient. Other reported symptoms included dysphagia, epistaxis, and nasal obstruction. Changes in voice quality occur as a result of mass compression or tumor infiltration of the vagus nerve at the base of the skull. Liver cancer metastasis to the nasopharynx should be considered in the metastatic workup of patients with a history of liver cancer and a nasopharyngeal mass.

Liver Cancer Metastasis to Cervical Lymph Nodes

Despite the applicability of various surveillance programs for early detection of liver cancer,[54] and although metastasis in affected patients is primarily hematogenous with lymphatic spread being mostly toward abdominal and peritoneal lymph nodes, a review of the literature revealed several cases of cervical lymphadenopathy in patients with HCC. In 2000, Kowk Lau et al reported a 67-year-old man who presented with a right upper extremity numbness and an enlarged right supraclavicular lymph node. CT of the chest and abdomen showed diffuse mediastinal lymphadenopathy, hepatomegaly, and a hepatic lesion in the left lobe. Excision of the supraclavicular lymph node was performed, and immunostaining confirmed the diagnosis of metastatic HCC.[55] In 2003, Thorburn et al described 2 cases of supraclavicular lymphadenopathy in patients with HCC. The first was a 67-year-old man who presented with weight loss, jaundice, and edema of the ankle. On examination, he was found to have right supraclavicular lymph node enlargement in addition to hepatomegaly. Ultrasonography of the abdomen showed a lobulated cirrhotic liver and a mass in the left lobe. Fine-needle aspiration of the suspected cervical lymph node confirmed the presence of metastatic HCC. The second case was a 72-year-old woman with a known history of biliary cirrhosis, who also presented with a right supraclavicular enlarged lymph node. CT showed multiple mediastinal lymphadenopathies and heterogeneous liver masses. Fine-needle aspiration of the supraclavicular lymphadenopathy revealed metastatic HCC.[56] In 2003, Seyfettin et al described a 75-year-old man with a history of hepatitis B, who presented with abdominal pain and right cervical lymphadenopathy. Ultrasound of the abdomen showed splenomegaly and an enlarged liver with heterogenous consistency. The diagnosis of HCC was supported by hepatic arteriogram.[57] In 2012, Kobayashi et al reported a 64-year-old man who presented with left cervical lymphade-

nopathy in the absence of lymphadenopathy elsewhere in the body. Viral serology was positive for hepatitis C. Fine-needle aspiration of the cervical lymph node revealed poorly differentiated carcinoma. Metastatic workup using PET and CT of the abdomen revealed high uptake in the liver, with the presence of multiple nodules. In addition, the patient had elevated tumor markers for HCC which further confirmed the diagnosis of liver cancer with cervical metastasis.[58] In 2014, Irrapa et al reported a 49-year-old man who presented with a right cervical lymph node (4 × 3 cm) in addition to weight loss and weakness. On evaluation, he was found to be positive for hepatitis B and to have multiple hepatic lesions and peritoneal lymphadenopathy. Biopsy of the cervical lymph node confirmed the diagnosis of metastatic HCC.[59]

In all of these cases, dysphonia was not described as a symptom in the clinical presentation of affected patients. Nevertheless, given the anatomical course of the right recurrent laryngeal nerve in the neck, as well as the left recurrent laryngeal nerve in the neck and chest, HCC metastatic cervical lymphadenopathy should be included in the differential diagnosis of neoplasia-induced vocal fold paralysis. A change in voice quality in patients with history of HCC should raise the suspicion of a cervical metastatic lesion.

In conclusion, dysphonia is rare in patients with liver metastasis to the head and neck. When present, a mass-induced alteration in vocal tract anatomy, and/or compression/invasion of the recurrent laryngeal nerve or vagus along its course at the base of skull or neck, should be investigated. Surgery followed by radiation therapy, with or without targeted therapy, are usually the treatment options. Alternatively, patients may be managed with transarterial chemotherapy or radioembolization.

Dysphonia in Patients With Liver Cancer and Mediastinal Metastasis

Metastasis to the mediastinum in patients with liver cancer occurs. The estimated prevalence is between 4% and 5%, with solitary lesions occurring in less than 1% of cases.[60-66] When present, laryngeal function may be affected because of the course of the recurrent laryngeal nerve in proximity to the para-aortic and peritracheal lymph nodes. Based on a pathology study that included 490 patients with HCC, the para-aortic and mediastinal lymph nodes were involved in 64% and in 25% of the subgroup of patients with distant lymph node metastasis ($n = 91$ cases).[67] A thorough review of the literature revealed several case reports of mediastinal metastasis in HCC; many of the patients presented with dysphonia, dysphagia, and/ or upper airway symptoms. In 1989, Naka-gawa et al reported a 54-year-old man who presented with cough 3½ years after hav-ing had surgical resection of HCC. Hema-tologic examination revealed elevation in α-fetoprotein, and radiologic images of the chest showed mediastinal widening. Explo-ration of the chest with lymph node dissec-tion revealed a large metastatic mediastinal mass, the treatment of which resulted in improvement of symptoms. No histopath-ologic examination was described in that report.[68] In 1993, Yamashita et al reported a 58-year-old man, previously diagnosed with HCC, who presented with dysphonia secondary to unilateral vocal fold paralysis. CT of the chest showed a fibroadipose tissue mass in the paratracheal groove on the right side. Resection and microscopic examina-tion of that mass revealed metastatic HCC.[69] In 2009, Uchinami et al reported a 52-year-old man, diagnosed previously with HCC, who was found to have an isolated solitary mediastinal lymphadenopathy on follow-up CT of the chest, in addition to another lymphadenopathy in proximity to the com-mon hepatic artery. The patient underwent surgical resection of these lymph nodes, which proved to be metastatic HCC.[70] In 2010, Shoji et al described another patient with HCC who presented with metastatic cardiophrenic lymphadenopathy. Through a mini-thoracotomy, the lymph node was dissected off the cardiophrenic area. Histo-pathologic examination confirmed the pres-ence of extrahepatic metastasis.[71] In 2013, Suzumura et al reported a 75-year-old man with HCC who was found on follow-up to have an enhancing mediastinal lesion. The suspected lymph node was resected using video-assisted thoracic surgery, and the pathologic examination was consistent with metastatic HCC.[62] In 2013, Chen re-ported a 71-year-old man, diagnosed with HCC, who presented with hoarseness and left vocal fold paralysis 2 years following treatment with hoarseness and left vocal fold paralysis. Images of the chest showed a mediastinal mass close to the aorta. The mass was aspirated under endosonography, and histopathologic examination proved it to be metastatic HCC.[64] In 2016, Xu et al reported a 30-year-old man with a history of HCC who presented with back pain and dysphonia. CT of the chest and abdomen showed multiple intrahepatic lesions with lymphadenopathies in the peritoneum, cla-vicular areas, and mediastinum, particularly around the aortic arch. Aspiration biopsy of the right supraclavicular lymph node con-firmed the diagnosis of metastatic HCC.[66] In 2016, Tanaka et al described a 40-year-old woman, with a previous history of HCC and hepatectomy, who presented with dyspho-nia and difficulty in swallowing. Radiologic images of the chest showed a subaortic mass that was resected using video assistance. Histopathologic examination was consis-tent with lymph node metastatic HCC.[72] In

2018, Taniguchi et al reported a 66-year-old man who, despite several treatment courses with transarterial chemoembolization, developed a mediastinal recurrence discovered on follow-up with FDG-PET, together with elevation of α-fetoprotein. The patient was treated successfully with video-assisted thoracic surgery.[73]

In summary, patients with HCC and mediastinal metastasis may be asymptomatic or may present with voice and swallowing complaints secondary to compression or invasion of the recurrent laryngeal nerve along its course in the mediastinum. A high index of suspicion is needed to make the diagnosis. Immunostaining and the use of tissue markers are helpful in confirming the metastatic nature of the lesion. Affected patients usually have poor survival despite aggressive treatment.

Laryngeal Metastasis in Patients With Hepatic Carcinoma

Laryngeal involvement in patients with malignancies is well-recognized in the literature. The metastasis is usually hematogenous given the scarcity of lymphatics in the laryngeal framework. The spread usually occurs via the systemic circulation and rarely through a retrograde flow of blood through the vertebral venous plexus.[41] In patients with HCC, tumor invasion of the hepatic venous circulation often leads the tumor emboli to the right side of the heart and into the pulmonary circulation. In an autopsy study by Kacynski et al, portal and hepatic vein invasion were noted in 41% of patients with HCC. Lymphogenous spread from liver cancer to the larynx and neck is less common, as most lymphatic spread is limited to abdominal and peritoneal lymph nodes.[67]

Metastasis to the larynx can occur either in isolation or in conjunction with other extrahepatic metastatic lesions. A careful review of the literature revealed only 4 case reports of laryngeal/pharyngeal metastasis in patients with HCC. In a review by Ferlito et al on metastatic laryngeal malignancies, melanoma and renal carcinoma were the most common primary neoplasias metastasizing to the larynx in 36.7% and 13.3% of cases, respectively. Other less common primary neoplasias described in that report were breast carcinoma and adenocarcinoma of unspecified origin. Only one case of gallbladder carcinoma metastasis to the larynx was reported among 200 cases that were included, but no case of HCC was reported.[41] In 1990, Nambu et al was the first to report a patient with hepatocellular carcinoma and metastasis to the larynx. The lesion originated from the subglottis and had a papillomatous appearance.[74] In 1995, Kacynzki et al performed an autopsy study on 490 patients with hepatocellular carcinoma and reported involvement of the epipharynx in only 1 case. In their clinical-pathologic study, lymph nodes, lungs, and skeleton were the most common metastatic sites in 42%, 18%, and 17% of cases, respectively.[67] In 2002, Nobili et al reported a 73-year-old man diagnosed previously with HCC and kidney metastasis, who presented 3 years following treatment with laryngeal discomfort. On laryngeal examination, the patient had a pedunculated lesion originating from the lingual surface of the epiglottis. Histopathologic examination confirmed the diagnosis of a liver metastatic tumor. The authors discussed the routes of metastasis to the larynx and the sites most commonly affected.[75] In 2011, Hinojar-Gutiérrez et al reported a 55-year-old man who presented with a hard and painless neck mass of 8-months' duration. Laryngeal examination and CT of the neck showed a ventricular tumor that invaded the thyroid cartilage and had spread to extralaryngeal structures. Initial biopsy using fine-needle aspiration was suggestive of Hurtle cell carcinoma, based on which the patient underwent total laryngectomy and thyroidectomy. Further histologic analysis and immunostaining of the surgical specimen showed evidence of trabeculated structures that stained positively for hepatocyte-specific antibody and CD10. The patient was diagnosed with metastatic laryngeal hepatocarcinoma. Metastatic workup using serology testing and radiologic images confirmed the presence of well-differentiated carcinoma.[76]

Based on this, laryngeal metastasis, although rare, should not be excluded in the metastatic workup of patients presenting with history of liver carcinoma and a suspicious laryngeal mass. Based on numerous reports, advanced stage of the disease (stage III), vascular invasion, multinodular tumors, involvement of both lobes of the liver, and poor differentiation are clinical-pathologic features highly associated with distant metastasis.[67,77] A high index of suspicion is needed to make the diagnosis because dysphonia may not be a presenting complaint. The laryngeal site affected most commonly is the supraglottis, followed by the subglottis. A deep biopsy and histochemical staining are crucial in differentiating metastatic HCC from other lesions.

Treatment-Induced Dysphonia in Patients With Liver Cancer

Despite the advances in surgical techniques and oncologic treatment, liver cancer remains the third leading cause of mortality worldwide, second to colon and lung cancers.[1] Various treatment modalities have been described in the literature, with sur-

gical resection and/or liver transplantation being probably the best options. Alternatively, patients may undergo interventional treatments such as transarterial chemoembolization or radioembolization, cryoablation, and stereotactic body radiotherapy.[78] Other options include systemic therapies. Several chemotherapy regimens are used, among which are 5-FU, oxaliplatin and leucovorin (FOLFOX), and gemcitabine and oxaliplatin (GEMOX).[79] In patients with resistance to chemotherapy, targeted therapy using antiangiogenic treatment such as tyrosine kinase inhibitors is advocated.[80] The choice of therapy depends on the stage of the disease, size of the tumor, presence or absence of metastatic lesions, and general health of the patient. In patients with an advanced stage of the disease, extrahepatic metastasis, and recurrences following surgical intervention, a combination of therapies and tailored management strategies are adopted.[78]

Treatment-induced dysphonia in patients with HCC is not common except in patients on chemotherapy, or those who have intubation injuries during surgery, as well as those with systemic debilitation. Dysphonia has been reported primarily in patients on chemotherapy and/or tyrosine kinase inhibitors, namely, sorafenib. In a retrospective analysis by De Simone et al that included 7 patients with HCC recurrence who were treated with a combination of everolimus and sorafenib, the authors reported hoarseness in 28.6% of cases, in addition to other side effects such as hypothyroidism in 14.3%,[81] which also can cause dysphonia. In another review by Fu et al on the adverse effects of multitarget tyrosine kinase inhibitors, hoarseness was reported in 2.2% of patients treated with sorafenib. The study included 115 patients with gastrointestinal cancer, among whom 57 had HCC.[82] The occurrence of dysphonia in other patients with liver cancer on treatment can be attributed to the known chemotherapy-induced metabolic changes, weight loss, and dehydration. In the study by De Simone et al, asthenia and diarrhea were reported in 42.8% and 28.6% of cases, respectively.[81] Similarly, in the study by Fu et al, diarrhea was reported in 24.4% of cases.[82] Given the paramount role of body metabolism and hydration in phonation, these described side effects undoubtedly affect voice. Diarrhea also causes dysphonia by preventing consistent abdominal muscle contraction, which is necessary for support of phonation. Hydration, be it local or systemic, is a major determinant of vocal fold vibration. Several acoustic and aerodynamic measures may be affected by loss or shifts of body fluids, the most important of which is phonatory threshold pressure, the correlate of phonatory effort. Patients on chemotherapy who experience extensive diarrhea and vomiting are at a greater risk of developing voice fatigue and an inability to project the voice.[83,84] Moreover, dehydration-induced thickening of laryngeal secretions results in increased jitter and friction of the vocal folds during phonation.[85,86] A thorough review on chemotherapy and voice can be found in the literature.[87] Dysphonia in patients with liver cancer and on systemic therapy may be secondary to the use of tyrosine kinase inhibitors. Antiangiogenic therapy not only deters tumor vascular formation but also may impair the blood supply to the vocal fold cover. In a large review by Erika et al on the adverse effects of antiangiogenic therapy, the authors reported dysphonia in almost 1 out of 3 cases.[88] Dysphonia has been attributed to vocal fold ischemic changes, as adverse events from antiangiogenic medications. Hartl et al described the vocal fold changes as whitish mucosal lesions that impair vocal fold vibration and lead to change in voice quality.[89,90] Dysphonia in patients

with liver cancer and on treatment also may be secondary to therapy-induced body fatigue. Voice is a reflection of well-being, and it is negatively affected in patients who suffer body fatigue during the course of their treatment. In a review of the factors related to quality of life in patients with liver cancer and on various treatment modalities, Li et al reported worsening in physical function for 1 month following liver resection or radiofrequency ablation. History of alcohol intake and prior infection with hepatitis C affected the physical outcome as well.[91] In another study by van Roekel et al on 53 patients who underwent radioembolization, fatigue and pain were commonly reported. The authors emphasized the decline in quality of life for a few weeks after treatment.[92]

In summary, treatment-induced dysphonia occurs in patients with liver cancer. When present, special attention to dehydration and body fluids is recommended, as well as attention to general body function and fatigue. In patients receiving sorafenib and complaining of hoarseness, a laryngeal examination to rule out vocal fold mucosal necrosis is essential. Professional voice users with liver cancer need special attention given the devastating impact of dysphonia on their quality of life.

References

1. American Cancer Society. Key statistics about liver cancer. Updated 2019. Accessed November 20, 2019. https://www.cancer.org/cancer/liver-cancer/about/what-is-key-statistics.html
2. Yang JD, Hainaut P, Gores GJ, Amadou A, Plymoth A, Roberts LR. A global view of hepatocellular carcinoma: trends, risk, prevention and management. *Nat Rev Gastroenterol Hepatol*. 2019;16(10):589–604.

3. Ghouri YA, Mian I, Rowe JH. Review of hepatocellular carcinoma: epidemiology, etiology, and carcinogenesis. *J Carcinog*. 2017; 16:1–9.

4. Mohammadian M, Mahdavifar N, Mohammadian-Hafshejani A, Salehiniya H. Liver cancer in the world: epidemiology, incidence, mortality and risk factors. *WCRJ*. 2018;5(2):e1082.

5. Parkin DM, Bray F, Ferlay J, Pisani P. Global cancer statistics, 2002. *CA Cancer J Clin*. 2005;55(2):74–108.

6. American Cancer Society. What is liver cancer? Updated April 1, 2019. Accessed December 1, 2019. https://www.cancer.org /cancer/liver-cancer/about/what-is-liver -cancer.html

7. Welzel TM, Graubard BI, Quraishi S, et al. Population-attributable fractions of risk factors for hepatocellular carcinoma in the United States. *Am J Gastroenterol*. 2013;108 (8):1314–1321.

8. Parkin DM. The global health burden of infection-associated cancers in the year 2002. *Int J Cancer*. 2006;118(12):3030–3044.

9. Williams JH, Phillips TD, Jolly PE, Stiles JK, Jolly CM, Aggarwal D. Human aflatoxicosis in developing countries: a review of toxicology, exposure, potential health consequences, and interventions. *Am J Clin Nutr*. 2004;80(5):1106–1122.

10. Strosnider H, Azziz-Baumgartner E, Banziger M, et al. Workgroup report: public health strategies for reducing aflatoxin exposure in developing countries. *Environ Health Perspect*. 2006;114(12):1898–1903.

11. Bressac B, Kew M, Wands J, Ozturk M. Selective G to T mutations of p53 gene in hepatocellular carcinoma from southern Africa. *Nature*. 1991;350(6317):429–431.

12. Liu Y, Chang CC, Marsh GM, Wu F. Population attributable risk of aflatoxin-related liver cancer: systematic review and meta-analysis. *Eur J Cancer*. 2012;48(14): 2125–2136.

13. Chen CJ, Chen CW, Wu MM, Kuo TL. Cancer potential in liver, lung, bladder and kidney due to ingested inorganic arsenic in drinking water. *Br J Cancer*. 1992;66(5):888–892.

14. Tsuda T, Babazono A, Yamamoto E, et al. Ingested arsenic and internal cancer: a historical cohort study followed for 33 years. *Am J Epidemiol*. 1995;141(3):198–209.

15. Cao Y, Giovannucci EL. Alcohol as a risk factor for cancer. *Semin Oncol Nurs*. 2016; 32(3):325–331.

16. Bagnardi V, Blangiardo M, La Vecchia C, Corrao G. A meta-analysis of alcohol drinking and cancer risk. *Br J Cancer*. 2001;85(11): 1700–1705.

17. Turati F, Galeone C, Rota M, et al. Alcohol and liver cancer: a systematic review and meta-analysis of prospective studies. *Ann Oncol*. 2014; 25(8):1526–1535.

18. Younossi ZM, Koenig AB, Abdelatif D, Fazel Y, Henry L, Wymer M. Global epidemiology of nonalcoholic fatty liver disease— meta-analytic assessment of prevalence, incidence, and outcomes. *Hepatology*. 2016; 64(1):73–84.

19. Larsson SC, Wolk A. Overweight, obesity and risk of liver cancer: a meta-analysis of cohort studies. *Br J Cancer*. 2007;97(7):1005–1008.

20. Lee Y-CA, Cohet C, Yang Y-C, Stayner L, Hashibe M, Straif K. Meta-analysis of epidemiologic studies on cigarette smoking and liver cancer. *Int J Epidemiol*. 2009;38(6):1497–1511.

21. Koh W, Robien K, Wang R, Govindarajan S, Yuan J, Yu M. Smoking as an independent risk factor for hepatocellular carcinoma: the Singapore Chinese Health Study. *Br J Cancer*. 2011;105(9):1430–1435.

22. Fedirko V, Trichopolou A, Bamia C, et al. Consumption of fish and meats and risk of hepatocellular carcinoma: the European Prospective Investigation into Cancer and Nutrition (EPIC). *Ann Oncol*. 2013;24(8): 2166–2173.

23. Sawada N, Inoue M, Iwasaki M, et al. Consumption of n-3 fatty acids and fish reduces risk of hepatocellular carcinoma. *Gastroenterology*. 2012;142(7):1468–1475.

24. Talamini R, Polesel J, Montella M, et al. Food groups and risk of hepatocellular carcinoma: a multicenter case-control study in Italy. *Int J Cancer*. 2006;119(12):2916–2921.

25. Kurahashi N, Inoue M, Iwasaki M, et al. Vegetable, fruit and antioxidant nutrient

consumption and subsequent risk of hepatocellular carcinoma: a prospective cohort study in Japan. *Br J Cancer*. 2009;100(1): 181–184.

26. La Vecchia C, Negri E, Decarli A, D'avanzo B, Franceschi S. Risk factors for hepatocellular carcinoma in northern Italy. *Int J Cancer*. 1988;42(6):872–876.

27. Kowdley KV. Iron, hemochromatosis, and hepatocellular carcinoma. *Gastroenterology*. 2004;127(5 Suppl 1):S79–S86.

28. Dimitroulis D, Damaskos C, Valsami S, et al. From diagnosis to treatment of hepatocellular carcinoma: an epidemic problem for both developed and developing world. *World J Gastroenterol*. 2017;23(29):5282–5294.

29. Katyal S, Oliver JH 3rd, Peterson MS, Ferris JV, Carr BS, Baron RL. Extrahepatic metastases of hepatocellular carcinoma. *Radiology*. 2000;216(3):698–703.

30. Natsuizaka M, Omura T, Akaike T, et al. Clinical features of hepatocellular carcinoma with extrahepatic metastases. *J Gastroenterol Hepatol*. 2005;20(11):1781–1787.

31. Sawabe M, Nakamura T, Kanno J, Kasuga T. Analysis of morphological factors of hepatocellular carcinoma in 98 autopsy cases with respect to pulmonary metastasis. *Acta Pathol Jpn*. 1987;37(9):1389–1404.

32. Tanaka O, Kanematsu M, Kondo H, et al. Solitary mediastinal lymph node metastasis of hepatocellular carcinoma: MR imaging findings. *Magn Reson Imaging*. 2005;23(1):111–114.

33. Lee SM, Kim HS, Lee S, Lee JW. Emerging role of ^{18}F-fluorodeoxyglucose positron emission tomography for guiding management of hepatocellular carcinoma. *World J Gastroenterol*. 2019;25(11):1289–1306.

34. Cho E, Jun CH, Kim BS, Son DJ, Choi WS, Choi SK. 18F-FDG PET CT as a prognostic factor in hepatocellular carcinoma. *Turk J Gastroenterol*. 2015;26(4):344–350.

35. Lugli A, Tornillo L, Mirlacher M, Bundi M, Sauter G, Terracciano LM. Hepatocyte paraffin 1 expression in human normal and neoplastic tissues: tissue microarray analysis on 3,940 tissue samples. *Am J Clin Pathol*. 2004;122(5):721–727.

36. Lee JM, Park KM, Lee SY, Choi J, Hwang DW, Lee YJ. Metastasis of hepatocellular carcinoma to the ovary: a case report and review of the literature. *Gut Liver*. 2011;5(4): 543–547.

37. Young RH, Gersell DJ, Clement PB, Scully RE. Hepatocellular carcinoma metastatic to the ovary: a report of three cases discovered during life with discussion of the differential diagnosis of hepatoid tumors of the ovary. *Hum Pathol*. 1992;23(5):574–580.

38. D'Antonio A, Caleo A, Caleo O, Addesso M, Boscaino A. Hepatocellular carcinoma metastatic to the kidney mimicking renal oncocytoma. *Hepatobiliary Pancreat Dis Int*. 2010;9(5):550–552.

39. Michalaki V, Zygogianni A, Kouloulias V, Balafouta M, Vlachodimitropoulos D, Gennatas CG. Muscle metastasis from hepatocellular carcinoma. *J Cancer Res Ther*. 2011;7(1): 81–83.

40. Tunc B, Filik L, Tezer-Filik I, Sahin B. Brain metastasis of hepatocellular carcinoma: a case report and review of the literature. *World J Gastroenterol*. 2004;10(11):1688–1689.

41. Ferlito A, Caruso G, Recher G. Secondary laryngeal tumors: report of seven cases with review of the literature. *Arch Otolaryngol Head Neck Surg*. 1988;114(6):635–639.

42. Uehara K, Hasegawa H, Ogiso S, et al. Skip lymph node metastases from a small hepatocellular carcinoma with difficulty in preoperative diagnosis. *J Gastroenterol Hepatol*. 2003;18(3):345–349.

43. Nagy JA, Brown LF, Senger DR, et al. Pathogenesis of tumor stroma generation: a critical role for leaky blood vessels and fibrin deposition. *Biochim Biophys Acta*. 1989;948(3): 305–326.

44. Greenstein A, Witherspoon R, Iqbal F, Coleman H. Hepatocellular carcinoma metastasis to the maxilla: a rare case. *Aust Dent J*. 2013;58(3):373–375.

45. Pires FR, Sagarra R, Corrêa ME, Pereira CM, Vargas PA, Lopes MA. Oral metastasis of a hepatocellular carcinoma. *Oral Surg Oral Med Oral Pathol Oral Radiol Endod*. 2004; 97(3):359–368.

46. Maiorano E, Piattelli A, Favia G. Hepatocellular carcinoma metastatic to the oral mucosa: report of a case with multiple gingival localizations. *J Periodontol*. 2000;71(4): 641–645.

47. Li R, Walvekar RR, Nalesnik MA, Gamblin TC. Unresectable hepatocellular carcinoma with a solitary metastasis to the mandible. *Am Surg*. 2008;74(4):346–349.

48. Sundberg J. Vocal tract resonance. In: Sataloff RT. *Professional Voice: The Science and Art of Clinical Care*. 4th ed. San Diego, CA: Plural Publishing; 2017;309–328.

49. Raphael BN, Sataloff RT. Increasing vocal effectiveness. In: Sataloff RT. *Professional Voice: The Science and Art of Clinical Care*. 4th ed. San Diego, CA: Plural Publishing; 2017;1201–1212.

50. Kattepur AK, Patil DB, Krishnamoorthy N, et al. Isolated nasopharyngeal metastasis from hepatocellular carcinoma. *Int J Surg Case Rep*. 2014;5(3):115–117.

51. Guo S, Wang Y. A case of hepatocellular carcinoma in an elder man with metastasis to the nasopharynx. *Int J Clin Exp Pathol*. 2015; 8(5):5919–5923.

52. Lou LL, Zhang Y, Huang X, et al. Solitary nasopharynx metastasis from hepatocellular carcinoma after liver transplantation: a case report. *Medicine*. 2019;98(7):e14368.

53. Jonas S, Bechstein WO, Steinmüller T, et al. Vascular invasion and histopathologic grading determine outcome after liver transplantation for hepatocellular carcinoma in cirrhosis. *Hepatology*. 2001;33(5):1080–1086.

54. Harris PS, Hansen RM, Gray M, Massoud OI, McGuire BM, Shoreibah MG. Hepatocellular carcinoma surveillance: an evidence based approach. *World J Gastroenterol*. 2019; 25(13):1550–1559.

55. Lau KK, Wong KW, Ho WC, Lai TS, Lee KC, Leung TW. Hepatocellular carcinoma presenting with right supraclavicular lymph node metastasis and superior mediastinal syndrome. *Liver*. 2000;20(2):184–185.

56. Thorburn D, Sanai FM, Ghent CN. Hepatocellular carcinoma presenting as right supraclavicular lymphadenopathy. *Can J Gastroenterol*. 2003;17(10):605–606.

57. Köklü S, Arhan M, Kuksal A, Ülker A, Temucin T. An unusual presentation of hepatocellular carcinoma. *Int J Gastrointest Cancer*. 2003;34(2–3):63–65.

58. Kobayashi K, Himoto T, Tani J, et al. A rare case of hepatocellular carcinoma accompanied by metastasis of a cervical lymph node. *Intern Med*. 2012;51(4):381–385.

59. Madabhavi I, Patel A, Choudhary M, Anand A, Panchal H, Parikh S. Right cervical lymphadenopathy: a rare presentation of metastatic hepatocellular carcinoma. *Gastroenterol Hepatol Bed Bench*. 2014;7(3):177–182.

60. Yang Y, Nagano H, Ota H, et al. Patterns and clinicopathologic features of extrahepatic recurrence of hepatocellular carcinoma after curative resection. *Surgery*. 2007;141(2):196–202.

61. Yuen MF, Ahn SH, Chen DS, et al. Chronic hepatitis B virus infection: disease revisit and management recommendations. *J Clin Gastroenterol*. 2016;50(4):286–294.

62. Suzumura K, Hirano T, Kuroda N, et al. Solitary mediastinal metastasis of hepatocellular carcinoma treated by video-assisted thoracic surgery: report of a case. *Gen Thorac Cardiovasc Surg*. 2013;61(11):651–654.

63. Hung JJ, Lin SC, Hsu WH. Pancoast syndrome caused by metastasis to the superior mediastinum of hepatocellular carcinoma. *Thorac Cardiovasc Surg*. 2007;55(7):463–465.

64. Chen CC, Yeh HZ, Chang CS, et al. Transarterial embolization of metastatic mediastinal hepatocellular carcinoma. *World J Gastroenterol*. 2013;19(22):3512–3516.

65. Oh SY, Seo KW, Jegal Y, et al. Hemothorax caused by spontaneous rupture of a metastatic mediastinal lymph node in hepatocellular carcinoma: a case report. *Korean J Intern Med*. 2013;28(5):622–625.

66. Xu L, Xue F, Wang B, et al. Hoarseness due to lymph node metastasis of hepatocellular carcinoma: a case report. *Oncol Lett*. 2016; 12(2):918–920.

67. Kaczynski J, Hansson G, Wallerstedt S. Metastases in cases with hepatocellular carcinoma

in relation to clinicopathologic features of the tumor. An autopsy study from a low endemic area. *Acta Oncol.* 1995;34(1):43–48.

68. Nakagawa K, Nakahara K, Ohno K, Matsumura A, Kawashima Y. Mediastinal dissection of hepatocellular carcinoma with bilateral hilar and mediastinal lymph node metastasis. *Kyobu Geka.* 1989;42(10):857–860.

69. Yamashita R, Takahashi M, Kosugi M, Kobayashi C, Annen Y. A case of metastatic hepatocellular carcinoma of the superior mediastinum. *Nihon Kyobu Geka Gakkai Zasshi.* 1993;41(4):709–713.

70. Uchinami H, Abe Y, Kikuchi I, et al. A case of surgical treatment for solitary lymph node recurrence of hepatocellular carcinoma simultaneously developed in the mediastinum and abdominal cavity. *Nihon Shokakibyo Gakkai Zasshi.* 2009;106(7):1049–1055.

71. Shoji F, Shirabe K, Yano T, Maehara Y. Surgical resection of solitary cardiophrenic lymph node metastasis by video-assisted thoracic surgery after complete resection of hepatocellular carcinoma. *Interact Cardiovasc Thorac Surg.* 2010;10(3):446–447.

72. Tanaka H, Yamazaki N, Watanabe H, Nakade M. Solitary mediastinal lymph node metastasis from hepatocellular carcinoma. *Kyobu Geka.* 2016;69(3):207–209.

73. Taniguchi M, Hyodo M, Tezuka K, et al. Metachronous solitary mediastinal lymph node metastases of hepatocellular carcinoma treated by video-assisted thoracic surgery twice: report of a case. *Asian J Endosc Surg.* 2018;11(1):64–67.

74. Nambu T, Shinohara M, Takada A, Suzuki K, Koyama Y, Irie G. A case of icteric hepatoma with laryngeal metastasis and coexisting pancreatic cancer. *Gan No Rinsho.* 1990; 36(4):515–520.

75. Nobili S, SA Cunha A, Gontier R, Rullier A, Saric J. Métastase épiglottique d'un carcinome hépatocellulaire: a propos d'un cas. *Gastroentérologie clinique et biologique.* 2002;26(10):940–941.

76. Hinojar-Gutiérrez A, Nieto-Llanos S, Mera-Menéndez F, Fernández-Contreras ME, Mendoza J, Moreno R. Laryngeal metastasis as first presentation of hepatocellular carcinoma. *Rev Esp Dig (Madrid).* 2011;103(4): 222–224.

77. Abe T, Furuse J, Yoshino M, et al. Clinical characteristics of hepatocellular carcinoma with an extensive lymph node metastasis at diagnosis. *Am J Clin Oncol.* 2002;25(3): 318–323.

78. Lurje I, Czigany Z, Bednarsch J, et al. Treatment strategies for hepatocellular carcinoma—a multidisciplinary approach. *Int J Mol Sci.* 2019;20(6):E1465.

79. American Cancer Society. Embolization therapy for liver cancer. Updated 2019. Accessed December 1, 2019. https://www.cancer.org/cancer/liver-cancer/treating/embolization-therapy.html

80. European Association for the Study of the Liver. EASL Clinical Practice Guidelines: management of hepatocellular carcinoma. *J Hepatol.* 2018;69(1):182–236.

81. De Simone P, Crocetti L, Pezzati D, et al. Efficacy and safety of combination therapy with everolimus and sorafenib for recurrence of hepatocellular carcinoma after liver transplantation. *Transplant Proc.* 2014;46(1): 241–244.

82. Fu Y, Wei X, Lin L, Xu W, Liang J. Adverse reactions of sorafenib, sunitinib, and imatinib in treating digestive system tumors. *Thorac Cancer.* 2018;9(5):542–547.

83. Sivasankar M, Leydon C. The role of hydration in vocal fold physiology. *Curr Opin Otolaryngol Head Neck Surg.* 2010;18(3):171–175.

84. Solomon NP, DiMattia MS. Effects of a vocally fatiguing task and systemic hydration on phonation threshold pressure. *J Voice.* 2000;14(3):341–362.

85. Hartley NA, Thibeault SL. Systemic hydration: relating science to clinical practice in vocal health. *J Voice.* 2014;28(5):652.e1–652.e20.

86. Leydon C, Sivasankar M, Falciglia DL, Atkins C, Fisher KV. Vocal fold surface hydration: a review. *J Voice.* 2009;23(6):658–665.

87. Mattioni J, Opperman DA, Solimando DA, Sataloff RT. Cancer chemotherapy: an over-

view and voice implications: In Sataloff RT. *Professional Voice: The Science and Art of Clinical Care.* 4th ed. San Diego, CA: Plural Publishing; 2017:1137–1140.

88. Saavedra E, Hollebecque A, Soria JC, Hartl DM. Dysphonia induced by anti-angiogenic compounds. *Invest New Drugs.* 2014;32(4): 774–782.

89. Hartl DM, Ferté C, Loriot Y, et al. Dysphonia induced by vascular endothelium growth factor/vascular endothelium growth factor receptor inhibitors. *Invest New Drugs.* 2010; 28(6):884–886.

90. Hartl DM, Bahleda R, Hollebecque A, Bosq J, Massard C, Soria JC. Bevacizumab-induced laryngeal necrosis. *Ann Oncol.* 2012;23(1):276–278.

91. Li IF, Huang JC, Chen JJ, Wang TE, Huang SS, Tsay SL. Factors related to the quality of life in liver cancer patients during treatment phase: a follow-up study. *Eur J Cancer Care.* 2019;28(6):e13146.

92. van Roekel C, Smits ML, Prince JF, Bruijnen RC, van den Bosch MA, Lam MG. Quality of life in patients with liver tumors treated with holmium-166 radioembolization. *Clin Exp Metastasis.* 2020;37(1):95–105.

Index